DATE DUE

2001638	8/05/94

Psychiatry and Advanced Technologies

Psychiatry and Advanced Technologies

Editor

Luigi Ravizza, M.D.
Director, Psychiatric Department
University of Turin
Turin, Italy

Co-Editors

Filippo Bogetto M.D., and **Enrico Zanalda, M.D.**
Psychiatric Department
University of Turin
Turin, Italy

Raven Press New York

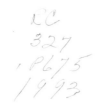

Raven Press, Ltd., 1185 Avenue of the Americas, New York, New York 10036

Made in the United States of America

Library of Congress Cataloging-in-Publication Data

Psychiatry and advanced tecnologies / editor, Luigi Ravizza ; co-
   editors, Filippo Bogetto and Enrico Zanalda.
        p.   cm.
   Includes bibliographical references.
   ISBN 0-7817-0003-5
   1. Biological psychiatry—Technological innovations—Congresses.
2. Psychiatry—Data processing—Congresses. I. Ravizza, Luigi.
II. Bogetto, Filippo. III. Zanalda, Enrico.
   [DNLM: 1. Brain—physiology—congresses. 2. Brain—radionuclide
imaging—congresses. 3. Brain Mapping—congresses. 4. Medical
Informatics—congresses. 5. Mental Disorders—genetics—congresses.
WL 335 P9749 1993]
RC327.P675   1993
616.89—dc20
DNLM/DLC
for Library of Congress   92-48413
                                                              CIP

9 8 7 6 5 4 3 2 1

Preface

During recent decades, modern psychiatry has achieved the same degree of cultural and scientific dignity as other branches of medicine, although it should be remembered that psychiatry must consider relational and psychodynamic problems in addition to those caused by biologic aberrations. The present position of psychiatry within the general field of neurosciences was made possible by biologic research that confirmed the ancient hypothesis, first suggested by Hippocrates and more recently by Kraepelin, Bleuler, and others, of the biologic genesis of mental disorders in their many manifestations. A relationship has now been identified between psychopathologic expression and dysfunctions of the neurotransmitter systems that mediate various psychic activities: cognitive functions, affective states, behavior, and personality.

All over the world, investigators from different disciplines, such as neuropharmacology, biochemistry, molecular biology, genetics, psychiatry, neurology, and psychoneuroendocrinoimmunology, have become fascinated with research in neuroscience that offers the hope of improving the quality of human life.

The American Congress has declared the decade 1990–2000 as the "brain decade"; this shows a far-sighted attention to scientific progress. In the United States, neuroscientists have carried out an ambitious program that involves the most important research institutes, with the aim of improving our knowledge of brain functions and of mental disorders. In this volume, particular attention will be given to those disorders that compromise personality in more serious ways, such as Alzheimer's disease, schizophrenia, and depression.

During the past few decades, the aminergic hypothesis has been proposed as a pathogenetic factor for affective and schizophrenic disorders, and has led to a better comprehension of the disorder and of the mechanism of action of psychotropic drugs. More recently, obsessive–compulsive disorders have been related to a hypofunction of the serotoninergic system; this hypothesis is supported by the surprising therapeutic efficacy of selective 5-HT-reuptake–blocker antidepressants such as clomipramine, fluoxetine, and fluvoxamine, now commonly known as antiobsessionals.

With regard to generalized anxiety disorder, some recent studies have shown a significant decrease of peripheral-benzodiazepine receptors in lymphocytes. These data, which still require confirmation, may suggest the presence in the brain of endogenous ligands for benzodiazepines.

The need to improve the validity of psychiatric diagnoses has led to the introduction of brain imaging: computerized electroencephalographic and brain functional maps in neurophysiology and CAT, RMN, single photon emission computer tomography, and positron emission tomography in neuro-radiology. Apart from organic mental disorders, such as Alzheimer's disease, multi-infarct dementia, Parkinson's disease, and other forms of dementia, these advanced technologies are now also used in the study of schizophrenic psychoses, depression, and obsessive–compulsive disorder. These new techniques are useful not only for identification of structural brain abnormalities but also for imaging of regional brain functions, for examination of local cerebral metabolism and blood flow, and for exploration of specific receptor dysfunctions. The results obtained from recent studies seem to indicate that new imaging technologies will represent the instruments of the future, especially if more specific and selective tracers can be developed.

Finally, it is important to stress the contribution of the rapid advances in computer science which have revolutionized the speed with which data processing and statistical analysis can be accomplished.

Although the scientific community is fully aware of the difficulties of research in neuroscience, it is determined to promote progress in this complex field. Advances in the development of new technologies such as PET, in molecular biology, and genetics, enable us to foresee even greater advances in the near future, which will lead to deeper understanding of the biologic correlations of mental disorders, and therefore to improved treatment of these disorders based on a more comprehensive knowledge of the side effects of psychotropic drugs and their mechanisms of action.

A large number of famous Italian and international scientists and clinicians have contributed to this volume, covering many fields of biologic research. We are also honored to have the opening contribution from Professor Costa e Silva, president of World Psychiatric Association and director of the Institute of Psychiatry of the University of Rio de Janéiro. We are deeply grateful to all of those whose presentations are included herein. In addition, we thank the pharmaceutical companies and individuals who cooperated in the organization of the meeting, the proceedings of which make up the context of this volume.

Luigi Ravizza, M.D.

Acknowledgment

This volume presents articles from the Congress Proceedings of the First International Meetings of Psychoneurobiology held September 25–28, 1990 in Saint Vincent (AO), Italy.

Contents

Contributors

A. C. Altamura
Professor of Psychiatry
Institute of Psychiatry
University of Cagliari
via Liguria, 13
09127 Liguria, Italy

E. Aronica, M.D.
Institute of Pharmacology
University of Catania
School of Medicine
viale Andrea Doria 6
95125 Catania, Italy

C. Asteggiano
Researcher
Neurology Department
University of Turin
via Cherasco 15
10126 Turin, Italy

T. A. Ban
Professor
Department of Psychiatry
Vanderbilt University
A-2215 Medical Center North
Nashville, Tennessee 37232

C. Benkelfat, M.D.
Section on Clinical
  Neuropharmacology
Laboratory of Clinical Science
National Institute of Mental Health
Bethesda, Maryland 20892
Current: Assistant Professor
Department of Psychiatry
McGill University
1033 Pine Avenue West
Montreal, Quebec H3A-1A1, Canada

P. Benna
Researcher
Neurology Department
University of Turin
via Cherasco 15
10126 Turin, Italy

B. Bergamasco
Professor
Neurology Department
University of Turin
via Cherasco 15
10126 Turin, Italy

F. Bernardi, M.D.
Department of Neurosciences
University of Cagliari
via Porcell 4
09124 Cagliari, Italy

C. Bianco, M.D.
Neurology Department
University of Turin
via Cherasco 15
10126 Turin, Italy

G. Biggio
Professor
Department of Experimental Biology
Chair of Pharmacology
University of Cagliari
via Palabanda 12
09123 Cagliari, Italy

E. Bo, M.D.
Neurology Department
University of Turin
via Cherasco 15
10126 Turin, Italy

A. Bocchetta, M.D.
Department of Neurosciences
University of Cagliari
via Porcell 4
09124 Cagliari, Italy

P. Boyer
Director of Research
Paris V University
100 rue de la Santé
75014 Paris, France

D. Brandeis, Ph.D.
Department of Child and Adolescent
  Psychiatry
University of Zurich
CH-8028 Zurich, Switzerland

P. Bucci
Department of Psychiatry
First Medical School
University of Naples
L.go Madonna delle Grazie 1
80138 Naples, Italy

A. Bussi, M.D.
USSL 32
Department of Psychiatry
Treviglio (BG), Italy

C. Burrai, M.D.
Department of Neurosciences
University of Cagliari
via Porcell 4
09124 Cagliari, Italy

P. L. Canonico
Professor
Chair of Pharmacology
University of Pavia
School of Dentistry
Pavia, Italy

P. Carrera
Master in Biology
Research Assistant
Department of Molecular Biology
Scientific Institute San Raffaele
University of Milan
via L. Prinetti 29
20127 Milan, Italy

G. Casabona, M.D.
Institute of Pharmacology
University of Catania
School of Medicine
viale Andrea Doria 6
95125 Catania, Italy

F. Catapano
Department of Psychiatry
First Medical School
University of Naples
L.go Madonna delle Grazie 1
80138 Naples, Italy

C. Cavallini, M.D.
Resident in Clinical Psychiatry
Scientific Institute San Raffaele
Clinical Psychiatry III
University of Milan
via L. Prinetti 29
20127 Milan, Italy

L. Cavicchioli
Senior Researcher
Fidia Research Laboratories
via Ponte della Fabbrica 3/A
35031 Abano Terme (PD), Italy

R. M. Cohen, M.D., Ph.D.
Chief, Section on Clinical Brain
  Imaging
Laboratory of Cerebral Metabolism
National Institute of Mental Health
Bethesda, Maryland 20892

C. Colombo, M.D.
Human Biology Unit
Psychiatric Branch
Department of Biomedical and
  Technological Sciences
University of Milan Medical School
Scientific Institute San Raffaele
via Prinetti 29
20127 Milan, Italy

A. Concas
Associate Professor
Department of Experimental Biology
Chair of Pharmacology
University of Cagliari
via Palabanda 12
09123 Cagliari, Italy

L. Conti
Associate Professor
Institute of Clinical Psychiatry
University of Pisa
via Roma 67
56100 Pisa, Italy

A. Copani, M.D.
Institute of Pharmacology
University of Catania
School of Medicine
viale Andrea Doria 6
95125 Catania, Italy

M. T. Coppola, M.D.
Institute of Psychiatry
University of Milan
Ospedale Maggiore-P. Guardia II
via Francesco Sforza 35
20122 Milan, Italy

R. Corona, Ph.D.
Central Laboratory
"San Giovanni di Dio" Hospital
via Ospedale 46
09124 Cagliari, Italy

P. Costa, M.D.
Neurology Department
University of Turin
via Cherasco 15
10126 Turin, Italy

J. A. Costa e Silva
Professor of Psychiatry
State University of Rio de Janéiro
Rua Getùlio das Neves, 22 CEP
22461 Rio de Janéiro, Brazil

T. H. Crook III, Ph.D.
Advanced Psychometrics Corporation
8311 Wisconsin Avenue
Bethesda, Maryland 20814-3126

R. Dal Toso
Senior Researcher
Fidia Research Laboratories
via Ponte della Fabbrica 3/A
35031 Abano Terme (PD), Italy

M. Del Zompo, M.D.
Department of Neurosciences
University of Cagliari
via Porcell 4
09124 Cagliari, Italy

C. De Leo
Biochemistry Technician
Psychiatry Department
University of Turin
via Cherasco 11
10126 Turin, Italy

M. Ferrari, M.D.
Research Vice-Chief of Molecular
    Biology Laboratory
Scientific Institute San Raffaele
University of Milan
via L. Prinetti 29
20127 Milan, Italy

P. Ferrero, M.D.
Neurology Department
University of Turin
via Cherasco 15
10126 Turin, Italy

M. B. First
Assistant Professor of Clinical
    Psychiatry
Columbia University
New York, New York
Research Psychiatrist
New York State Psychiatric Institute
722 West 168th Street
New York, New York 10032

S. Galderisi, M.D.
Department of Psychiatry
First Medical School
University of Naples
L.go Madonna delle Grazie 1
80138 Naples, Italy

O. Gambini, M.D.
Human Biology Unit
Psychiatric Branch
Department of Biomedical and
    Technological Sciences
University of Milan Medical School
Scientific Institute San Raffaele
via Prinetti 29
20127 Milan, Italy

A. A. Genazzani
Institute of Pharmacology
University of Catania
School of Medicine
viale Andrea Doria 6
95125 Catania, Italy

S. Giaquinto
Professor
St. John Baptist Hospital SMOM
via L. Dasti 7-14
00148 Rome, Italy

C. L. Grady, Ph.D.
Chief, Unit on Positron Emission
  Tomography
Laboratory of Neurosciences
National Institute on Aging
National Institutes of Health
Bethesda, Maryland 20892

M. Guazzelli
Researcher
Clinical Psychiatry I
University of Pisa
I-56100 Pisa, Italy

J. V. Haxby, Ph.D.
Chief, Unit on Neuropsychology
Laboratory of Neurosciences
National Institute on Aging
National Institutes of Health
Bethesda, Maryland 20892

B. Henggeler, Ph.D.
Brain Mapping Laboratory
Department of Neurology
University Hospital
Frauenklinikstrasse 26
8091 Zurich, Switzerland

H. Holcomb
University of Maryland Psychiatric
  Research Center
Baltimore, Maryland 20201
Johns Hopkins Medical Institution
Bethesda, Maryland

D. Kemali
Professor and Director
Department of Psychiatry
First Medical School
University of Naples
L.go Madonna delle Grazie 1
80138 Naples, Italy

J. L. Kennedy, M.D.
Assistant Professor
Department of Neurogenetics
The Clarke Institute of Psychiatry
University of Toronto
Toronto, Ontario, Canada

C. King
Section on Clinical Brain Imaging
Laboratory of Cerebral Metabolism
National Institute of Mental Health
Bethesda, Maryland 20892

M. Krug
Laboratory Chief
Institute of Neurobiology and Brain
  Research
Academy of Sciences
Magdeburg, Germany

D. Lampman, M.S.
Senior Physicist
NMR Advanced Technology Group
Picker International Inc.
Cleveland, Ohio 44143

D. Lehman
Professor
Brain Mapping Laboratory
Department of Neurology
University Hospital
Frauenklinikstrasse 26
8091 Zurich, Switzerland

A. Leon
Neuroscience Director
Fidia Research Laboratories
via Ponte della Fabbrica 3/A
35031 Abano Terme (PD), Italy

H. Loats, B.S., M.S.
Research Associate
Johns Hopkins Oncology
Westminster, Maryland 21157

M. Locatelli, M.D.
Human Biology Unit
Psychiatric Branch
Department of Biomedical and
  Technological Sciences
University of Milan Medical School
Scientific Institute San Raffaele
via Prinetti 29
20127 Milan, Italy

F. Macciardi, M.D., Ph.D.
Vice-Head, Section of Psychiatric
  Genetics
Department of Psychiatry
University of Milan Medical School
Scientific Institute San Raffaele
via Prinetti 29
20127 Milan, Italy

G. Maina, M.D.
Psychiatry Department
University of Turin
via Cherasco 11
10126 Turin, Italy

M. Maj
Professor Department of Psychiatry
First Medical School
University of Naples
L.go Madonna delle Grazie 1
80138 Naples, Italy

G. F. Marchesi
Professor and Director
Institute of Psychiatry
University of Ancona
L.go Capelli 1
60121 Ancona, Italy

P. L. Marconi, M.D.
III Psychiatric Clinic
University of Rome "La Sapienza"
Viale dell'Università 30
00185 Rome, Italy

C. Marino, M.D.
Resident in Clinical Psychiatry
Scientific Institute San Raffaele
Clinical Psychiatry III
University of Milan
via L. Prinetti 29
20127 Milan, Italy

E. Marotta, M.S.
Neurology Department
University of Turin
via Cherasco 15
10126 Turin, Italy

M. Martinez, Ph.D.
Researcher Geneticist
Department of Health and Human
  Services
National Institute of Mental Health
10-3N218
Bethesda, Maryland 20892

G. Massimetti
Researcher
Institute of Clinical Psychiatry
University of Pisa
via Roma 67
56100 Pisa, Italy

J. McNally, Ph.D.
Manager
NMR Advanced Technology Group
Picker International Inc.
Cleveland, Ohio 44143

M. Memo
Professor
Institute of Pharmacology and
  Experimental Therapeutics
University of Brescia
via Valsabbina 19
25124 Brescia, Italy

C. M. Michel, Ph.D.
Brain Mapping Laboratory
Department of Neurology
University Hospital
Frauenklinikstrasse 26
8091 Zurich, Switzerland

A. M. Milani
Biochemistry Technician
Psychiatry Department
University of Turin
via Cherasco 11
10126 Turin, Italy

B. Miller, M.D.
Associate Professor of Neurology
Harbor-UCLA Medical Center
Torrance, California 90509

C. Missale
Professor
Institute of Pharmacology and
    Experimental Therapeutics
School of Medicine
University of Brescia
via Valsabbina 19
25124 Brescia, Italy

A. Mucci, M.D.
Department of Psychiatry
First Medical School
University of Naples
L.go Madonna delle Grazie 1
80138 Naples, Italy

J. Murdoch, Ph.D.
Senior Physicist
NMR Advanced Technology Group
Picker International Inc.
Cleveland, Ohio 44143

D. L. Murphy, M.D.
Chief, Laboratory of Clinical Science
National Institute of Mental Health
Bethesda, Maryland 20892

A. Musazzi
Institute of Psychiatry
University of Milan
Ospedale Maggiore-P. Guardia II
via Francesco Sforza 35
20122 Milan, Italy

B. Nardi, M.D., Ph.D.
Assistant Professor
Institute of Psychiatry
University of Ancona
L.go Capelli 1
60121 Ancona, Italy

F. Nicoletti
Researcher
Institute of Pharmacology
University of Catania School of
    Medicine
Catania, Italy

T. R. Nordahl, M.D., Ph.D.
Section on Clinical Brain Imaging
Laboratory of Cerebral Metabolism
National Institute of Mental Health
Bethesda, Maryland 20892
Current: Department of Psychiatry
University of California/Davis
Davis, California

M. Paley, Ph.D.
Manager MRI Sequence Development
Picker International Inc.
Cleveland, Ohio 44143
Current: Principal Research Fellow in
    MRI
University College and Middlesex
    Schools of Medicine
The Middlesex Hospital
Mortimer Street
London W1N 8AA, England

P. Pancheri
Professor of Psychiatry
University of Rome "La Sapienza"
Viale dell'Università 30
00185 Rome, Italy

M. Pedditzi, M.D.
Department of Neurosciences
University of Cagliari
via Porcell 4
09124 Cagliari, Italy

D. Piacentini, M.D.
Clinical Vice-Chief
USSL 27
Department of Psychiatry
Zogno (BG), Italy

P. Pietrini
Clinical Psychiatry I
University of Pisa
I-56100 Pisa, Italy
Current: Senior Staff Fellow
Laboratory of Neurosciences
National Institute on Aging
National Institutes of Health
Bethesda, Maryland 20892

J. L. Rapoport
Chief, Child Psychiatry Branch
National Institute of Mental Health
National Institutes of Health
Bethesda, Maryland 20892

L. Ravizza
Professor and Director
Psychiatric Department
University of Turin
via Cherasco 11
10126 Turin, Italy

K. G. Reymann
Laboratory Chief
Institute of Neurobiology and Brain
  Research
Academy of Sciences
Magdeburg, Germany

V. Rinaldi, M.D.
USSL 27
Department of Psychiatry
Zogno (BG), Italy

T. Rippeon, M.S.
Staff Scientist
Loats Associates, Inc
Westminster, Maryland 21157

P. Rocca, M.D.
Psychiatry Department
University of Turin
via Cherasco 11
10126 Turin, Italy

S. Romanello
Junior Researcher
Fidia Research Laboratories
via Ponte della Fabbrica 3/A
35031 Abano Terme (PD), Italy

B. Ross, M.D.
Director, MR Spectroscopy
Huntington Medical Research
  Institutes
660 South Fair Oaks Avenue
Pasadena, California 91105

E. Sanna
Department of Experimental Biology
Chair of Pharmacology
University of Cagliari
via Palabanda 12
09123 Cagliari, Italy

G. Santoro
Department of Experimental Biology
Chair of Pharmacology
University of Cagliari
via Palabanda 12
09123 Cagliari, Italy

P. Sarteschi
Professor and Director
Clinical Psychiatry I
University of Pisa
I-56100 Pisa, Italy

M. Santi
Research Assistant Professor
Georgetown University Medical
  School
3900 Reservoir Rd NW
Washington, DC 20007

S. Scarone, M.D.
Associated Professor of Psychiatry
Psychiatric Branch
Department of Biomedical and
  Technological Sciences
University of Milan Medical School
Scientific Institute San Raffaele
via Prinetti 29
20127 Milan, Italy

M. B. Schapiro, M.D.
*Chief, Brain Aging and Dementia
  Section*
Laboratory of Neurosciences
National Institute on Aging
National Institutes of Health
Bethesda, Maryland 20892

P. H. Seeburg
Professor
Zentrum für Molekulare Biologie
Im Neuenheimer Feld 282
6900 Heidelburg, Germany

W. Semple, Ph.D.
Section on Clinical Brain Imaging
Laboratory of Cerebral Metabolism
National Institute of Mental Health
Bethesda, Maryland 20892
Current: Department of Psychiatry
Case Western Reserve University
Cleveland, Ohio

M. Serra
Researcher
Department of Experimental Biology
Chair of Pharmacology
University of Cagliari
via Palabanda 12
09123 Cagliari, Italy

S. Sigala
*Institute of Pharmacology and
  Experimental Therapeutics
  School of Medicine*
University of Brescia
via Valsabbina 19
25124 Brescia, Italy

G. Simson
Advanced Psychometrics Corporation
8311 Wisconsin Avenue
Bethesda, Maryland 20814-3126

E. Smeraldi
Professor of Psychiatry
Head, Department of Neuroscience
Scientific Institute San Raffaele
Clinical Psychiatry III
University of Milan
via L. Prinetti 29
20127 Milan, Italy

P. Spano
Professor
*Institute of Pharmacology and
  Experimental Therapeutics
  School of Medicine*
University of Brescia
via Valsabbina 19
25124 Brescia, Italy

S. E. Swedo, M.D.
Senior Investigator
Child Psychiatry Branch
National Institute of Mental Health
National Institutes of Health
Bethesda, Maryland 20892

G. Tacchini, M.D.
Institute of Psychiatry
University of Milan
Ospedale Maggiore-P. Guardia II
via Francesco Sforza 35
20122 Milan, Italy

C. Tamminga
*University of Maryland Psychiatric
  Research Center*
Baltimore, Maryland 20201

G. Toffano
Director of Research Laboratory
Fidia Research Laboratories
via Ponte della Fabbrica 3/A
35031 Abano Terme (PD), Italy

R. Torta
Researcher
Psychiatry Department
University of Turin
via Cherasco 11
10126 Turin, Italy

S. Vighetti
Graduate Technician
Neurology Department
University of Turin
via Cherasco 15
10126 Turin, Italy

A. Zadeik–Hipkins
Advanced Psychometrics Corporation
8311 Wisconsin Avenue
Bethesda, Maryland 20814-3126

A. Zanotti
Senior Researcher
Fidia Research Laboratories
via Ponte della Fabbrica 3/A
35031 Abano Terme (PD), Italy

Psychiatry and Advanced Technologies

Psychiatry and Advanced Technologies,
edited by L. Ravizza, F. Bogetto, and
E. Zanalda. Raven Press, Ltd.,
New York © 1993.

1

The Neurobiology of Mood Disorders: A Decade of Progress

Jorge Alberto Costa e Silva

*Department of Psychiatry, State University of Rio de Janeiro,
Rio de Janeiro, Brazil*

Investigation of the biology of mood disorders has generated a complex mixture of evidence from both animal and clinical research. It is important to recognize the limitations of that evidence. Speculation and model-building are just as important in biology as in other fields. However, the building blocks are subject to similar limitations as those found in primate research or phenomenology. Biologic information does not necessarily provide special insight into etiology.

Living systems are mercurial in their response to challenge. They adapt readily, and therefore our intrusion changes the nature of what we seek to observe. Clinical research into mental illness presents a particular problem in this regard. Yet, except for the primates, there are few, if any, adequate animal models of human mood disturbance. Hence clinical research, the detailed investigation of individuals with depression and mania, is essential. Two drawbacks are immediately apparent in this setting. First, we cannot hope to control all the necessary variables to provide precise research results. Second, to obtain biologic information we can sample only a limited number of tissues. For detailed metabolic information we must turn to the laboratory, particularly to the rat. However, here we invade the normal central nervous system (CNS), not one that is locked in melancholic withdrawal. Again, therefore, we face limitations. Cross-referencing and correlation of the information gathered in the clinical setting and in the laboratory is therefore vital if we are to advance our specific understanding of the biology of mood disorders.

SLEEP STUDIES

Insomnia has long been recognized as a central symptom of depression. Recent studies utilizing polysomnographic electroencephalograph (EEG) sleep recordings have demonstrated specific abnormalities in the sleep of most depressed patients. These abnormalities represent some of the best established biologic observations in depression.

Some studies report that rapid eye movement (REM) latency is most reduced in more severely depressed patients, and that REM latency differentiates primary from secondary depression (1). Shortened REM latency seems to be associated with primary and endogenous depression and has been used diagnostically to differentiate subgroups of depressed patients. However, short REM latency also appears to be present in certain other pathologic conditions (e.g., narcolepsy), and even at times in normal subjects. Interestingly, short REM latency appears to be present in those depressed patients who demonstrate nonsuppression on the dexamethasone suppression test (DST), and therefore shares with the DST both potential usefulness as a biologic marker and the same lack of specificity for depression demonstrated by the DST.

The sleep abnormalities observed in depressed patients are among the most consistent and important biologic findings in depression. Although they are not specific for depression, their consistent presence supports the hypothesis that there is a biology of depression and provides clues to the underlying pathophysiology. Although sleep studies are not yet practical for routine clinical use, the sleep abnormalities described provide strong support for the diagnosis of depression, and early data suggest that sleep parameters may be useful in the prediction of treatment response. If replicated, the finding that early changes in sleep parameters predict eventual response to tricyclic antidepressants may be of considerable clinical importance if it enables a correct choice of initial treatment and thereby shortens the time required for recovery from depressive episodes.

NEUROENDOCRINE STUDIES IN DEPRESSION

Cortisol

Many studies have now shown dysregulation of the hypothalamic–pituitary–adrenal axis (HPA), manifests primarily by cortisol hypersecretion, disinhibition of nocturnal secretion of cortisol, and loss of the normal circadian variation. Cortisol hypersecretion is probably the best established biochemical abnormality in depression. In certain studies, urinary free cortisol (UFC) values have enabled differentiation between depressed (both bipolar and unipolar) and manic patients and from normal subjects (2). In some studies, urinary and plasma cortisol values appear to correlate with the degree of depression, and the highest values are observed in psychotic depression (2). Cortisol levels also appear to correlate with cognitive abnormalities and ventricular enlargement on computed axial tomography (CAT) scans in depressed patients (3). Basic studies utilizing radiotagged hypothalamic corticotropin-releasing hormone (CRH) have documented a blunted adrenocorticotropic hormone (ACTH) response to CRH (despite hypercortisolism), providing evidence that the defect in depression is at the level of hypothalamus rather than the pituitary or adrenal gland (4).

Thyroid Abnormalities

Classical endocrinology has demonstrated clear psychiatric abnormalities, including depression, with both overt hypothyroidism and hyperthyroidism. Gold and colleagues (5) have also suggested that a subset (5–10%) of patients with depression or anergia could be said to have Grade II or III hypothyroidism. These patients would have been considered euthyroid if they had been worked up by traditional methods. This subclinical hypothyroidism is demonstrated only by basal increases in thyroid-stimulating hormone (TSH) or in an abnormal TSH response to thyrotropin-releasing hormone (TRH). These patients often have detectable levels of antimicrosomal thyroid antibodies, and Nemeroff et al. (6) have demonstrated that 20% of depressed patients consecutively admitted to a psychiatric hospital had antithyroid antibodies. Furthermore, lithium may induce antithyroid antibodies and patients who develop antithyroid antibodies are more likely to develop overt hypothyroidism when given lithium. However, at this point it is difficult to define the stages of subclinical hypothyroidism, to integrate these results with the data of blunted TSH responses, or to determine how both relate to psychiatric symptoms and treatment issues.

NEUROTRANSMITTER ABNORMALITIES

Norepinephrine

The modern study of the biologic aspects of depression began with the catecholamine hypothesis of mood disorders in the mid-1960s. Simply stated, this hypothesis proposed that at least some cases of depression were associated with a functional deficiency of norepinephrine (NE) at important synapses in the brain, whereas mania was hypothesized to involve increases in NE. The earliest evidence was indirect and was based on observations that the MAO-inhibiting antidepressants blocked an important pathway for NE metabolism and the tricyclic antidepressants prevented the metabolism of NE by blocking its reuptake into the presynaptic nerve terminal.

Dopamine

Although most of the original interest in the catecholamine theory of depression, as well as more recent studies, has centered largely on 5-HT (serotonin), there is increasing neurochemical and pharmacologic evidence that functional dopamine (DA) activity may be reduced in some depressed patients and increased in manic patients. The initial pharmacologic evidence implicating involvement of DA in depression involved studies that demonstrated modest antidepressant effects with the DA precursor L-dopa. It was particularly provocative that pretreatment levels of the principal DA metabolite, homovanillic acid (HVA), in cerebrospinal fluid predicted a favorable response to L-dopa.

Recently developed and relatively specific postsynaptic DA agonists have demonstrated even more obvious antidepressant activity for these agents. In a double-blind trial with piribedil, Post and colleagues (7) reported antidepressant effects in 12 of 16 patients and again, a low pretreatment level of HVA in cerebral spinal fluid (CSF) predicted greater clinical improvement. Subsequent trials with piribedil and bromocriptine (8) also reported antidepressant responses and occasional shifts into mania. Certainly, the demonstration of clear efficacy in large clinical trials of nomifensine, amineptine, and bupropion, which have prominent effects on DA systems, have further implicated the DA system in depression.

Serotonin

Interest in the potential role of serotonin (5-HT) abnormalities in the biochemistry of mood disorders has been second only to the catecholamines. Available evidence suggests that decreased 5-HT activity may either increase vulnerability to depression or be a causative factor. The wide distribution of 5-HT in the brain and its interaction with multiple other neurotransmitters enable it to function as an inhibitory influence on neuronal mechanisms and on behavior. Considerable evidence suggests that 5-HT is involved in those processes that appear to become abnormal in depression, e.g., mood, insomnia, short REM latency, disturbed circadian rhythms, abnormal neuroendocrine function, and abnormalities of libido. Several animal models of depression are also consistent with a hyposerotonergic hypothesis of depression.

Central Serotonin Receptors

Recently, there have been significant advances in our understanding of 5-HT biochemistry and physiology, and it now seems possible that not only the mood disorders but many other CNS disorders result from aberrations in the serotoninergic system, such as pain, various obsessive–compulsive disorders, obesity, schizophrenia, anxiety, sexual dysfunction, migraine, and various vasospastic disorders.

Much of the recent progress in 5-HT research was stimulated by the discovery of *multiple* 5-HT receptors and by the design of selective ligands (5-HT$_1$ has four separate classes: 1A, 1B, 1C, 1D + 5-HT$_2$ + 5-HT$_3$).

The fact that during the past several years the existence of multiple 5-HT receptors has become apparent provides new opportunities for drug discovery. The availability of drugs that are selective for certain 5-HT receptor subtypes is allowing characterization of 5-HT receptor physiology in animals. Moreover, as more clinical data are obtained with these new tools, we may be able to treat certain CNS diseases more effectively and may also gain a greater understanding of 5-HT receptor function throughout the body.

Acetylcholine

In 1972, Janowsky and colleagues (9) focused attention on the cholinergic system when they hypothesized that affective disturbances were related to relative imbalances between the brain adrenergic and cholinergic systems. They postulated that depression represented a relative cholinergic predominance, with mania thought to be an illness of relative adrenergic predominance. Most of the subsequent evidence has supported this model, and suggests at least some involvement of the cholinergic system in depression.

Muscarinic Receptors

Although several studies have suggested differences in muscarinic receptor binding between affective patients and normal subjects, this remains a controversial area. Nadi and colleagues (10) reported that fibroblasts grown in culture from affective disorder patients and their relatives had more muscarinic–cholinergic (QNB) binding sites than normal subjects. Furthermore, Meyerson and colleagues (11) reported increased muscarinic receptor-binding activity in the brains of patients who died by suicide as compared to those who died of other causes. However, recent studies from multiple groups have failed to find evidence of increased muscarinic binding, either in the brain or the periphery, in suicides. Because [^{123}I]-QNB is a high-affinity mixed muscarinic receptor ligand that allows imaging of the distribution of muscarinic receptor sites in the brain, single photon emission computed tomography (CT) (SPECT) may lead to the best understanding of the role of muscarinic receptors in the brain.

Some of the available evidence is consistent with the hypothesis that acetylcholine (ACh) may be involved in the etiology or expression of affective disorders. Although there is little direct biological evidence, the pharmacologic data suggest that ACh is involved in the induction of the symptoms of depression and perhaps in some of the biologic abnormalities (e.g., cortisol, sleep) observed in depression. It is even more likely that changes in the ACh system may either cause or interact with perturbations in other systems, most notably the noradrenergic system. The recent findings of enhanced cholinergic REM induction in volunteers with a family history of affective illness and the persistence of that abnormality in remitted patients suggest the importance of genetic factors and that cholinergic abnormalities may result in a predisposition to depression rather than being actively involved in "causing" depression. The ACh system interacts at both an anatomic and a pharmacologic level with the NE system to "modulate" changes in the adrenergic system. Muscarinic hypersensitivity might predispose to the development of depression in response to changes in the NE system secondary to adverse life experiences. This type of model is more consistent with a growing data base suggestive of the involvement of multiple brain neurotransmitters in depression and with evidence suggesting that biologic deficits in depression may be related to defective regulatory processes.

ELECTROLYTE STUDIES

Extensive studies of electrolyte metabolism, particularly of sodium metabolism in depression and mania, lend further support to the evidence for an increased state of neurophysiologic arousal in these states. Balance studies are difficult to interpret, however, and very demanding to perform for both patients and researchers. Therefore, when isotope dilution techniques became available which, together with a total body counter, made it possible to calculate changes in metabolically active sodium, there was a rapid switch to this new technique.

Coppen and Shaw (12), in studies that have been confirmed by most investigators, reported a significant shift of sodium into the cells during depression and mania. They calculated that such a shift would decrease the average resting potential of the nerve and concluded that the neurons of the depressed patient would be more excitable. The difference was of similar magnitude to the excitatory postsynaptic potential which initiates depolarization at the synapse. Hence, electrolyte studies also suggest a hyperexcitable state of the CNS during depressive illness.

GENETIC MARKERS

There has been remarkable success with restriction fragment length polymorphism (RFLP) strategies in the search for a gene associated with Huntington's disease. In theory, this technique could be utilized in affective illness. Bipolar illness may be relatively homogeneous; high-density families exist, and a large number of individuals are informative. The RFLP methodology involves the detection of different fragment lengths of DNA. DNA is then cut by bacterial enzymes (restriction endonucleases), which allow the visualization of specific fragments with radiographic techniques. It is then possible to study these specific fragments of DNA in an entire pedigree.

At present, more than one-third of the human genome has been mapped, and it is predicted that within the next few years mapping of the entire genome will be accomplished. With these techniques it is possible to search for a gene(s) associated with bipolar disorder. Preliminary evidence suggests that Chromosome 11 may contain the gene for bipolar illness.

Finally, we might ask: What is the significance of searching for trait or genetic markers? It would certainly be valuable if, in a high-density family with, for example, five siblings, we would be able to identify which sibling had an increased probability of developing depressive illness. This would allow early recognition of the developing illness by the individual and by the family. Early initiation of prophylactic treatment and the possibility of developing specific social support systems might help to prevent onset of the disease. It would also allow, for the first time, truly preventative investigations to be performed.

At present, although no thoroughly investigated and specific markers exist for mood disorders, there are a number of extremely promising candidates, and it is believed that this is a particularly fruitful area for further investigation.

POSITRON EMISSION TOMOGRAPHY IN DEPRESSION RESEARCH

Currently, positron emission tomography (PET) is the only technology that affords quantitative, three-dimensional imaging of various aspects of brain function. In most of the few PET studies of mood disorders performed thus far, cerebral glucose metabolism was investigated by the fluorodeoxyglucose method. The greatest diagnostic potential of PET was demonstrated in certain forms of organic depression, whereas metabolic abnormalities in major unipolar and bipolar depression were more subtle (albeit significantly different). Other PET tracers for investigation of transmitter systems are available but have not been systematically applied in depression research.

Many studies have indicated that psychiatric diseases are often associated with certain biochemical abnormalities, but conventional laboratory techniques have largely failed to identify the neuroanatomical structures involved or to determine the temporal relationship of mood and behavior to biochemical changes in the brain. Furthermore, despite detailed investigations, neither x-ray CT nor magnetic resonance imaging (MRI) of protons has provided specific insights into the etiology or anatomic locations affected in the various mental disorders. PET, by contrast, seems well suited to study of the pathophysiologic correlates of psychiatric syndromes because it is the only method that affords quantitative, three-dimensional imaging of several well-defined brain mechanisms. To date, however, its applications to psychiatric problems have been quite limited and most of the PET studies of mental disorders have focused on schizophrenia and, more recently, on anxiety and panic disorders, rather than on affective syndromes (13–15). Moreover, although mood disorders have a high rate of incidence and lend themselves to both comparative cross-sectional and longitudinal studies because of their commonly transient nature, the groups of patients analyzed usually have been small. Except for five patients who underwent PET measurements of cerebral oxygen consumption, blood flow, and volume (16), brain glucose metabolism was the physiological quantity assessed in all other PET studies of brain function in depression (13,17).

CONCLUSIONS

We performed a selective review of various biologic investigations in depression with a particular emphasis on findings that might have current or future clinical relevance. There is no coherent "biology" of depression at this point, nor is it likely that there will be in the near future. Research has tended to focus on one area to the exclusion of others, and this, coupled with the inherent complexity of the work, has prevented definitive elucidation of even single mechanisms: certainly, coherent relationships among areas of research have been impossible to date. However, as research in this area has expanded, areas of consensus have been formed and will be touched on throughout this volume.

Although such hints of convergence and basic explanations of biologic mechanisms in depression are exciting, more definitive understanding of these mechanisms probably awaits decades of further research. The practical and widespread clinical use of biologic factors also must probably be relegated to the future. Despite increasing confidence in certain findings, (particularly sleep changes, HPA axis abnormalities, and certain of the urinary and CSF measurements), none is ready for routine use by the clinician. The early, relatively uncritical use of the DST reflected both the great need for external and easily obtained measurements and the difficulties of translating these biologic measurements into routine practice.

The structural complexity of the CNS, its multiple chemical messengers, its detailed regulation, and its rapid response to challenge predict that manifest behavior is a function of many variables. We are only beginning to understand what mechanisms underlie the behaviors that are dominant in mood disorders. Although disturbed biogenic amine metabolism may represent a final common pathway to dysfunction, the amount of neurotransmitter in the synaptic cleft is only one of the many contributing variables. Pre- and postsynaptic regulatory mechanisms, including changes in receptor sensitivity, ionic shifts across neuronal membranes, changes in enzyme activity, variations in the balance between systems regulating opposing behaviors, are all known to be relevant factors. Certainly there must be many more. Therefore, theories based on the disturbance of a single variable are unlikely to serve us well in the future.

Basic studies in biochemical pharmacology support the concept that multiple mechanisms are employed by the brain in the regulation of specific behaviors.

A normally functioning serotonergic system may be necessary for the appropriate behaviors driven by the norepinephrine system to be expressed. If serotonin is diminished, then changes in the activity of norepinephrine neurons may result in aberrant behaviors, such as those found in mood disorders.

The highly consistent clinical findings that low levels of CSF 5-hydroxyindoleacetic acid (5-HIAA) occur in depressed persons (both during illness and often after recovery), that 5-HT and 5-HIAA in the brains of suicide victims are reduced, that methysergide (a general 5-HT antagonist) makes mania worse, and that tryptophan aids in speeding the recovery from acute mania all suggest, when considered in light of the animal studies, that the interaction between the two systems in the control of behavior is a fundamental one. Indeed, it appears certain that consideration of the dynamic interactions of brain mechanisms will become a central theme in our future understanding of the neurobiology of mood disorders. The components of such disorders can be understood only in their relationship to one another.

REFERENCES

1. Kupfer DJ, Foster FG, Reich L, Thompson KS, Weiss B. EEG sleep changes as predictors in depression. *Am J Psychiatry* 1976;133:622–6.
2. Rubinow DR, Post RM, Savard R, Gold PW. Cortisol hypersecretion and cognitive impairment in depression. *Arch Gen Psychiatry* 1984;41:279–83.
3. Kellner CH, Rubinow DR, Gold PW, Post RM. Relationship of cortisol hypersecretion to brain CT scan alterations in depressed patients. *Psychiatr Res* 1983;8:191–7.
4. Gold PW, Chrousos G, Kellner C, et al. Psychiatric implications of basic and clinical studies with corticotropin-releasing factor. *Am J Psychiatry* 1984;141:619–27.
5. Gold MS, Pottash ALC, Extein I, et al. Hypothyroidism and depression. Evidence from complete thyroid function evaluation. *JAMA* 1981;245:1919–22.
6. Nemeroff CB, Simon JS, Happerty JJ Jr, Evans DL. Antithyroid antibodies in depressed patients. *Am J Psychiatry* 1985;142:840–3.
7. Post RM, Gerner RH, Carman JS, et al. Effects of dopamine agonist piribedil in depressed patients. Relationship of pretreatment homovanillic acid to antidepressant response. *Arch Gen Psychiatry* 1978;35:609–15.
8. Silverstone T. Response to bromocriptine distinguishes bipolar from unipolar depression. *Lancet* 1984;1:903–4.
9. Janowsky DS, Kheled EL Yousef M, Daws JM, Sekerke HJ. A cholinergic-adrenergic hypothesis of mania and depression. *Lancet* 1972;2:632.
10. Nadi NS, Nurnberger JL Jr, Gershon ES. Muscarinic cholinergic receptors on skin fibroblasts in familiar affective disorder. *N Engl J Med* 1984;311:225–30.
11. Meyerson LR, Wennogle LP, Abel MS, et al. Human brain receptor alterations in suicide victims. *Pharmacol Biochem Behav* 1982;17:159–63.
12. Coppen AJ, Shaw DM. Mineral metabolism in melancholia. *BMJ* 1963;2:1439.

13. Buchsbaum MS, Cappelletti J, Ball R, et al. Positron emission tomographic image measurement in schizophrenia and affective disorders. *Ann Neurol* 1984;15(suppl 1):S157–65.
14. Volkow ND, Brodie JD, Wolf AP, et al. Brain organization in schizophrenia. *J Cereb Blood Flow Metab* 1986;6:441–6.
15. Mazziotta JC, Phelps ME, Phal JJ, et al. Reduced cerebral glucose metabolism in asymptomatic subject at risk for Huntington disease. *N Engl J Med* 1987;316:357–62.
16. Raichle ME, Mintun MA, Herscovitch P. Positron emission tomography with 15 oxygen radiopharmaceuticals. *Res Publ Assoc Res Nerv Ment Dis* 1985;63:51–9.
17. Baxter LR, Phelps ME, Mazziotta JC, et al. Cerebral metabolic rates for glucose in mood disorders. *Arch Gen Psychiatry* 1985;42:441–7.

Psychiatry and Advanced Technologies,
edited by L. Ravizza, F. Bogetto, and
E. Zanalda. Raven Press, Ltd.,
New York © 1993.

2

Brain Electric Fields and Classes of Thought

D. Lehmann, C.M. Michel, B. Henggeler, and D. Brandeis

Brain Mapping Laboratory, Neurology Department, University Hospital, 8091 Zurich, Switzerland

The target phenomena of psychiatry are the pathologic deviations of brain information processing, the deviations of thought and emotions. Thoughts and emotions are the private (subjective) aspects of complex brain processes whose subcomponents, such as molecules or single cells, cannot individually represent complete thoughts or emotions.

BRAIN ELECTRIC DATA IN PSYCHIATRY

One approach to the operationalization of these psychiatric target phenomena is the measurement of brain electric field data. The brain electric field appears particularly suited for biological measurements in psychiatry because (i) it reflects very sensitive and subtle changes in thought, emotions, and behavior (see, e.g., 1–3), (ii) it offers a time resolution that can reach fractions of seconds, which appears necessary to monitor brain information processing, (iii) it is noninvasive and harmless and therefore suited for continuous monitoring, and (iv) it can be described as a homogeneous entity, reminiscent of conscious thought. With electroencephalogram (EEG) time-series analysis (frequency band power and coherence, amplitudes, latencies), many studies have shown various relationships between psychiatric diagnostic criteria, symptoms, prognosis, and EEG/event-related potential (ERP) data (5–7). Typically in these reports, particular temporal frequency bands were identified that most sensitively reflected the psychiatric target phenomena.

BRAIN ELECTRIC FIELDS AND BRAIN FUNCTIONAL STATES

Our work has concentrated on EEG and ERP analysis strategies that exploit fully the information available in the space domain of the brain electric fields. The brain electric activity can be displayed as a series of momentary maps of the potential distribution (electric ''landscape'') on the scalp (8). Maps of different landscapes must be generated by the activity of different neuronal populations because these different populations probably execute different information processing tasks. Therefore, it can be assumed that different distributions (maps) of the brain electric field represent different functional brain activities such as steps, types, or contents of information processing. Thus, a given map landscape is suggested to manifest a particular global functional state that corresponds to a particular function of brain information processing. In more detail, the global functional state that is manifest in a map can be viewed as a mosaic of local functional states that reflect the large number of parallel processes active at each moment in time. However, we suggest that the global functional state as measured by the map landscape, just like consciousness on the subjective side, might be treated as an operational unity. It is interesting to consider that such a global state of the brain electric field may reflect the subjective homogeneity of a thought.

MODELING OF MOMENTARY FIELDS BY EQUIVALENT DIPOLE SOURCES

A momentary potential distribution map such as the electric ''landscape,'' which is measured simultaneously from many electrodes on the scalp, can be described by an equivalent electric dipole source whose location, orientation, and strength optimally account for the observed data. This time-domain method accounts for the observed potential distribution by a single (or more) equivalent dipole source(s) in terms of amplitudes. An equivalent source might therefore be fitted into each map of a long series, as done in magneto-metric encephalography (MEG) studies of spontaneous activity (9–13). If model sources for individual temporal frequency bands are desired, temporal frequency band passing is necessary before source modeling of the momentary maps.

Dipole Sources in the Frequency Domain

We have developed an alternate method (14) that accounts for entire epochs of multichannel EEG data after transformation into the frequency domain by a single (or more) equivalent dipole source in terms of phase angles (for each frequency point). We call this the FFT dipole approximation. (The underlying rationale is that a single sine wave source produces fields in which the phase differences between locations are only 0° and 180°.) After transformation of the data into the frequency domain and entering the results into a sine–cosine diagram for each frequency point, the method computes the best-fit line into each resulting constellation of entry points (Fig. 1). The

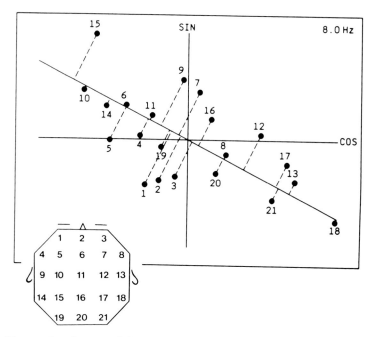

FIG. 1. Sine–cosine diagram of the 8.0-Hz point results of the Fourier transform of a 19-channel EEG epoch of 2 s. Best-fit straight line through the data entry constellation; this line minimizes the sum of the squared deviations (dotted) between the original entry locations and their orthogonal projections onto the straight line; the voltage values are the distances between projected points on the straight line vs. the chosen reference ("FFT dipole approximation" by a single generator in terms of phase angles). Electrodes 2 and 20 are interpolated.

entries are orthogonally projected onto the best-fit line and the projected locations are read out as a potential distribution map, the FFT dipole approximation map. When squared, this best-fit potential distribution map is the optimal approximation (15) of the original power map that is constructed from the transformed data (Fig. 2). The FFT dipole approximation potential distribution map can be used for computation of an equivalent dipole source in terms of amplitude distribution, using the conventional techniques.

SOURCE LOCALIZATION FOR EEG FREQUENCY BANDS

Different temporal EEG frequencies are known to predominate in grossly different brain functional states such as wakefulness and sleep. In wakefulness, frequencies in the 8- to 12-Hz band predominate, whereas in sleep, slower frequencies in the 1- to 7.5-Hz band are predominant. Nevertheless, the continuous EEG at all times shows contributions from all frequencies, varying in relative weight.

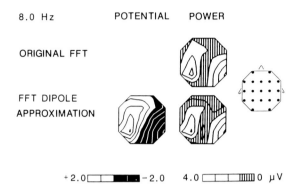

FIG. 2. Top: Original 8.0-Hz power map of the epoch treated in Fig. 1. **Bottom:** FFT dipole approximation potential distribution map (left) and the corresponding power map (right). Head seen from above, nose up. The "power" maps actually show square roots of power.

We have used the FFT dipole approximation technique to investigate the locations of the equivalent electric sources of the two major EEG frequency bands during relaxation in 13 normal subjects of 26 years mean age. Nineteen electrodes were used, and from each subject 10 artifact-free epochs of 2 s were collected at random intervals over 30 min. The FFT dipole approximations were computed and averaged for each subject, using a procedure that permutates the polarities of the members of the average to determine the combination with minimal standard deviation over approximations. For each frequency point of the average FFT dipole approximations, the three-dimensional equivalent single sources in terms of amplitude distribution was computed using the 3-shell option of the program "dipole" (BioLogic, Mundelein, IL, U.S.A.). For each subject, the x, y, and z coordinates of the source locations were averaged within the two frequency bands, 1 to 7.5 and 8 to 12 Hz. The mean band locations were averaged over subjects and tested for significance of differences using paired t tests ($n = 13$) in the three dimensions. The location of the equivalent source of the 1- to 7.5-Hz band was significantly more anterior ($p < 0.0001$) and deeper ($p < 0.002$) than that of the 8- to 12-Hz band; there was no difference in the lateral dimension. [On the basis of potential distribution studies, the "α" activity (8–12 Hz) has always been described as of occipital origin (16).]

SOURCES OF BRAIN ELECTRIC FIELDS DURING DIFFERENT TYPES OF THOUGHT

As a model for the electrophysiologic study of psychiatric problems, we investigated the equivalent dipole source locations that are associated with different types of thought. Because the major EEG frequency bands must be modeled by significantly different equivalent dipole sources, we analyzed the data separately for the 1- to 7.5- and 8- to 12-Hz EEG frequency bands.

Volunteer subjects in a quiet recording room reported their momentary thought briefly whenever a gentle prompt signal was sounded, while 19 EEG channels were continuously recorded. Thirty prompts were given at random to each subject, at least 2.5 min after the last prompt and after 20 s of artifact-free EEG had been observed, over about 1.5 h of recording. Twelve subjects (six men and six women, mean age 33.5, SD $\pm$ 6.1 years) were used. The collected reports were rated by two independent raters as belonging to "visual imagery thoughts" or "abstract thoughts" or to neither of these classes. "I just thought about that beach lunch we had last summer" is an example of a visual imagery thought, whereas "I thought about my teaching schedule this afternoon" is an abstract thought. About one-third of the reports were in each of the three categories, in agreement between two raters.

The 2-s EEG epochs immediately preceding the prompts were artifact-edited and subjected to the FFT dipole approximation. For each subject, mean FFT approximations were computed (with the optimizing permutation procedure) for all epochs belonging to the same report category. Then, the mean FFT dipole approximations were used for three-dimensional dipole source computation ("Dipole" program by BioLogic, 3-shell option). The obtained x, y, and z coordinates were averaged for each subject, within each of the two thought classes and within the two frequency bands, 1.0 to 7.5 and 8.0 to 12 Hz. In this way we obtained for each subject the x-y-z locations of the equivalent sources of the 1- to 7.5- and 8- to 12-Hz EEG frequency bands of the EEG epochs that were associated with "visual" and "abstract" thoughts.

The mean source locations over subjects (in the sagittal plane) for the two thought types and two frequency bands are shown in Fig. 3. The slow frequency sources again were more anterior and lower than the mean 8- to 12-Hz sources. "Abstract" type thoughts were associated with more anterior equivalent source mean locations than "visual imagery" thoughts in both frequency bands. The difference of the locations for abstract and visual types of thoughts, as tested with ANOVA, was significant in the 1- to 7.5-Hz band in the anterior–posterior dimension ($p < 0.02$) and not significant in the 8- to 12-Hz band. No significances were found in the vertical and lateral dimensions.

The present results establish that different neural populations were active during the production of thoughts of the "visual imagery" category and thoughts of the "abstract" category, since different electric field distributions must have been generated by at least partly different generators, one or many.

DISCUSSION

Our work on equivalent dipole source localization in the frequency domain for brain electric data in normal subjects has demonstrated that the different

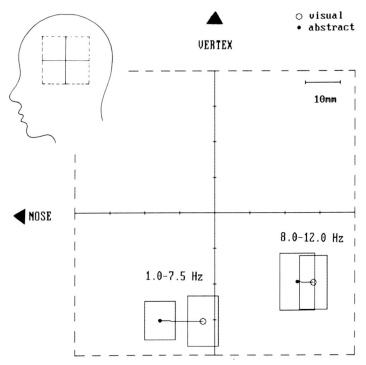

FIG. 3. Locations of the mean equivalent dipole generator sources of the 1- to 7.5-Hz and the 8- to 12-Hz EEG frequency band, for repeated epochs of 2 s (19 channel recordings) associated with momentary thoughts of the "visual imagery" type (circles) and of the "abstract" type (dots). Means and SE (rectangles) over the results of twelve normal subjects. Head seen from the left, nose left, top up; spherical head model; its center (origin of the coordinate system) is at 10% above the preauricular zero point of the 10/20 system. The anterior–posterior difference between source locations of the two thought types was significant in the 1- to 7.5-Hz band.

temporal frequency bands of brain electric fields are generated by different neuronal populations, suggesting that long-lasting global functional states, such as sleep and waking, are subserved by different brain structures; it is conceivable that these structures might be active simultaneously in all functional states, albeit with different weights.

The study of equivalent dipole sources of brain electric activity during different types of thoughts (visual imagery vs. abstract) demonstrated that for the slow-frequency band between 1 and 7.5 Hz the equivalent dipole sources showed significantly different localizations. Even though the reliability of absolute location is open (17) and concerns problems that need not be discussed here, our data clearly show that different neuronal populations are active when thoughts of these two different types are produced. The differences of source locations between thought classes were worked out using short data epochs of no more than 2 s duration, and were common over subjects. This makes it reasonable to hope that it will be possible to match a catalogue of thought classes with a catalogue of brain functional states for healthy subjects that can be used to search for the deviations that lead to psychopathology in psychiatric patients.

ACKNOWLEDGMENT

This work was supported in part by the Swiss National Science Foundation, the EMDO Foundation, the Hartmann–Muller Foundation, the Sandoz Foundation for Medical–Biological Research, and the Gertrud-Ruegg-Foundation. We appreciate the collaboration of Mr. B.A. Kofmel, M.A., during the data collection.

REFERENCES

1. Ehrlichman H, Wiener MS. EEG asymmetry during covert mental activity. *Psychophysiology* 1980;17:228–35.
2. Grass P, Lehmann D, Meier B, Meier CA, Pal I. Sleep onset: factorization and correlations of spectral EEG parameters and mentation rating parameters. *Sleep Res* 1987;16:231.
3. Koukkou M, Lehmann D. Dreaming: the functional state shift hypothesis, a neuropsychophysiological model. *Br J Psychiatry* 1983;142:221–31.
4. Itil TM, Shapiro DM, Schneider SJ, Francis IV. Computerized EEG as a predictor of drug response in treatment resistant schizophrenics. *J Nerv Ment Dis* 1981;169:629–37.
5. Koukkou M. EEG states of the brain, information processing, and schizophrenic primary symptoms. *Psychiatr Res* 1982;6:235–44.
6. Shagass C, Roemer RA, Straumanis JJ, Josiassen RC. Combinations of evoked potential amplitude measurements in relation to psychiatric diagnosis. *Biol Psychiatry* 1985;20:701–22.
7. John ER, Pritchep LS, Fridman J, Easton P. Neurometrics: computer-assisted differential diagnosis of brain dysfunctions. *Science* 1988;239:162–9.
8. Lehmann D. Multichannel topography of human alpha EEG fields. *Electroenceph Clin Neurophysiol* 1971;31:439–44.
9. Vvedensky VL, Ilmonieni RJ, Kajola MJ. Study of the alpha rhythm with a 4-channel SQUID magnetometer. *Med Biol Engin Comput* 1986;(suppl 23, part 1):11–2.
10. He B, Musha T, Ye W, Nakajima Y, Homma S. The dipole tracing method and its application to human alpha wave. In: Tsutsui J, ed. *EEE topography*. Shinagawa (Tokyo): Neuron Publishers, 1987:10–17.
11. He B, Ye W, Musha T. Equivalent dipole tracing of human alpha activities. *IEEE Eng Med Biol Soc* 1989;1217–8.
12. Narici L, Romani GL. Neuromagnetic investigation of synchronized spontaneous activity. *Brain Topogr* 1989;2:19–30.
13. Williamson SJ, Kaufman L. Advances in neuromagnetic instrumentation and studies of spontaneous brain activity. *Brain Topogr* 1989;2:129–54.
14. Lehmann D, Michel CM. Intracerebral dipole source localization for FFT power maps. *Electroenceph Clin Neurophysiol* 1990;76:271–6.
15. Michel CM, Henggeler B, Lehmann D. Correlation between original and single-dipole approximated power maps. *Brain Topogr* 1990;3:255–6.
16. Adrian ED, Yamagiwa K. The origin of the Berger rhythm. *Brain* 1935;58:323–51.
17. Cohen D, Cuffin BN, Yunokuchi K, et al. MEG versus EEG localization test using implanted sources in the human brain. *Ann Neurol* 1990;28:811–7.

Psychiatry and Advanced Technologies,
edited by L. Ravizza, F. Bogetto, and
E. Zanalda. Raven Press, Ltd.,
New York © 1993.

3

Electroencephalography Mapping in the Study of Schizophrenia

L. Ravizza, *C. Asteggiano, R. Torta, *S. Vighetti,
and G. Maina

*Department of Psychiatry and *Department of Neurology, University of Turin,
10126 Turin, Italy*

We studied the resting electroencephalography (EEG) in 10 Type I schizophrenic patients and 8 normal controls. EEG was analyzed as maps of both absolute power and relative power in frontal, temporocentral, and parieto-occipital regions. Patients with schizophrenia had decreased α activity, which was not specific to the frontal region. Schizophrenic patients also had increased frontal left-sided θ activity, which was not statistically significant. We hope to confirm these preliminary data with a larger sample group.

INTRODUCTION

The main aim of our EEG studies on schizophrenic disorders was to determine whether or not there is any basic difference in brain bioelectrical activity between schizophrenic patients and normal subjects. EEG studies demonstrated that over 30% of the schizophrenic patients exhibited baseline bioelectrical measurements that were outside the limit of normal variations. Only a few of these findings were confirmed by different studies such as, for example, more slow activity (θ and δ) and a decrease of fast α.

EEG brain mapping appears to provide much new information about bioelectrical activity in schizophrenia and is a useful technique to identify topographical differences. The development of this technique has also led to various attempts to classify schizophrenic patients according to bioelectric variables. In line with this strategy are studies that try to relate different clinical variables to baseline bioelectric variables or patterns. The criteria for the clinical subtyping of the disorder have been numerous. For example, one of the most simple attempts was to determine whether or not there is any basic difference in EEG mapping between acute and chronic schizophrenics. No significant findings have been confirmed by different studies according to this subclassification, except for an increased variability of bioelectric potentials (1).

Correlation analysis has also been applied to examine the relationship of EEG measurements to each of the principal schizophrenic symptoms. For example, delusions and hallucinations were correlated with bioelectric patterns of passage from high frequencies to slow frequencies in centroparietal regions (2). In accordance with the reports of other authors regarding the association between thought disorders and bioelectric variables, an increase of δ and β waves seems to be more evident in the dominant hemisphere of subjects with a high rate of these symptoms (3).

From this standpoint, many other clinical variables have been studied, such as the onset of the disorder (early or late) and the response to drug treatment. The very few important studies that have examined EEG mapping variables as predictors of neuroleptic responsiveness reported different baseline characteristics in association with a favorable or poor clinical response to drug treatment. One of the most confirmed characteristics was the presence of a typical slow α wave in patients who are nonresistant to treatment with neuroleptic agents (4,5).

Several studies have examined the topographic differences in baseline EEG among the subtypes of schizophrenia that are proposed by the World Health Organization (ICD-9 and ICD-10) or the American Psychiatric Association (DSM-III and DSM-III-R). In these cases, complex clinical features were classified according to precise diagnostic criteria for examination in comparison to EEG measurements. Another attempt to subtype schizophrenic disorders is based on the positive/negative symptoms distinction (Type I and Type II schizophrenia): this seems to be, in our opinion, the most important subclassification of schizophrenia to be used in biologic research, as it is based on a very simple but fundamental distinction of the disorder. Type I schizophrenia, for example, seems to be associated, with decreased strength in α and β waves and increased θ and δ (6). During tests of neuropsychological activation, it has been found that Type II schizophrenic patients do not exhibit an increase of β frequencies in frontal areas (7).

The present report focuses on recent and preliminary EEG mapping studies conducted in our laboratory on patients with schizophrenia.

SUBJECTS AND METHODS

Subjects

The experimental group comprised 10 psychiatric patients (6 men and 4 women, age range 33.6 ± 7.5 years) from the Psychiatric Clinical Department of the University of Turin, Italy. All patients had never been medicated or had been withdrawn from medication at least 4 weeks before the study.

They were chosen according to the following criteria: diagnosis of schizophrenia according to DSM-III-R criteria and diagnosis of Type I schizophrenia according to Crow; 20–60 years old, right-handed, Italian as native language, no history of epilepsy and organic brain damage, and no familial history of epilepsy; drug washout of 4 weeks minimum; Scale for Assessment of Positive Symptoms (SAPS) > 25.

The control group was made up of eight healthy volunteers, matched for sex (four men and four women, age range 33.2 ± 3.2 years) and cultural level to the sample group. All were right-handed and there was no positive history of epilepsy or organic brain damage.

Clinical Evaluation

Complete medical, psychiatric, and psychopharmacologic records were collected for both groups. The schizophrenic patients were also evaluated with the following rating scales: the Brief Psychiatric Rating Scale (BPRS), the Scale for Assessment of Negative Symptoms (SANS), and the SAPS.

EEG Recording and Mapping

The EEGs were recorded while subjects were seated in a resting condition, with eyes closed. Electrodes were attached with standard procedures at all 19 International 10–20 System locations (Fp1, Fp2, F7, F3, Fz, F4, F8, T3, C3, Cz, C4, T4, T5, P3, Pz, P4, T6, 01, 02) and they were referenced to linked ears (A1 + A2).

The unipolar EEG was recorded for 15 min at least. Selection of epochs (2 s) for subsequent spectral analysis was done by visual inspection to exclude those containing artifacts. A spectral analysis of the selected epochs was made and the estimates were combined into frequency bands corresponding to δ (0.4–3.9 Hz), θ (4.0–7.0 Hz), α (7.1–12.9 Hz), and β_1 (13–15.5 Hz). These EEG maps dealt with both absolute power and relative power that were analyzed in frontal, temporocentral, and parieto-occipital regions. We used for the study a "Brain Surveyor" from BASIS Trade (Verona, Italy).

To compare the baseline differences in absolute and relative power between groups the Mann–Whitney U test was used.

RESULTS

Regarding the clinical characteristics of the sample group, we found a mean age of onset of the disorder of 22.5 ± 6.1 years, a mean duration of the illness of 4.6 years, and a mean education level of 12.4 years (the mean education level in the control group was 14.1 years). Concerning their symptomatology, we found the following rating scale total scores: BPRS 39.2 ±

TABLE 1. *Diagnosis (according to DSM-III-R) and rating scale total scores of the schizophrenic patients*

Patient	Diagnosis	BPRS	SAPS	SANS
1	Paranoid	39	35	10
2	Paranoid	32	29	12
3	Disorganized	36	28	08
4	Disorganized	45	37	07
5	Undifferentiated	44	46	09
6	Disorganized	40	45	10
7	Paranoid	42	45	10
8	Undifferentiated	35	39	14
9	Disorganized	40	35	12
10	Paranoid	39	32	11

4.0; SAPS 37.1 $\pm$ 6.6; and SANS 10.3 $\pm$ 2.05. The results of clinical and psychopathologic evaluations are shown in Table 1.

Concerning the relationship between the clinical conditions and the baseline bioelectric variables, we present here only the preliminary data; they can be considered as findings indicative of a trend that must be confirmed by other data. In comparison to the healthy volunteer group, the group of schizophrenic patients showed: a significantly decreased α activity; a slight increase of θ activity in the left frontal area, although this finding is not statistically significant; no significant difference in δ activity; and no significant difference in β activity. Table 2 shows these differences in EEG relative

TABLE 2. *Baseline differences in relative power between schizophrenic and controls; p values from the Mann–Whitney U test*

	α	β	θ	δ
Fp1	0.05		*	
Fp2	0.05			
F7				
F8	0.05		*	
F3				
Fz			*	
F4				
T3	0.05			
T4	0.05			
C3				
C4				
Cz				
P3	0.05			
P4	0.05			
T5				
T6				
Pz				
O1	0.05			
O2	0.05			

* Not statistically significant.

power between the two groups examined are from the statistical point of view.

DISCUSSION

A dominant frequency in the α range was found in the normal control group. In contrast, the schizophrenic patients had reduced α frequency. This is, at present, the only statistically significant finding of our study. On one hand, this is in contrast to studies that found this reduction in α frequency in schizophrenia associated with cerebral ventricular enlargement (8); our sample group was made up of Type I schizophrenic patients, who should not have such brain abnormalities. On the other hand, our findings are in partial agreement with those authors who believe that the α reduction in schizophrenia is related to some particular clinical subtypes of the disorder, such as the disorganized and the undifferentiated (9). In our group of Type I schizophrenic patients, there were four disorganized and two undifferentiated. This group is too small for statistical analysis, although it will be interesting to evaluate this point with a larger group.

Concerning the increased slow activities that some studies have reported in schizophrenia (diffused or in frontal regions) (10,11), our data do not appear to confirm this. We found slightly increased θ activity in the left frontal area of schizophrenia patients, but this will have to be confirmed because it is not yet statistically significant. If it remains unconfirmed, this could mean that specific EEG abnormalities are not frequent in Type I schizophrenia and that there are no baseline EEG differences between this subtype of the disorder and the normal controls. On the other hand, it could also mean that Type I schizophrenia represents too heterogeneous a disorder that must be subclassified before any specific on bioelectric alterations or abnormalities can be correlated.

REFERENCES

1. Itil T, Shapiro DM, Herrmann WM, Schultz W, Morgan V. The system for EEG parametrization and classification of physiotropic drugs. *Pharmacopsychiat Neuropsychopharmacol* 1979;12:4–9.
2. Stevens HE, Livermore A. Telemetered EEG in schizophrenia. *J Neurol Neurosurg Psychiatry* 1982;45:385–95.
3. Serafetidines EA. EEG laterla asymmetries in psychiatric disorders. *Biol Psychiatry* 1984; 19:237–46.
4. Itil TM, Shapiro D, Schneider SJ, Francis IB. Computerized EEG: predictor of outcome in schizophrenia. *J Nerv Ment Dis* 1981;169:629–637.
5. Martucci N, Manna V. EEG elettroencefalogramma computerizzato. In: AAVV, eds. 'Diagnostica per immagini nell'invecchiamento cerebrale'. *Promopharma* 1988:73–86.
6. Guenther W, Davous P, Godet JL, Guillibert E, Breitling D, Rondot P. Bilateral brain dysfunction during motor activation in Type II schizophrenia measured by EEG mapping. *Biol Psychiatry* 1988;23:295–311.

7. Williamson PC, Kutcher SP, Cooper PW, et al. Psychological, topographic EEG, and CT scan correlates of frontal lobe function in schizophrenia. *Psychiatr Res* 1989;29:137–49.
8. Karson CM, Coppola R, Daniel DG, Weinberger DR. Computerized EEG in schizophrenia. *Schizophr Bull* 1988;14:193–7.
9. Colombo C, Gambini O, Macciardi F, et al. Alpha reactivity in schizophrenia and in schizophrenic spectrum disorders; demographic, clinical and hemispheric assessment. *Int J Psychophysiol* 1989;7:47–54.
10. Morihisa JM, Duffy FM, Wyatt RJ. Brain electrical activity mapping (BEAM) in schizophrenic patients. *Arch Gen Psychiatry* 1983;40:719–28.
11. Karson CM, Coppola R, Morihisa JM, Wienberger DR. Computed electroencephalographic activity mapping in schizophrenia. *Arch Gen Psychiatry* 1987;44:514–7.

Psychiatry and Advanced Technologies,
edited by L. Ravizza, F. Bogetto, and
E. Zanalda. Raven Press, Ltd.,
New York © 1993.

4

Computed Electroencephalography Mapping and Event-Related Potentials in Pre- and Post-treatment Schizophrenic Patients

S. Galderisi, A. Mucci, P. Bucci, F. Catapano, M. Maj, and D. Kemali

Department of Psychiatry, First Medical School, University of Naples, 80138 Naples, Italy

Research concerning the possible biological correlates of schizophrenia has greatly been hindered by discrepancies in the findings. Recently, the possibility that schizophrenia represents a mixture of different entities, instead of a single disease, has been carefully reconsidered by many authors (1–3), and it has been concluded that research in biological psychiatry may be fostered by the identification of more "homogeneous" clinical groups in which common biologic aspects are more likely to be found. During the last decade, dichotomic models have been proposed, such as paranoid/nonparanoid, poor/good premorbid adjustment, but points of controversy have arisen for each of them (4–6). More recently, great attention has been devoted to the positive/negative dichotomy in which the two subtypes can be differentiated on a clinical, pathophysiological, and prognostic basis (2,3). However, many authors have reported difficulties in the identification, within their schizophrenic samples of predominantly "positive" or "negative" clinical pictures, stating that very often clinicians deal with "mixed" subtypes. Moreover, a lack of stability within the same patient, of the positive and negative symptoms has been found in follow-up studies (7). In addition, the prognostic value of such a dichotomy has been questioned, as some studies have shown that negative symptoms may predict either a good or a poor outcome, depending on their occurrence during the acute or chronic phase of the illness (8,9).

Although not exempt from pitfalls (10), a more promising approach to the identification of schizophrenic subgroups with homogeneous biological characteristics may be based on responsiveness to neuroleptics, as suggested by neuroanatomical (11), biochemical (12,13), and neurophysiological findings (14).

In the present study, the results of both computed electroencephalography (CEEG) mapping and an event-related potential (ERP) investigation are reported and discussed as promising tools in the identification of biological correlates of response to treatment in schizophrenic patients.

CEEG STUDY

Methods

The CEEG mapping study was carried out in 20 DSM-III-R (15) schizophrenic patients, 7 women and 13 men, age range between 19–37 years (mean ± SD, 25.65 ± 4.84), a duration of illness ranging from 0.6–17 years (mean ± SD, 5.01 ± 4), and age at onset from 16–26 years (mean ± SD, 20.9 ± 2.8). Patients were subtyped according to both DSM-III-R and Andreasen's criteria (16). Following DSM-III-R criteria 12 were paranoid, 4 disorganized, 3 undifferentiated, and 1 catatonic. Six patients met Andreasen's criteria for positive, 2 for negative, and 12 for mixed schizophrenia.

Eighteen patients completed a washout period of at least 15 days (45 days for long-acting neuroleptics) before entering the study, and two were drug-naive. The control group included 21 healthy subjects matched with patients for age, sex, and handedness.

A baseline (day 0) resting EEG was recorded from all subjects. Patients were then administered a single oral dose of haloperidol and EEGs were recorded after 1, 3, 6, and 8 h. Treatment with haloperidol was continued for 4 weeks (with dosage increased weekly up to 7 mg/day) and further EEG recordings were obtained weekly. No other central nervous system (CNS) effective drugs were allowed during this period. Extrapyramidal side effects in three patients required anticholinergic treatment (biperiden, 4 mg/day) which was always discontinued 2 days before EEG recordings.

EEG was recorded from 16 unipolar leads of the 10–20 System; the HZI BFM system (17) was used for A/D conversion and Fast Fourier transform of the EEG signal. Eight frequency bands were considered (δ, 1.3–3.5 Hz; θ_1, 3.7–5.5 Hz; θ_2, 5.7–7.5 Hz; α_1, 7.7–9.5 Hz; α_2, 9.7–12.5 Hz; β_1, 12.7–15 Hz; β_2, 15.2–26 Hz; β_3, 26.2–35 Hz). Further methodological details can be found elsewhere (18).

Clinical evaluation was done on the basis of psychiatric interviews, at day 0 and then weekly. Andreasen's Scales for the Assessment of Positive (SAPS) and Negative (SANS) Symptoms were used for symptom ratings.

Baseline CEEG characteristics and changes induced by acute and chronic haloperidol administration were studied in relationship to patients' responsiveness to treatment. Patients were considered "responders" when a 50% reduction of the global score on SAPS + SANS was observed after 28 days of treatment.

For comparisons between groups the Mann–Whitney U test was used; changes induced by treatment were assessed by the Wilcoxon–Wilcox test.

Results

Twelve patients (six men and six women) were responders (R) and eight (seven men and one woman) were nonresponders (NR). R and NR were not different for age, education, and duration of illness, but NR showed a significantly younger age at onset (mean ± SD, 19.5 ± 1.6) than R (mean ± SD, 22.4 ± 2.6; $p < 0.01$).

As to clinical evaluation, notwithstanding a predominance of negative symptoms in NR, no significant baseline difference was observed between responders and nonresponders on psychopathologic ratings. After 28 days of treatment, a significant reduction of total scores on both SANS and SAPS was observed in R; in NR a significant reduction of the total score on SAPS was observed, whereas negative symptoms were almost unchanged (Fig. 1).

When baseline CEEGs of the two subgroups were compared, R showed higher α_2, β_1, and β_2 amplitude (Fig. 2), less θ_2 and α_1 as well as more α_2 and β_1 relative power than NR (Fig. 2).

In addition to the baseline differences, R and NR showed different patterns of CEEG changes after haloperidol administration. Only results concerning changes observed in the sixth hour after drug administration and in the twenty-eighth day of treatment will be reported.

Both subgroups exhibited a decrease of δ and an increase of β amplitude, but while in R a significant increase of θ_2 and α_1 was found, no change of θ_2 and a decrease of α_1 was observed in NR (Fig. 3). Relative power results were similar (Fig. 4). After 28 days of treatment, CEEG modifications could be observed only in patients with a favorable clinical response, whereas almost no change was observed in nonresponders (Tables 1 and 2).

ERP STUDY

Methods

The ERP study was carried out in 18 DSM-III, right-handed schizophrenic patients, 14 men and 4 women, 11 paranoid, 4 undifferentiated, 3 residual,

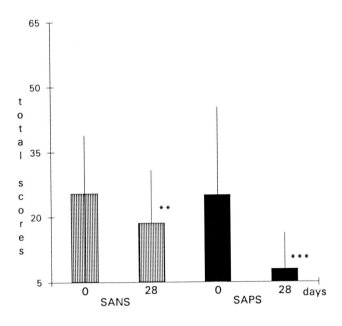

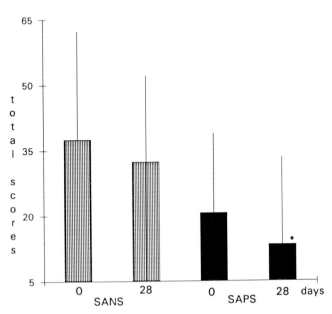

FIG. 1. Total scores on Andreasen's Scales for the Assessment of Negative (SANS) and Positive (SAPS) Symptoms in responders **(top)** and nonresponders **(bottom)** on days 0 (end of the washout period) and 28. * $p < 0.04$; ** $p < 0.01$; *** $p < 0.003$.

AMPLITUDE

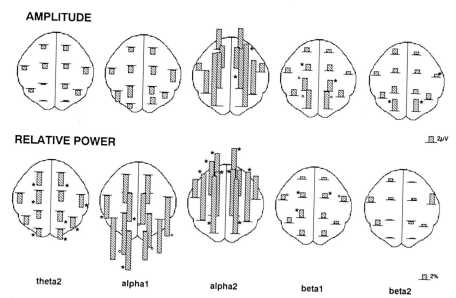

RELATIVE POWER

◳ 2μV

| theta2 | alpha1 | alpha2 | beta1 | beta2 |

FIG. 2. Mean differences between baseline EEGs of responders and nonresponders. In the drawing the frontal poles are shown upward, the right side at reader's right. Upward bars indicate an increase in responders. * $p < 0.05$; ° $p < 0.01$.

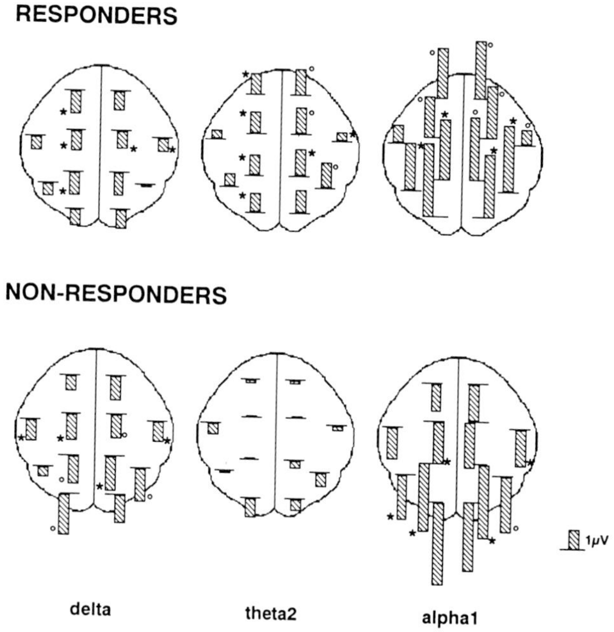

RESPONDERS

NON-RESPONDERS

◳ 1μV

| delta | theta2 | alpha1 |

FIG. 3. Mean differences in amplitude between EEG recorded 6 h after a single dose of haloperidol and at baseline. In the drawing the frontal poles are shown upward, the right side at reader's right. Upward bars indicate an increase in the sixth hour recording. * $p < 0.05$; ° $p < 0.01$.

TABLE 1. *Changes in band amplitude observed in responders after 28 days of haloperidol treatment:* p *values from Wilcoxon–Wilcox tests*

Frequency bands	Leads											
	F_3	F_4	T_3	T_4	T_5	T_6	C_3	C_4	P_3	P_4	O_1	O_2
δ												
θ_1 ↑						0.008						
θ_2 ↑	0.006	0.006	0.03	0.04		0.008	0.008	0.008	0.01	0.03		
α_1 ↑	0.006	0.006			0.04	0.04	0.04	0.04	0.02		0.04	
α_2											0.04	
β_1 ↓												
β_2												
β_3 ↓		0.01		0.03		0.006		0.01		0.006		0.02

TABLE 2. *Changes in band amplitude observed in nonresponders after 28 days of haloperidol treatment:* p *values from Wilcoxon–Wilcox tests*

Frequency bands	Leads											
	F_3	F_4	T_3	T_4	T_5	T_6	C_3	C_4	P_3	P_4	O_1	O_2
δ												
θ_1												
θ_2												
α_1												
α_2												
β_1 ↑			0.05		0.04							
β_2 ↑					0.02							
β_3												

RESPONDERS

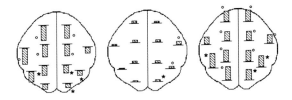

NON-RESPONDERS

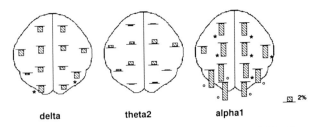

delta   theta2   alpha1

FIG. 4. Mean differences in relative power between EEG recorded 6 h after a single dose of haloperidol and at baseline. In the drawing the frontal poles are shown upward, the right side at reader's right. Upward bars indicate an increase in the sixth hour recording.* $p < 0.05$; ° $p < 0.01$.

with an age range between 20 and 44 years (mean ± SD, 29.89 ± 7.33), and a duration of illness ranging from 0.6 to 23 years (mean ± SD, 7.08 ± 6.84). The washout period was the same as in the CEEG study. The 11 paranoid patients were retested after 28 days of haloperidol treatment (daily dosage up to 7 mg).

The control group included 23 healthy controls, 19 men and 4 women, comparable with patients for age, handedness, and education. Eleven of them were the control group for the retested patients.

ERPs were recorded during a visual target detection task, in which stimuli were same or different-name consonant pairs (respectively, target, T and nontarget, NT). The stimuli were tachistoscopically presented to the right or to the left visual field, and subjects were required to press a button at the appearance of a T stimulus on the screen.

The Comprehensive Psychopathological Rating Scale (CPRS) (19) was used for symptom ratings. Patients were considered responders when a 50% reduction of the CPRS global score was observed. Further methodological details on ERP recording and analysis are reported elsewhere (20,21).

ERP components were identified by means of the Principal Component Analysis. Differences between groups, as well as visual field and treatment effects, were evaluated by means of ANOVA followed by Dunnett's post-hoc test.

Results

Healthy controls showed faster reaction time ($p < 0.0005$) and larger P520 ($p < 0.01$) for stimuli presented to the right visual field (RVF). Schizophrenic subjects did not exhibit a RVF advantage either on reaction time or P520 amplitude. When compared with healthy controls, patients showed a reduction of the P360, P520 and slow wave (SW) only for stimuli presented to the RVF (Fig. 5), suggesting the presence of hemispheric lateralization abnormalities in schizophrenia.

After 28 days of treatment, a partial recovery of these ERP abnormalities was observed (Fig. 6). Such a normalization did not parallel clinical improvement, since in 57.1% of the patients it could be observed earlier than symptom remission. On the other hand, it could not be considered independent from psychopathological changes, as it was not observed in treatment-resistant patients.

DISCUSSION

According to our findings, significant neurophysiological differences exist between R and NR after haloperidol treatment.

For CEEG parameters, a baseline comparison between R and NR showed a predominance of fast α and β activity in R and more θ_2 and slow α in NR. A decrease of fast activities and an increase of slow α have previously been observed in therapy-resistant schizophrenics (14,22). Interestingly, a

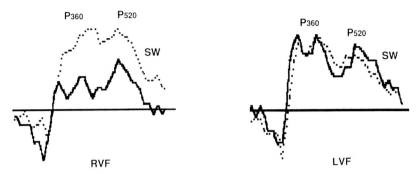

FIG. 5. Grand mean waveforms of schizophrenic patients (——) and controls (----) for stimuli presented to the right visual field (RVF) and left visual field (LVF). Significant reduction of P360 and slow wave (SW) in schizophrenic patients ($p < 0.01$) for the RVF stimuli.

relationship between slow α and enlarged lateral ventricles in schizophrenic patients has been reported (23,24). In this connection, it is worth mentioning that an increased size of the lateral ventricles has frequently been found in drug-resistant schizophrenic patients (25). Therefore, the predominance of slow α in the EEG of drug-free schizophrenic patients may allow the identification of a subgroup of therapy-resistant patients in which morphological abnormalities are more likely to be found.

Results from our study show that CEEG differences between R and NR were not confined to their baseline profiles but involved their respective patterns of drug-induced changes. For the acute haloperidol administration, an opposite pattern of changes for the slow α band (increase in R, decrease in NR) was found and after 4 weeks of treatment the CEEG profile of R was

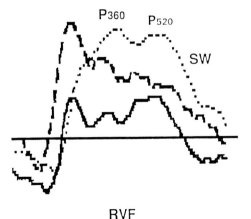

FIG. 6. Grand mean waveforms of pre- (——), post-treatment (----) schizophrenic patients and normal controls (----) showing significant increase of P360 and slow wave (SW) in post-treatment schizophrenic patients vs. pretreatment schizophrenic patients ($p < 0.05$).

dramatically changed with respect to their baseline, whereas no modification was observed in NR.

Unlike the CEEG indices, baseline clinical variables did not differentiate between the two subgroups.

Our ERP results, although preliminary for the small size of the sample, are in line with previous reports (26), and suggest an association between LPC amplitude normalization and response to treatment.

In conclusion, the present study supports the view that electrophysiological indices, in association with the evaluation of treatment response, represent powerful tools in the identification of different biological subtypes within diagnostic categories.

REFERENCES

1. Strauss JS, Carpenter WT Jr, Bartko JJ. The diagnosis and understanding of schizophrenia, Part III: speculation on the processes that underlie schizophrenic symptoms and signs. *Schizophr Bull* 1974;1:61–9.
2. Crow TJ. Molecular pathology of schizophrenia: more than one disease process? *BMJ* 1980; 280:1–9.
3. Andreasen NC, Olsen SA, Dennert JW, Smith MR. Ventricular enlargement in schizophrenia: relationship to positive and negative symptoms. *Am J Psychiatry* 1982;139:297–302.
4. Wyatt RJ, Potkin SG, Kleinman JE, Weinberger DR, Luchins DJ, Jeste DV. The schizophrenia syndrome. Examples of biological tools for subclassification. *J Nerv Ment Dis* 1981; 169:100–12.
5. Goldstein MJ. Premorbid adjustment, paranoid status, and pattern of response to phenothiazine in acute schizophrenia. *Schizophr Bull* 1970;3:24–37.
6. Klorman R, Strauss JS, Kokes RF. Some biological approaches to research on premorbid functioning in schizophrenia. *Schizophr Bull* 1977;3:226–39.
7. Johnstone E, Owens D, Frith C, Crow TJ. The relative stability of positive and negative features in chronic schizophrenia. *Br J Psychiatry* 1986;150:60–4.
8. Kay SR, Fiszbein A, Lindenmayer JP, Opler LA. Positive and negative syndromes in schizophrenia as a function of chronicity. *Acta Psychiatr Scand* 1986;74:507–18.
9. Kay SR, Singh MM. The positive-negative distinction in drug-free schizophrenic patients. Stability, response to neuroleptics, and prognostic significance. *Arch Gen Psychiatry* 1989; 46:711–18.
10. Csernansky JG, Kaplan J, Hollister LE. Problems in the classification of schizophrenics as neuroleptic responders and nonresponders. *J Nerv Ment Dis* 1985;173:325–31.
11. Weinberger DR, Bigelow LB, Kleinman JE, Klein ST, Rosenblatt JE, Wyatt RJ. Cerebral ventricular enlargement in chronic schizophrenia. An association with a poor response to treatment. *Arch Gen Psychiatry* 1980;37:11–3.
12. Pickar D, Labarca R, Doran AR, et al. Longitudinal measurement of plasma homovanillic acid levels in schizophrenic patients. *Arch Gen Psychiatry* 1986;43:669–76.
13. Petrie EC, Faustman WO, Moses JA, Lombrozo L, Csernansky JG. Correlates of rapid neuroleptic response in male patients with schizophrenia. *Psychiatry Res* 1989;33:171–7.
14. Itil TM, Marasa MS, Saletu B, Davis S, Mucciardi N. Computerized EEG: predictor of outcome in schizophrenia. *J Nerv Ment Dis* 1975;160:188–203.
15. American Psychiatric Association (APA). *DSM-II-R: diagnostic and statistical manual of mental disorders.* 3rd edition, revised. Washington, DC: American Psychiatric Association, 1987.
16. Andreasen NC, Olsen SA. Negative vs. positive schizophrenia: definition and validation. *Arch Gen Psychiatry* 1982;39:789–94.
17. Itil TM, Shapiro DM, Eralp E, Akman A, Itil KZ, Garbizu C. A new brain function diagnostic unit, including the dynamic brain mapping of computer analyzed EEG, evoked potentials

and sleep (a new hardware/software system and its application in psychiatry and psycho-pharmacology). *New Trends Exp Clin Psychiatry* 1985;1:107–77.

18. Galderisi S, Mucci A, Mignone ML, Maj M, Kemali D. CEEG mapping in drug-free schizophrenics—Differences from healthy subjects and changes induced by haloperidol treatment. *Schizophr Res* 1992;6:15–24.

19. Asberg M, Montgomery SA, Perris C, Schalling D, Sedvall G. The comprehensive psycho-pathological rating scale. *Acta Psychiatr Scand* 1978;271(suppl):5–27.

20. Galderisi S, Maj M, Mucci A, Monteleone P, Kemali D. Lateralization patterns of verbal stimuli processing assessed by reaction time and event-related potentials in schizophrenic patients. *Int J Psychophysiol* 1988;6:167–76.

21. Kemali D, Galderisi S, Maj M, Mucci A, Di Gregorio M. Lateralization patterns of event-related potentials and performance indices in schizophrenia: relationship to clinical state and neuroleptic treatment. *Int J Psychophysiol* 1991;10:225–30.

22. Itil TM, Shapiro DM, Schneider SJ, Francis IB. Computerized EEG as a predictor of drug response in treatment resistant schizophrenics. *J Nerv Ment Dis* 1981;169:629–37.

23. Kemali D, Galderisi S, Maj M. EEG correlates of clinical heterogeneity of schizophrenia. In: Giannitrapani D, Murri L, eds *The EEG of mental activities*. Basel: Karger, 1988: 169–181.

24. Karson CN, Coppola R, Daniel DG. Alpha frequency in schizophrenia: an association with enlarged cerebral ventricles. *Am J Psychiatry* 1988;145:861–4.

25. Smith RC, Baumgartner R, Ravichandran GK, et al. Lateral ventricular enlargement and clinical response in schizophrenia. *Psychiatry Res* 1985;14:241–53.

26. Duncan CC, Perlstein WM, Morihisa JM. The P300 metric in schizophrenia: Effects of probability and modality. In: Johnson R Jr, Rohrbaugh JW, Parasuraman R, eds. *Current trends in event-related potential research (EEG suppl. 40)*. Amsterdam: Elsevier, 1987: 670–4.

Psychiatry and Advanced Technologies,
edited by L. Ravizza, F. Bogetto, and
E. Zanalda. Raven Press, Ltd.,
New York © 1993.

5

Validity of the Event-Related Potentials from Auditory Stimuli in Neuropsychiatric Disorders

C. Bianco, P. Benna, P. Costa, E. Bo, E. Marotta,
S. Vighetti, *L. Ravizza, and B. Bergamasco

*Institute of Clinical Neurology and *Institute of Psychiatry, University of Turin,
10126 Turin, Italy*

In clinical neurophysiology the evoked potentials are employed as an objective test of afferent function in patients with neurological and sensory disorders (1). Nevertheless, certain components of evoked potentials seem to be associated with cognitive processes, and their use enables investigation of how the sensory information is utilized by the subject examined (2–4). Evoked potentials can be separated into two sets of components: stimulus-related (exogenous) components, which represent an obligate neuronal response to a given stimulus and are sensitive to the physical characteristics of the stimulus, and event-related (endogenous) components, which are dependent on the information content of the stimulus and appear only when a subject "attends" to stimuli (and then, only when a stimulus has meaning for the subject). Stimulus-related potentials are employed in nervous conduction studies (such as detection of subclinical lesions, monitoring), and event-related potentials in the assessment of cognitive functions. These differences suggest an associate utilization of both evoked responses in clinical practice, because afferent and cognitive disorders can coexist; for example, in a previous study (Bianco et al., 1986, personal communication) we demonstrated altered stimulus-related potentials in Alzheimer's disease, where severe alterations of the endogenous potentials had been also described (5–7).

The P300 or P3 component (so called because of its latency) of the event-related brain potential has been studied extensively since its discovery by Sutton et al. (8). It is a large positive wave, maximal over the midline central and parietal regions, with a latency of 300 ms or greater, depending on stimulus and subject parameters. The P3 can be elicited with a stimulus of any modality. The most commonly used method to obtain the P3 is referred to as the "oddball" paradigm. This involves the presentation of unexpected or infrequent stimuli ("rare," "target"), randomly interspersed among more frequent stimuli ("frequent," "nontarget"). In most studies, the unexpected stimuli differ from the more common stimuli in terms of frequency or intensity. A P3 will be seen following the target but not the nontarget stimuli. P3 consists of multiple peaks (P300 complex); among them, the main subcomponents P3a and P3b are elicited, respectively, after an infrequent stimulus (P3a, earlier), or by attending to a task-relevant stimulus (P3b). The generator site of the P3 is not known with certainty. Postulated generators of the P300 in the human include the frontal cortex, the centroparietal cortex, the temporal cortex, specifically auditory cortex, multiple subcortical sites, the hippocampal formation, and the thalamus (6). The P300 response has been associated with a variety of cognitive functions, including information delivery, orienting, signal detection, stimulus evaluation time, and decision making. The latency of P300 is considered to be a measure of the speed of cognition, and the amplitude is affected by the probability of occurrence of the target stimulus. The latency of P300 negatively correlates with amplitude, as demonstrated by Polich (9). In normal populations the latency increases with age, whereas the amplitude is slightly affected. In addition, several subjective factors may affect the P300, including the subject's level of attention and the relative difficulty of the task. Snyder et al. (10) reported no substantial differences in the scalp distribution of P300 elicited by auditory, visual, and somatosensory stimulations.

There is classic evidence that the subject must be awake, alert, and cooperative to obtain the P300. Although a relevant-task situation is often used to produce the P300, a variety of reports have demonstrated that P3-like wave forms also can be obtained with procedures that do not employ an active, intentional discrimination task (11–13). In 1989, Polich (14) demonstrated that the P3 component produced by an auditory passive sequence appears to mimic reliably the event-related potentials (ERPs) obtained from an active discrimination task, suggesting that this may be a useful and reliable means of eliciting the P3 ERP in subject populations or experimental situations in which an active discrimination task cannot be performed.

The data implicating P300 as a correlate of the speed of information processing (15,16) have made it a likely candidate for indexing slowed cognitive function in normal elderly subjects, as well as for altered mental functions in patients with neurologic and psychiatric disorders, such as dementia, schizophrenia, and depression. Several authors (3,17–20) found significantly prolonged P300 latencies in dementia, suggesting that P300 latency can provide a sensitive and perhaps specific test for differentiating dementia from other cognitive disorders of the elderly, such as depression or pseudodementia (21). In addition to the more promising studies mentioned above, there are a series of more pessimistic studies concerning the clinical utility of

TABLE 1. *Methods for eliciting the P3 response used in our laboratory*

Auditory binaural stimulation
  Frequent stimuli: tone bursts, frequency 1,000 Hz
  Rare (target) stimuli: tone bursts, frequency 2,000 Hz
Stimulus
  Intensity 80 dB HL, duration 100 ms, slope 4 ms
Interstimulus interval 1 s
Filters 0.3–53 Hz
Stimulation series
  First, 100 frequent stimuli
  Second, passive oddball paradigm with 15% target tones
  Third, active oddball paradigm with 15% target tones

the P3 in dementia (22–24). In schizophrenia, multiple investigators have reported a lower amplitude of P3 compared with the controls (19,25,26), whereas most of these studies have not reported a change in P3 latency. Similar findings have been reported for depressed patients (19,24,26,27).

In our practice, the P3 response is usually recorded by an auditory oddball paradigm as illustrated in Table 1. In 1986 we carried out a study on P300 response in depression (Bianco et al., personal communication). We recorded the P300 event-related response by auditory oddball paradigm in 20 patients (14 women, 6 men, age range 40–66 years, mean 56.5) with major depression according to the DSM-III criteria. At the time of investigation, all the subjects had been free of therapy for at least 30 days. The data collected (Table 2) were compared with an age-matched control group of 20 subjects (12 women, 8 men, mean age 60.125 years, range 50–78). The absolute values of P300 amplitude and latency with both passive and active paradigms did not significantly differ between the patient group and the control group. Nevertheless, the depressed patients showed a significant reduction in increasing amplitude of P300 ("amplitude gain") after the active discrimination task, when compared with passive paradigms, in accord with the impairment of initiative and "surprise" in this disease.

In our opinion, in confirmed cognitive disorders P300 studies cannot replace an accurate psychometric evaluation because the information obtained with these methods is inadequate. On the other hand, their utility in the assessment of some diseases without clinical evidence of cognitive deficits

TABLE 2. *Auditory P300 response in depressed patients*

	Absolute amplitude μV (SD)	"Gain" amplitude μV (SD)	Latency ms (SD)
Patients	8.04 (2.94)	3.45 (2.99)*	366.79 (44.66)
Controls	10.51 (5.31)	7.01 (3.72)	340.73 (61.06)

* $p < 0.01$ vs. controls.

TABLE 3. *Auditory P300 and P3-like responses in cirrhotic patients*

	P300	P3-like
Latency ms (SD)		
Controls	317.06 (22.50)	314.65 (27.75)
Total patients	358.54 (40.40)***	348.14 (38.38)**
Postinfectious	393.11 (22.95)****	367.25 (27.16)***§
Alcoholics	348.46 (39.01)**	342.57 (39.82)*
Amplitude μV (SD)		
Controls	16.84 (6.37)	11.71 (5.23)
Total patients	12.48 (7.55)*	9.05 (4.75)*
Postinfectious	15.27 (7.44)	9.54 (4.25)
Alcoholics	11.67 (7.54)*	8.90 (4.96)*

* $p < 0.05$ vs. controls; ** $p < 0.01$ vs. controls, *** $p < 0.001$ vs. controls, **** $p < 0.0001$ vs. controls, § $p < 0.001$ vs. alcoholics.

might be established to determine if some modifications of the P300 response are present and if they may be related to an early cognitive impairment.

In line with this aim, in recent years we have investigated different patient populations (data above), as follows: chronic liver disease (suspected toxic/metabolic cerebral damage), to demonstrate subclinical signs of hepatic encephalopathy (Bianco et al., 1989, 1991, personal communication) on the basis of some previous reports (28,29), and primary generalized epilepsy (absence of cerebral damage on neuroimaging, with subjective history but no clinical evidence of moderate cognitive dysfunction) to confirm the presence of cognitive damage and its possible relationship to antiepileptic medication (Bianco et al., 1989, personal communication).

EXPERIMENT 1

Forty cirrhotic patients (30 men, 10 women, age range 30–59 years, mean 41.35) were subjected to auditory P300 recording; 25 were alcohol abusers and 15 had a postinfectious cyrrhosis. The control group consisted of 30 healthy subjects (20 men, 10 women, age range 25–60 years, mean 40.85). The results are shown in Table 3. In the patients the P300 latency was significantly prolonged, more so in the postinfectious cirrhotic patients. In addition, the alcohol abusers also showed smaller P300 amplitudes with respect to both controls and other patients.

EXPERIMENT 2

Auditory P3 responses following both passive and active paradigms were recorded in 20 patients (age range 17–39 years, mean 27.62) suffering from primary generalized epilepsy. They were chronically treated with a single antiepileptic medication, phenobarbital ($n = 10$) or sodium valproate ($n = $

TABLE 4. *Auditory P300 and P3-like responses in epileptic patients*

Latency ms (SD)	P300	P3-like
Controls	308.31 (22.09)	293.12 (22.62)
Total patients	339.11 (30.43)*	330.46 (27.15)**
Valproate	322.00 (37.98)	310.62 (15.67)
Phenobarbital	346.72 (25.23)**	339.38 (26.91)***

Amplitude: no significant differences.
* $p < 0.05$ vs. controls, ** $p < 0.01$ vs. controls, *** $p < 0.001$ vs. controls.

10), with plasma drug levels in the normal range. All the subjects complained of loss of concentration and memory and of behavioral changes. In these patients we found prolonged latencies of passive and particularly of active P3 responses with respect to an age-matched control group, whereas the amplitudes did not significantly differ (Table 4).

These findings seem to confirm that some alterations of the P3 response (particularly its latency) can represent a sensitive tool for detection of some subclinical cognitive dysfunctions. Nevertheless, as mentioned above, it also appears that these alterations are consistent among different cases, and therefore they can demonstrate only a slowing in cognitive processing without defining the degree. Moreover, the consideration of event-related responses requires great accuracy in collection of data and evaluation of the results, with particular regard to the age range of the patients examined, controls, and statistical comparison.

Although at present there is clear evidence of the usefulness of P300 in awake subjects, more questions arise about the same responses (P3-like) elicited by passive paradigms. Polich (14) suggested their use in patients who are unable to perform an active discrimination task; we believe that this may be of particular interest in patients with severe alterations of consciousness. In fact, the majority of reports concerning neurophysiologic assessment of patients in coma have centered only on stimulus-related responses and provide no information about stimulus processing (event-related activity). Therefore, we attempted to perform serial recordings of the P3-like response using the auditory passive oddball paradigm in a group of 25 patients, age range 16–50 years, with severe and prolonged traumatic coma. Our aims were, first, to determine if P3-like activity could be elicited in these patients and, second, if elicitable, to establish the relationship between P3-like activity and clinical outcome in serial investigations. As discussed above (Bianco et al., 1990, personal communication), in 68% of patients ($n = 17$) it was possible to record a P3-like response at the first examination (performed within 48 h after the acute trauma), whereas this response was absent in 8. In later recordings (performed weekly), the P3-like response varied, appearing in five patients and disappearing in four. In the remaining patients it continued to be present ($n = 13$) or absent ($n = 3$). Comparison of these data with the clinical outcome showed a good recovery of consciousness for patients in whom the P3-like response was initially present or appeared later, and whereas a poor outcome when P3-like response was initially absent or later disappeared.

The patients with a good clinical outcome also underwent recording of the auditory P300 and P3-like response following both passive and active discrimination tasks after discharge. In these subjects we found prolonged latencies of P300 (349.9 ms, SD 49.34, $p < 0.001$) and P3-like (341.85 ms, SD 58.39, $p < 0.01$) as compared with an age-matched control group (P300 latency 312.91 ms, SD 19.40; P3-like latency 306.03 ms, SD 24.11).

The reliability of the P3-like response evoked by passive paradigms in coma and its relationship to clinical outcome has been recently confirmed in other reports (30,31). In normal subjects, Polich (14) ascribed these events to a more rudimentary level of cognitive processing than the classic P300 response. The presence (or absence) of a P3-like response in comatose patients might be interpreted as preservation (or loss) of these rudimentary cognitive processes in coma, and this in turn may be related to the clinical outcome. However, because the relationship between this response and the cognitive outcome after coma is still unclear, the real meaning of the P3-like response as an endogenous cognitive event is still open to question.

REFERENCES

1. Starr A. Sensory evoked potentials in clinical disorders of the nervous system. *Annu Rev Neurosci* 1978;1:103–27.
2. Donchin E. Event-related brain potentials: a tool in the study of human information processing. In: Begleiter H, ed. *Evoked potentials and behavior.* New York: Plenum Press, 1979,13–88.
3. Goodin DS, Squires KC, Starr A. Long latency event-related components of the auditory evoked potential in dementia. *Brain* 1978;101:635–48.
4. Onofrj MC, Nobilio D, Pace AM, et al. Valutazione clinica della componente P300 ottenuta con paradigma uditivo "odd-ball". *Riv It EEG Neurofisiol Clin* 1988;11:183–214.
5. Goodin DS. Event-related (endogenous) potentials. In: Aminoff MJ, ed. *Electrodiagnosis in clinical neurology,* 2nd ed. New York: Churchill Livingstone, 1986:575–95.
6. Oken BS. Endogenous event-related potentials. In: Chiappa KH, ed. *Evoked potentials in clinical medicine,* 2nd ed. New York: Raven Press, 1989:563–92.
7. Onofrj MC, Gambi D, Del Re ML, et al. Mapping of event-related potentials to auditory and visual odd-ball paradigms in patients affected by different forms of dementia. *Eur Neurol* 1991;31:259–69.
8. Sutton S, Braren M, Zubin J, John ER. Evoked potential correlates of stimulus uncertainty. *Science* 1965;150:1187–8.
9. Polich J. Normal variation of P300 from auditory stimuli. *Electroencephalogr Clin Neurophysiol* 1986;65:236–40.
10. Snyder E, Hillyard SA, Galambos R. Similarities and differences among the P3 waves to detected signals in three modalities. *Psychophysiology* 1980;17:112–22.
11. Aleksandrov IO, Maksimova NE. P300 and psychophysiological analysis of the structure of behavior. *Electroencephalogr Clin Neurophysiol* 1985;61:548–58.
12. Glover AA, Onofrj MC, Ghilardi MF, Bodis–Wollner I. P300-like potentials in the normal monkey using classical conditioning and an auditory "oddball" paradigm. *Electroencephalogr Clin Neurophysiol* 1986;65:231–5.

13. Pineda JA, Foote SL, Neville HJ. Long-latency event-related potentials in squirrel monkeys: further characterization of wave form, morphology, topography, and functional properties. *Electroencephalogr Clin Neurophysiol* 1987;67:77–90.
14. Polich J. P300 from a passive auditory paradigm. *Electroencephalogr Clin Neurophysiol* 1989;74:312–20.
15. Kutas M, McCarthy G, Donchin E. Augmenting mental chronometry: the P300 as a measure of stimulus evaluation time. *Science* 1977;197:792–5.
16. Magliero A, Bashore TR, Coles MGH. Donchin E. On the dependence of P300 latency on stimulus evaluation processes. *Psychophysiology* 1984;21:171–86.
17. Syndulko K, Hansch EC, Cohen SN, et al. Long latency event-related potentials in normal aging and dementia. In: Courjon J, Mauguiere F, Revol M, eds. *Clinical application of evoked potentials in neurology.* New York: Raven Press, 1982:279–85.
18. Pfefferbaum A, Ford JM, Wenegrat BG, Roth WT, Kopell BS. Clinical application of the P3 component of event-related potentials. I. Normal aging. *Electroencephalogr Clin Neurophysiol* 1984;59:85–103.
19. Pfefferbaum A, Wenegrat BG, Ford JM, Roth WT, Kopell BS. Clinical application of the P3 component of event-related potentials: II. Dementia, depression and schizophrenia. *Electroencephalogr Clin Neurophysiol* 1984;59:104–24.
20. Maurer K, Ihl R, Dierks Th. Topographie der P300 in der Psychiatrie. II. Kognitive P300-Felder bei Demenz. *EEG-EMG* 1988;19:26–9.
21. Giedke H, Thier P, Balz J. The relationship between P300 latency and reaction time in depression. *Biol Psychol* 1981;13:31–4.
22. Slaets JPJ, Fortgens R. On the value of P300 event-related potentials in the differential diagnosis of dementia. *Br J Psychiatry* 1984;145:652–6.
23. Neshige R, Barrett G, Shibasaki H. Auditory long latency event-related potentials in Alzheimer's disease and multi-infarct dementia. *J Neurol Neurosurg Psychiatry* 1988;51:1120–5.
24. Patterson JV, Michalewski HJ, Starr A. Latency variability of the components of auditory event-related potentials to infrequent stimuli in aging, Alzheimer-type dementia, and depression. *Electroencephalogr Clin Neurophysiol* 1988;71:450–60.
25. Baribeau–Braun J, Picton TV, Gosselin JY. Schizophrenia: a neurophysiological evaluation of abnormal information processing. *Science* 1983;219:874–6.
26. Maurer K, Dierks T. Topographie der P300 in der Psychiatrie. I. Kognitive P300-Felder bei Psychosen. *EEG-EMG* 1988;19:21–5.
27. El Massioui F, Lesèvre N. Attention impairment and psychomotor retardation in depressed patients: an event-related potential study. *Electroencephalogr Clin Neurophysiol* 1988;70:46–55.
28. Weissenborn K, Scholz M, Hinrichs H, Wiltfang J, Schmidt FW, Kunkel H. Neurophysiological assessment of early hepatic encephalopathy. *Electroencephalogr Clin Neurophysiol* 1990;75:289–95.
29. Davies MG, Rowan MJ, Macmathuna P, Keeling PWN, Weir DG, Feely J. The auditory P300 event-related potential: an objective marker of the encephalopathy of chronic liver disease. *Hepatology* 1990;12:688–94.
30. Yingling CD, Hosobuchi Y, Harrington M. P300 as a predictor of recovery from coma. *Lancet* 1990;336:873.
31. Gott PS, Rabinowicz AL, De Giorgio CM. P300 auditory event-related potentials in nontraumatic coma. Association with Glasgow Coma Score and awakening. *Arch Neurol* 1991;48:1267–70.

Psychiatry and Advanced Technologies,
edited by L. Ravizza, F. Bogetto, and
E. Zanalda. Raven Press, Ltd.,
New York © 1993.

6

Clinical and Electroencephalography Mapping Investigations in Acute and Remission Schizophrenic Patients

Gian Franco Marchesi and Bernardo Nardi

Institute of Psychiatry, University of Ancona, 60121 Ancona, Italy

Since the classical studies of Berger (1), much research has attempted to identify the presence and significance of alterations of bioelectric patterns in patients with schizophrenia. Such alterations observed with traditional electrophysiologic methods were seen, according to various researchers, in 20–60% of the patients studied. The alterations tend to be more evident in severe, chronic cases and in patients with a positive family history, especially the catatonic subtype. However, such alterations are not specific (i.e., less bioelectric organization, less evidence of α activity, poor interhemispheric symmetry, lower differentiation between anterior and posterior regions) but depend on a different functional behavior of the central nervous system (CNS) (2–7).

According to many studies, drugs that act on the various psychological functions and on the corresponding behavioral aspects can induce alterations in electroencephalogram (EEG) patterns (i.e., low activity or fast activity increase, appearance of epilepsy-like symptoms), both after a single administration of drug and after steady-state levels are achieved (8–11). The recent introduction of computed EEG (CEEG), which enables cerebral EEG maps (EEGM) to be obtained, has provided an important new tool for scientific study of the pathogenic mechanisms of schizophrenia. In particular, this technique may better define the quantitative and topographic alterations observed. EEG mappers have attempted to elucidate these alterations in different schizophrenic subgroups and, especially, in two particular syndromes (12–14). The first syndrome shows a predominance of positive symptoms (i.e., hallucinations, delusions, bizarre behaviour, formal positive thought disturbances). The second consists mainly of negative symptoms (i.e., affective flattening, alogia, avolition and apathy, anedonia and social withdrawal, and altered attention). This negative syndrome appears to be characterized not only by different pathophysiologic mechanisms but also by the presence of anatomic functional correlations [frequent alterations are shown by computed tomography (CT) and magnetic resonance imaging (MRI) particularly ventricular enlargement], by the response to therapy (lower efficacy of neuroleptic drugs), and by the prognosis (more severe clinical course, leading to a "pseudodemential" status).

Recently, many studies have been published concerning modifications of electrophysiologic parameters in patients with schizophrenia (2–5,15–17). Such data confirm the complexity (and probably the heterogeneity) of pathophysiologic and developmental processes in schizophrenia. The observed modifications in biologic parameters have once again stimulated interest in the psycho-organic aspects of schizophrenia, although this does not reduce the etiologic and pathogenetic importance of the psychosocial aspects.

In previous reports concerning schizophrenic patients (2–7,15,16) patients with schizophrenia, as compared with control subjects, exhibited alterations such as less reactivity of α rhythm (with a tendency to spread to anterior regions), greater pressure of slow activity (δ and θ) in the frontotemporal regions, lower reduction of α activity in the central regions during cognitive tasks, and more stability of the β/α ratio passing from psychosensorial rest to distressing cognitive–affective tasks.

The aim of our investigation was to evaluate the presence of any relationships between clinical (consequent to neuroleptic medication) and bioelectric EEGM modifications.

SUBJECTS AND METHODS

Fifteen patients (nine men, mean age 30 years, range 19–45 years; six women, mean age 32 years, range 24–42 years) were evaluated. They were selected from a larger group of schizophrenic patients observed in the Clinical Psychiatry Department of the University of Ancona, Ancona, Italy. Inclusion criteria were as follows: a diagnosis of chronic schizophrenia, no medication for at least 2 months before hospital admission, absence of mental involution or other mental and neurologic disorders, hospital admission due to an acute exacerbation.

The diagnosis of schizophrenia was made according to the American Psychiatric Association's diagnostic criteria of DSM-III-R (18). Positive and negative symptoms were evaluated both after admission and before discharge. Such evaluations were done by the same psychiatrist who made the initial clinical evaluation. The Scale for the Assessment of Positive Symptoms (SAPS) and the Scale for the Assessment of Negative Symptoms (SANS) were used for this purpose (12).

During hospitalization (mean length of stay 20 ± 5 days), patients were medicated with neuroleptics (mean dose 6 mg haloperidol and 100 mg clorpromazine/day).

Patients underwent EEGM during psychosensorial rest (PSR: supine in a bed, eyes closed, relaxed) after admission and before discharge under the same conditions (laboratory, technicians, work-up). The first EEGM recording was performed 24 h after neuroleptic medication; this enabled us to compare the modifications of bioelectric patterns during the acute and remission phases of schizophrenia, avoiding the need to consider the differences between nonmedication and acute medication conditions. It is well known that neuroleptics can induce EEG modifications within 3 h after medication (8,9,11). The first recording was performed when each patient was in an acute clinical phase of psychopathology.

Bioelectric patterns were recorded with 19 electrodes, according to the 10–20 International System (Fp1, Fp2, F7, F3, Fz, F4, F8, T3, C3, Cz, C4, T4, T5, P3, Pz, P4, T6, O1, O2), with average reference montage, and were analyzed with a "Brain Surveyor" from Basis Trade (Verona, Italy). Each subject underwent an EEGM recording for at least 5 min; EEGM patterns were recorded on a hard disk according to standard EEG criteria with a rejection threshold of 127 μV. An electro-oculogram was also recorded to exclude eye artifacts.

After a recording was done, all 19-channel electric patterns were analyzed on the monitor and each 2-s epoch containing artifacts was excluded. The remaining record was analyzed with a spectral analysis program. Employing such a program, EEGM were obtained for each frequency band (δ 1–4 Hz; θ 4–8 Hz; α 8–12 Hz; β 12–31 Hz), according to standard criteria (19). The EEGM obtained dealt with: (i) absolute power (the average amount of EEG activity in each frequency band, measured in μV^2 and irrespective of the amount of EEG activity in other frequency bands), and (ii) relative power (quotient between power in one frequency band and total power across all bands, expressed as a percentage). Furthermore, both absolute and relative power were analyzed in frontal (F: Fp1, Fp2, F7, F3, Fz, F4, F8), temporocentral (TC: T3, C3, Cz, C4, T4), and parieto–occipital (PO: T5, P3, Pz, P4, T6, O1, O2) regions.

For every patient, acute and remission maps were compared for each frequency band. In addition, electrophysiologic modifications were analyzed, taking into consideration the clinical and psychodiagnostic (SAPS, SANS) data.

RESULTS

The results of the clinical and psychodiagnostic evaluation are shown in Table 1. Twelve patients had the paranoid type of schizophrenia (seven men, five women) and three had the undifferentiated type (two men, one woman).

TABLE 1. Scale for the Assessment of Positive Symptoms (SAPS) and Scale for the Assessment of Negative Symptoms (SANS) scores

Patient	Gender	Clinical diagnosis	SAPS				SANS				
			Hallucination	Delusion	Bizzare behavior	Posit. form thought d.	Affect. flatten	Alogia	Avolit.	Anhedon. asocial.	Attention impairment
BN	F	Paranoid	0/0	5/4	0/0	5/4	2/2	3/3	2/2	3/3	1/1
MA	M	Paranoid	4/1	4/1	1/1	2/1	1/1	1/1	1/1	3/1	1/1
SP	F	Paranoid	5/2	5/4	2/2	3/3	2/2	2/2	2/1	3/2	2/1
NF	F	Paranoid	5/0	4/1	4/1	4/1	4/2	3/2	4/1	3/2	3/2
PC	M	Paranoid	4/3	4/1	3/2	2/1	1/1	1/1	3/2	3/2	1/1
SS	M	Paranoid	5/4	4/3	3/2	0/0	2/2	1/1	3/3	2/2	2/2
SA	F	Paranoid	5/3	5/3	5/3	3/3	0/0	0/0	2/2	2/2	1/1
GS	M	Paranoid	4/2	5/3	5/3	2/2	2/2	2/2	2/2	3/3	1/1
GF	M	Paranoid	3/2	5/4	3/2	4/3	0/0	0/0	2/1	2/2	1/1
ER	M	Paranoid	5/2	5/3	3/2	3/0	3/2	1/0	3/2	3/2	0/0
BA	M	Paranoid	3/0	5/3	2/0	0/0	2/2	2/2	1/0	2/2	3/1
BM	F	Paranoid	1/0	5/3	5/2	2/0	2/0	1/1	0/0	2/2	0/0
GM	M	Undiffer.	0/0	0/0	2/0	2/2	4/3	4/3	4/4	4/4	1/1
GG	M	Undiffer.	4/2	4/2	2/2	2/1	1/1	2/1	3/2	2/2	3/3
MA	F	Undiffer.	5/3	5/5	5/4	5/3	3/3	3/3	4/4	4/5	2/1

5, Severe; 4, marked; 3, moderate; 2, mild; 1, doubtful; 0, absent. For each item, the first value refers to the evaluation made after hospitalization, the second value to evaluation made before discharge.

On SAPS and SANS, all the patients showed both positive and negative symptoms, but with a different percentage. In six cases (GS, MA, SA, GF, BA, BMG) there was a marked prevalence of positive symptoms and in one case (GM) of negative symptoms.

During hospitalization, more marked improvements were seen in positive symptoms as compared with negative symptoms. As shown in Table 1, two patients (BN, SS) with paranoid schizophrenia and two patients (GM, MA) with undifferentiated schizophrenia did not demonstrate any evident improvement during their hospitalization.

Qualitative analysis of EEGM concerning the topographic distribution of the spectral bands (absolute and relative power) during acute exacerbation of schizophrenia showed the two principal patterns (Figs. 1–4). The first was a "normal-like" spectral band distribution (prevalence of β activity in anterior regions, α activity in posterior regions, and absence of remarkable slow activity). EEGM performed before discharge in these patients (BA, GF, ER, GS) showed little change with regard to increased α and/or β activity. The second pattern was characterized by the presence of slow activity, especially in anterior regions, often associated with less α activity (with respect to the normal range) in posterior regions (remaining patients). In this second pattern, three patients (GG, SA, SS) exhibited only a few changes, often limited to one or two frequency bands; in the others, evident changes between the two EEGM records (i.e., less slow activity and/or more fast activity) were seen, varying according to the individual patient. The most important changes were a reduction of δ activity (especially in frontal regions) and/or an increase of α activity (in parieto-occipital and sometimes in frontal regions).

In seven cases (BA, BM, GG, MA, NF, SA, SS) with either the first or second pattern, the initial EEGM showed α activity in both posterior and anterior regions, with little reactivity to a visual arrest reaction. In these patients, the EEGM performed before discharge showed persistence or an increase of anterior α activity, in accordance with our previous reports on schizophrenics (17). All patients with the undifferentiated type of schizophrenia had the second pattern, whereas the patients with paranoid schizophrenia had either the first or the second pattern.

Concerning quantitative analysis of EEGM patterns, both absolute and relative power for each spectral band were analyzed in F, TC, and PO regions. The results are shown in Table 2 (absolute power) and Table 3 (relative power). In many cases (but not in all), there was a reduction of slow activity (δ and θ) and/or an increase of fast activity (α and β) in the second EEGM recording made before discharge (D) compared with the first EEGM recording made after hospitalization (H).

Analysis of Pearson correlation coefficients (Table 5), considering the mean group values, showed a positive and statistically significant correlation between the reduction of δ and θ activity and the increase of α and β relative

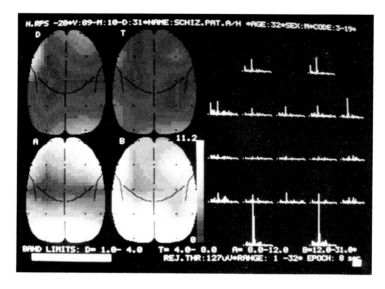

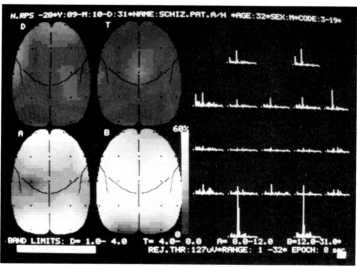

FIG. 1. EEG mapping of a schizophrenic patient in acute exacerbation (A, "normal-like" pattern). **Top:** Absolute power maps; **bottom:** relative power maps. On the right are power spectra for each EEGM channel. D, δ; T, θ; A, α; B, β.

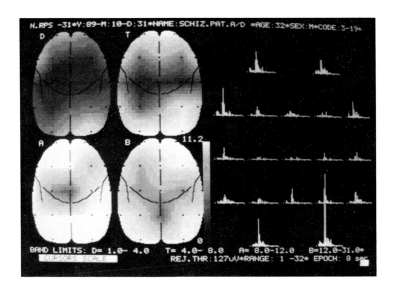

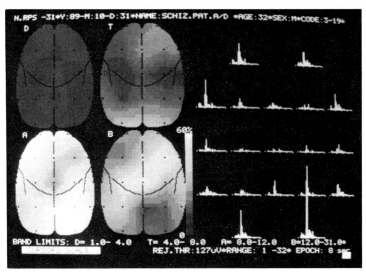

FIG. 2. EEG mapping of a schizophrenic patient in remission (A, "normal-like" pattern). **Top:** Absolute power maps; **bottom:** relative power maps. On the right are power spectra for each EEGM channel. D, δ; T, θ; A, α; B, β.

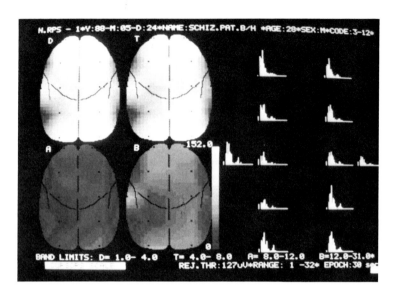

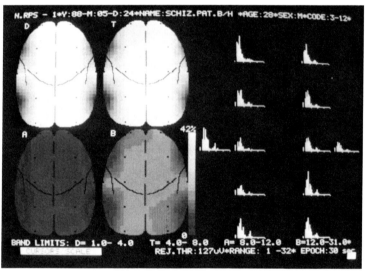

FIG. 3. EEG mapping of a schizophrenic patient in acute exacerbation (B, "slow" pattern). **Top:** Absolute power maps; **bottom:** relative power maps. On the right are power spectra for each EEGM channel. D, β; T, θ; A, α; B, β.

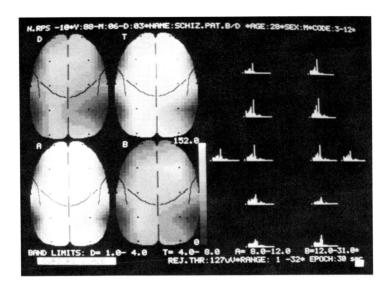

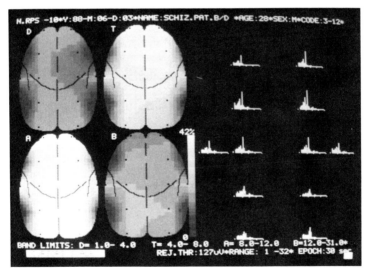

FIG. 4. EEG mapping of a schizophrenic patient in remission (B, "slow" pattern). **Top:** Absolute power maps; **bottom:** relative power maps. On the right are power spectra for each EEGM channel. D, δ; T, θ; A, α; B, β.

TABLE 2. Absolute power at EEGM

	δ						θ					
	F		TC		PO		F		TC		PO	
Patient	H	D	H	D	H	D	H	D	H	D	H	[
BN	30.3	10.0	3.2	16.0	9.8	3.6	6.5	2.7	1.6	2.6	2.8	
MA	115.0	64.7	119.0	62.2	102.8	61.3	65.4	128.8	90.3	115.0	89.2	8.
SP	2.8	3.5	1.3	5.6	1.6	2.2	1.1	1.9	0.7	1.0	0.9	
NF	3.1	3.1	2.3	1.8	1.2	1.4	1.5	2.1	1.3	1.3	1.8	:
PC	283.0	122.4	229.0	91.7	202.1	76.6	192.5	59.4	166.0	44.5	151.4	3(
SS	5.6	7.9	2.2	6.0	4.1	6.1	4.1	3.8	2.1	4.0	4.0	
SA	6.3	5.0	1.9	2.3	4.4	3.5	4.7	4.7	2.5	2.0	4.4	
GS	3.0	4.7	1.3	2.0	2.3	4.8	2.1	9.0	1.6	3.6	2.1	1
GF	3.0	2.0	2.5	1.2	2.9	1.5	3.4	2.4	1.7	1.5	1.9	
ER	3.0	3.7	1.8	1.5	1.9	2.0	1.7	2.1	1.1	1.7	1.1	
BA	4.2	9.2	1.4	7.8	5.8	8.6	4.2	4.4	3.0	3.8	8.4	
BM	4.7	3.7	2.5	2.4	2.9	2.3	3.5	2.2	1.9	2.3	3.0	
GM	11.1	15.6	4.8	4.2	4.8	7.2	3.1	4.9	2.1	3.6	4.5	
GG	134.0	108.0	101.4	102.8	102.1	84.4	179.0	203.0	176.5	182.1	144.4	15:
MA	19.0	73.5	6.5	16.3	11.0	16.0	5.2	35.8	1.8	2.9	4.3	

F, frontal; TC, temporocentral; PO, parieto-occipital.
H, at initial hospitalization; D, at discharge.

TABLE 3. Relative power (%) at EEGM

	δ						θ					
	F		TC		PO		F		TC		PO	
Patient	H	D	H	D	H	D	H	D	H	D	H	[
BN	58.5	26.7	34.7	14.5	50.5	15.6	15.5	10.5	17.5	11.6	14.5	9
MA	41.2	16.0	37.0	16.0	38.0	17.7	26.2	34.7	28.0	29.7	33.0	25
SP	37.7	26.5	31.1	30.6	30.8	28.6	14.8	20.1	15.6	20.3	17.0	20
NF	19.5	11.2	30.5	12.2	9.0	4.7	14.5	8.2	14.2	9.0	12.0	7
PC	48.5	45.5	44.5	40.0	40.5	31.2	32.7	22.0	32.0	19.0	29.7	15
SS	22.7	25.0	16.2	25.2	18.0	20.5	17.7	13.5	15.7	15.2	16.7	13
SA	13.0	10.0	9.7	13.7	10.2	8.2	10.7	10.7	13.2	11.2	10.5	8
GS	15.5	10.0	12.6	7.6	9.1	7.6	11.2	20.1	12.8	13.3	8.3	22
GF	31.1	26.0	27.3	24.1	24.0	28.5	24.4	32.0	20.1	28.3	12.3	27
ER	13.4	16.0	12.0	9.7	14.7	10.1	7.7	8.5	7.3	10.3	8.7	6
BA	9.7	18.2	10.2	16.7	6.2	7.5	10.7	8.5	15.5	10.0	9.7	6
BM	29.0	13.2	29.5	27.1	27.1	22.6	22.5	13.4	20.1	20.5	25.8	15
GM	21.0	18.3	17.0	9.6	7.6	8.6	6.7	6.7	6.7	7.5	6.7	5
GG	20.5	15.2	16.7	13.7	15.2	13.2	27.5	29.0	24.5	24.7	21.7	25
MA	41.0	60.5	35.0	55.5	30.5	32.7	13.0	11.0	9.2	12.7	10.7	10

F, frontal; TC, temporocentral; PO, parieto-occipital.
H, at initial hospitalization; D, at discharge.

the δ, θ, α, and β frequency bands

α						β					
F		TC		PO		F		TC		PO	
H	D	H	D	H	D	H	D	H	D	H	D
2.2	3.4	0.7	2.6	2.3	8.5	4.5	9.9	3.2	11.2	4.8	11.7
40.0	154.0	49.2	144.0	38.7	159.0	72.4	67.4	84.3	78.2	58.1	65.8
0.7	1.1	0.4	0.5	0.9	1.2	2.8	4.1	4.5	2.0	1.9	2.6
3.3	12.7	2.2	5.1	14.0	30.5	2.5	6.7	2.5	5.0	2.8	7.25
84.6	132.6	86.9	30.5	119.0	62.7	72.8	76.7	74.6	80.3	95.9	107.6
9.1	9.3	5.6	4.5	13.5	22.1	5.9	6.2	3.4	4.8	3.9	5.8
11.2	10.0	5.5	3.6	44.7	43.1	21.3	24.1	9.0	8.7	12.9	15.1
6.5	10.9	2.6	10.9	49.1	49.1	6.2	12.8	6.1	8.6	7.9	13.4
2.6	1.1	2.0	0.8	9.9	1.3	3.6	2.0	2.9	1.7	3.4	1.3
1.7	3.6	1.4	3.2	1.6	11.0	13.1	13.4	9.3	8.9	6.6	11.1
22.9	22.0	7.7	11.7	9.2	13.9	7.5	12.4	6.2	11.2	16.6	23.9
2.2	1.9	1.2	1.2	2.9	6.1	5.6	8.7	2.6	3.3	2.7	4.2
12.8	15.1	6.8	21.2	45.2	107.1	17.5	30.5	14.3	25.5	28.1	59.9
244.1	250.2	230.3	299.5	366.7	282.0	150.4	174.7	158.8	170.7	126.2	122.9
4.2	11.6	3.1	2.8	15.3	41.8	7.5	5.6	7.9	3.9	13.4	9.2

the δ, θ, α, and β frequency bands

α						β					
F		TC		PO		F		TC		PO	
H	D	H	D	H	D	H	D	H	D	H	D
7.7	15.1	8.5	13.0	8.5	21.8	18.2	46.7	35.2	60.0	26.0	50.8
14.0	37.0	15.2	38.2	13.5	42.0	25.5	15.2	26.2	20.2	21.7	19.5
8.8	20.1	7.3	8.8	10.5	10.0	32.7	39.2	36.1	32.8	33.6	36.5
31.5	52.7	24.5	40.5	53.0	61.7	24.0	29.2	28.5	37.2	21.2	27.5
14.0	11.7	16.5	12.7	18.7	18.5	12.5	27.5	14.0	34.7	18.7	44.0
37.0	35.2	44.0	27.2	49.7	50.7	24.5	25.0	26.0	28.5	18.2	17.2
26.5	24.2	28.5	22.7	49.0	44.7	49.0	55.2	47.2	52.2	31.7	41.7
37.2	49.0	20.5	44.3	44.5	57.8	33.4	29.7	51.0	42.1	35.6	23.0
18.7	13.8	17.8	27.5	32.5	25.1	26.2	26.4	29.0	27.5	26.3	25.1
7.6	15.3	9.7	18.0	14.5	31.6	67.0	60.0	66.3	60.0	58.7	56.0
60.0	46.0	40.7	35.7	63.5	62.7	20.2	26.7	33.2	36.7	21.5	23.2
14.2	11.5	11.6	11.8	22.6	22.8	35.5	49.4	33.8	35.5	25.3	37.5
31.2	30.8	24.5	33.3	41.2	37.6	43.5	50.4	51.7	54.8	47.7	57.0
35.0	35.5	42.0	42.0	49.0	46.7	22.7	25.0	22.0	23.5	18.7	20.0
14.2	18.7	15.2	13.0	24.0	50.5	31.5	9.2	39.7	18.5	36.0	16.2

activity observed at the time of discharge (δ/α, $p = 0.004$; θ/β, $p = 0.009$). These data indicate that at the time of discharge the patients exhibited significant electrophysiologic improvement (i.e, shifting of their slow frequency bands to the faster ones).

To study the relationships between EEGM data and the clinical evolution of schizophrenia with regard to hospitalization and discharge, a comparison was made between differences in SAPS and SANS scores and in relative power percentages. As shown in Table 4, relative power of slow activity was reduced and fast activity was increased in many but not all of the patients in whom a significant reduction of positive symptoms was also indicated by SAPS. Less evident were the relationships between negative symptoms (SANS) and electrophysiologic data.

In general, the patients with the first EEGM pattern had mild pathology or evident positive symptoms rapidly controlled by therapy. The other patients (the second EEGM pattern) had a very heterogeneous clinical picture.

Finally, a statistical analysis of the correlation coefficient between psychodiagnostic and relative power data was made.

As shown in Table 5, there was no significant correlation between mean group EEGM improvement on the one hand and SAPS and SANS on the other. In fact, the best correlation was found between relative α mean power and the mean of SAPS + SANS ($p = 0.074$), whereas the correlation coefficients between α power and SAPS or SANS were $p = 0.082$ and $p = 0.105$, respectively. The correlation between δ activity and SAPS or SANS was even less significant. As shown in Fig. 5, all patients who exhibited a psycho-

TABLE 4. *Comparison scores between clinical modifications (SAPS, SANS), and δ, θ, α, and β relative power at EEGM*

Patient	SAPS	SANS	SAPS + SANS	δ	θ	α	β
BN	2	0	2	−29.0	−5.4	10.4	26.0
MA	7	2	9	−22.2	1.0	24.9	−6.1
SP	4	3	7	−4.6	4.4	4.1	2.0
NF	14	8	22	−13.6	−5.4	15.3	6.7
PC	6	2	8	−5.6	−12.6	−2.1	20.3
SS	3	0	3	4.6	−2.8	−5.8	1.0
SA	6	0	6	−0.3	−1.3	−4.1	7.1
GS	6	0	6	−4.0	7.8	16.3	−8.4
GF	4	1	5	−1.3	10.1	−11.0	−0.8
ER	9	6	15	−1.5	0.6	11.0	−5.3
BA	7	1	8	5.4	−3.7	−6.6	−2.8
BM	8	2	10	−7.6	−6.2	−0.8	9.3
GM	2	2	4	−3.0	−0.3	1.6	6.5
GG	5	3	8	−3.4	1.7	−0.6	1.7
MA	5	−2	3	−14.1	0.5	2.6	−21.1

All values indicate the differences at discharge compared with hospitalization. For SAPS and SANS, positive values indicate a clinical improvement; for EEGM, negative values in delta and theta activity and positive values in α and β activity indicate an electrophysiologic improvement.

TABLE 5. *Pearson correlation coefficients and their statistical significance among improvement scores (at discharge, with respect to hospitalization) in positive and negative symptoms (SAPS and SANS scales), and relative power in spectral bands* δ, θ, α, *and* β

	δ	θ	α	β
SAPS	−0.0377	−0.2385	0.3780	−0.1312
	p = 0.447	p = 0.196	p = 0.082	p = 0.321
SANS	0.0022	−0.1521	0.3441	0.1603
	p = 0.497	p = 0.294	p = 0.105	p = 0.284
SAPS + SANS	−0.0212	−0.2156	0.3920	0.0004
	p = 0.470	p = 0.220	p = 0.074	p = 0.499
δ	—	0.1829	−0.6540	−0.2385
		p = 0.257	p = 0.004	p = 0.196
θ	0.1829	—	0.0586	−0.6001
	p = 0.257		p = 0.418	p = 0.009
α	−0.6540	0.0586	—	−0.1268
	p = 0.004	p = 0.418		p = 0.326
β	−0.2385	−0.6001	−0.1268	—
	p = 0.196	p = 0.009	p = 0.326	

[a] n = 15.

diagnostic improvement (SAPS + SANS) of not less than 7 points also showed a reduction in the relative power of slow activity (δ + θ) and an increase of fast activity (α + β), although such a modification did not respond to a linear correlation. There was an exception in only one patient (BA), in whom slow activity did not significantly change (as his δ increase was counterbalanced by a θ decrease) and his fast activity decreased. Furthermore, the patient (BN) who had the worst correlation (low SAPS, good EEGM improvement) during hospitalization demonstrated delusional thought without any evident hallucinations. Obviously, this reduced the improvement scores on SAPS.

DISCUSSION AND CONCLUSIONS

During hospitalization, a reduction of positive symptoms (SAPS) was more evident as compared with negative symptoms (SANS). These data are in agreement with recent results of many authors concerning the increased activity of neuroleptic medication on positive symptoms of schizophrenia (10,11,13,14,20,21), although there are also dissenting reports (14).

Regarding EEGM, patients with paranoid schizophrenia showed a "normal-like" or "slow" pattern, whereas patients with undifferentiated schizophrenia showed only the second pattern. This result is in agreement with the hypothesis that schizophrenia is a heterogeneous syndrome with regard to its electrophysiologic correlations, and that there are no pathognomonic patterns, even though some alterations (such as slow activity in frontal regions) have often been described in many patients (2–7).

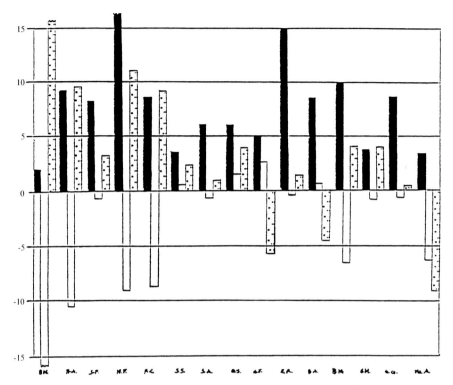

FIG. 5. Modifications in the patients investigated concerning SAPS + SANS scores (*dark columns*), slow activity relative power (*white columns*), and fast activity relative power (*dotted columns*). Improvement at discharge with respect to hospitalization is given both by positive dark columns (for SAPS + SANS) and dotted columns (for α + β activity) and by negative white columns (δ + θ activity).

Electrophysiologic patterns of the spectral bands showed, in many cases, a reduction of slow activity (more δ than θ) and/or an increase of fast activity (especially α). Such modifications were not due to a difference between the drug-free and medication conditions, because the first EEGM was recorded when clinical exacerbation was present and neuroleptics had been administered for at least 24 h. Therefore, both EEGM patterns, recorded for every patient after hospitalization and before discharge, are an expression of functional aspects related to the pharmacodynamic effects of the therapy and to the clinical changes in neurophysiologic systems.

The alterations observed (i.e., presence of slow activity, especially in anterior regions, less bioelectrical organization, less evidence of α activity with lower differentiation between anterior and posterior regions) can be considered a functional electrophysiologic expression of clinical impairment. A topographic analysis of the differences at the time of discharge showed that slow activity was reduced, especially in frontal regions, not only according to other EEG data (3,21) but also according to data concerning other functional investigations of brain activity (i.e., improvement in the reduction of cerebral metabolism on PET and of blood flow at SPECT (5).

Not all clinical (in particular, psychodiagnostic) and EEGM improvements were in agreement; however, in some patients there was a good relationship between a reduction of slow activity and an increase of fast activity on the one hand and an improvement of scores at SAPS and SANS on the other. In other cases there was neither EEGM nor psychodiagnostic improvement. The fact that a significant correlation was not present in any case (as shown by mean group analysis) can be explained, first, by the fact (previously mentioned) that schizophrenia is a very complex and heterogeneous syndrome. Therefore, the psychodiagnostic scales, the clinical evaluations, and the electrophysiologic investigations can explore neurophysiologic and behavioral aspects that do not entirely coincide. For example, no significant correlation between any specific symptom (i.e., the presence of hallucinations or delusions) and EEGM patterns was seen. Furthermore, among the many works published on EEGM in schizophrenia, the heterogeneous results obtained may be due not only to differences in the workup employed by the authors (17) but also to interindividual differences resulting from specific neurophysiologic patterns. Moreover, not even the same operative–functional system may be involved in all patients, even though they may have very similar symptoms. Our results are in agreement with data that point out the complexity of schizophrenia. Both genetic and environmental factors are important in the clinical picture and in producing the onset and maintenance of symptoms (10). Finally, the fact that clinical and electrophysiologic improvement are both present, but not in the same manner, in every patient (and not in linear correlation) demonstrates the utility of many different diagnostic approaches, especially those that explore functional aspects. In addition, in all of our patients, when one of the two aspects investigated (psychopathologic and electrophysiologic) improved the other always improved (even if only partially).

It is important to remember that the classification of schizophrenia is still linked to clinical judgment and that psychodiagnostic tests (such as SAPS and SANS) are made on the basis of a specialized evaluation. Therefore, the usefulness of an EEGM investigation in studying the clinical course and in improving the prognosis of patients with schizophrenia treated with neuroleptics is linked to the necessity of obtaining an "objective" evaluation parameter.

The absence of specific pathognomonic electrophysiologic patterns but, paradoxically, the presence of significant qualitative and quantitative EEGM alterations (which indicate a different mechanism in information processing not only during verbal or visual–spatial tasks but also under basal resting conditions) is in agreement with the hypothesis that schizophrenia is not a homogeneous disorder but a real syndrome. Furthermore, the changes seen after modifications of the clinical picture in the same patient suggest a resettlement of the "operative–functional systems" (22) of the brain during verbal and nonverbal data processing (23). This emphasizes the clinical value of an intraindividual and longitudinal study over time, rather than an interindividual transverse characterization of the alterations. An intraindividual longitudinal EEGM study over time can provide better understanding of all aspects of schizophrenia. For this purpose, we are expanding the number of schizophrenic patients to be studied and we intend to study them over a longer period.

In conclusion, our data show the following: (i) In patients with schizophrenia hospitalized during an acute exacerbation, there were many EEGM alterations, the most common of which were the presence of slow activity in the frontal regions, the absence or reduction of α activity in the PO regions, and also the presence of α activity in the anterior regions. (ii) In remission, patients usually (but not always) showed an improvement in their EEGM pattern (reduction of slow activity, increase of fast activity). (iii) The mean group values show a statistically significant positive correlation between the reduction of δ and θ activity and the increase of α and β activity observed at the time of clinical discharge. (iv) EEGM improvement is not directly correlated with clinical improvement studied by psychodiagnostic scales for positive and negative symptoms (SAPS and SANS).

Therefore, EEGM can be a useful tool to study clinical changes and to improve prognostic criteria. The presence of several electrophysiologic modifications (with a large interindividual variability) in patients treated with neuroleptic agents confirms the importance of an intraindividual study. Finally, EEGM not only confirms the value of functional neuroimaging investigations (and can integrate metabolic and flow data obtained by PET and SPECT) but can be recommended on the basis of its practicality, low operating cost, and the absence of dangerous side effects.

ACKNOWLEDGMENT

We thank Marisa Del Papa and Maria Ida Giuli, neuropathophysiological technicians of the Clinical Psychiatry Dept., University of Ancona, for their help in carrying out the EEG mapping examinations; Dr. Raul Castagnani, engineer at the Data Analysis Center, University of Ancona, for his cooperation in the statistical analysis of our data; and William J. Montesano, Jr., State University of New York at Buffalo for his assistance in reviewing the text.

REFERENCES

1. Berger H. Ueber das Elektrenkephalogram des Manschen. *Arch Psychiatr Nervenkr* 1929; 87:527–41.

2. Kemali D, Vacca L, Marciano F, Celani T, Nolfe G, Iorio G. Computerized EEG in schizo-phrenics. *Neuropsychobiology* 1980;6:260–7.
3. Morihisa JM, Duffy FH, Wyatt RJ. Brain electrical activity mapping (BEAM) in schizo-phrenic patients. *Arch Gen Psychiatry* 1983;40:719–28.
4. Prichep LS, John ER, Chabot R. Neurometric EEG in the evaluation of psychiatric patients. *J Clin Neurophysiol* 1987;4:235–6.
5. Buchsbaum MS, Wu JC, Guich S. EEG mapping and positron emission tomography in schizophrenia. In: Kemali D, ed. *I International symposium on neurophysiological corre-lates of psychopathological conditions*. Capri, 1988;8.
6. Marchesi GF, Nardi B, Pannelli G. Psychosensorial and cognitive EEG mapping in acute and remitted schizophrenic syndromes. *Neuropsychobiology* 1992;25:69.
7. Marchesi GF, Nardi B, Trovarelli I, Paciaroni G, De Rosa M, Borioni S. EEG mapping e sindromi schizofreniche. In: Volterra V, ed. New trends in schizophrenia. Santa Maria a Vico: Centro Praxis, 1990:109–19.
8. Pockberger H, Rappelsberger P, Petsche H. Thau K, Kufferle B. Computer assisted EEG topography as a tool in the evaluation of actions of psychoactive drugs in patients. *Neuro-psychobiology* 1984;12:183–7.
9. Itil TM, Itil KZ. The significance of pharmacodynamic measurements in the assessment of bioavailability and bioequivalence of psychotropic drugs using CEEG and dynamic brain mapping. *J Clin Psychiatry* 1986;47:20–7.
10. Kaplan HI, Sadock BM. *Synopsis of psychiatry*. Baltimore: Williams & Wilkins, 1988.
11. Bellantuono C, Tansella M. *Gli psicofarmaci nella pratica terapeutica*. Roma: Il Pensiero Scientifico, 1989.
12. Andreasen NC. *Scales for the assessment of negative and positive symptoms*. Iowa City: University of Iowa, 1981.
13. Crow TJ. Two syndromes in schizophrenia. *Trends Neurosci* 1982;351:4.
14. Kemali D, Maj M. Farmacoterapia della schizofrenia. Limiti dell'approccio tradizionale e possibili orientamenti futuri. *Neurol Psichiat Scienze Umane* 1989;9(suppl):208–23.
15. Flor–Henry P, Koles ZJ. Statistical quantitative EEG studies of depression, mania, schizo-phrenia, and normals. *Biol Psychol* 1984;19:257–79.
16. Nardi B, Pettinelli M, Trovarelli I, Paciaroni G, Marchesi GF. Presupposti teorici ed appli-cazioni cliniche delle mappe elettroencefalografiche cerebrali (MEEG) nei disturbi mentali. *Riv Psichiatr* 1988;23:34–42.
17. Nardi B, De Rosa M, Magari S, Marchesi GF. Applicazioni dell'EEG mapping nello studio dei disturbi mentali: problematiche e prospettive. *Riv Ital EEG Neurofisiol Clin* 1989;12: 29–40.
18. American Psychiatric Association. *Diagnostic and statistical manual of mental disorders (DSM-II-R)*. 3rd rev. Washington, DC: American Psychiatric Association, 1987.
19. Nuwer MR. Quantitative EEG: techniques and problems of frequency analysis and topo-graphic mapping. *J Clin Neurophysiol* 1988;5:1–43.
20. Harnryd C, Bjerkenstedt L, Bjork K, et al. Clinical evaluation of sulpiride in schizophrenic patients. A double-blind comparison with chlorpromazine. *Acta Psychiatr Scand* 1984;69: (suppl):7–30.
21. Galderisi S, Mucci A, Mignone ML, Milici N, Bucci P. Brain mapping and haloperidol treatment monitoring. In: Kemali D, ed. *Biological indexes and psychopathological dimen-sions*. Naples, 1990.
22. Luria AR. *Higher cortical functions in man*. New York: Basic Books, 1980.
23. Giannitrapani D, Murri L, eds. *The EEG of mental activities*. Basel: Karger, 1988.

Psychiatry and Advanced Technologies,
edited by L. Ravizza, F. Bogetto, and
E. Zanalda. Raven Press, Ltd.,
New York © 1993.

7

The Meaning of Physiological Computed Electroencephalography: A Statistical Approach

O. Gambini, M. Locatelli, C. Colombo, F. Macciardi, and S. Scarone

Psychiatric Branch, Department of Biomedical and Technological Sciences, University of Milan Medical School, Scientific Institute San Raffaele, 21027 Milan, Italy

One of the remaining difficulties that limits the utility of computed electroencephalography (EEG) in research is the complexity of analyzing the massive amounts of data generated by multiple electrode recordings (16 or more) for each frequency band under different experimental conditions (1). Furthermore, several controversies have recently emerged concerning the statistical treatment of the raw EEG values (both absolute and relative power) because of their non-normal distribution (2). Even if the raw data could be interpreted in a straightforward way, their non-Gaussian distribution would make the utilization of parametric statistics a problem (3). Following this reasoning, transformation of the raw data has recently been proposed as an obligatory step before any statistical approach is undertaken, to obtain a normal distribution (4). The log transformation of the relative value (X) according to the formula $Y = \log[X/(1 - X)]$ has recently shown good capacity for data normalization (5). Once normalized, the different statistical analyses can be carried out using the transformed EEG data. Statistical analysis of EEG data has primarily been made by means of t test, analysis of variance (ANOVA), and multiple analysis of variance (MANOVA), but these methods are not immune to criticism. The t test has frequently been used to compare both different groups of subjects and different conditions of the same group of subjects (6,7). In t test analysis and ANOVA, each derivation is treated separately and its application cannot be considered completely correct because pairs of electrodes leads are not independent of each other (i.e., the recordings from the leads must be regarded as contemporary events). A further possibility is MANOVA, which permits the simultaneous analysis of all variables (derivations and conditions). Nevertheless, this choice can be inappropriate when a very large number of variables are to be analyzed together (i.e., 16 derivations, 8 frequency bands, several conditions). In this case, a larger number of subjects is needed. Unfortunately when the number of variables is very large some results appear to be significant by chance (1). An alternative choice proposed (8) is factor analysis (FA), a generalized procedure for generating and defining dimensional space among a relatively large group of variables that is used primarily for data reduction (9). This means that FA locates a smaller number of valid dimensions or factors. It thus enables us to see whether some common underlying relationships exist among data, such that the data can be rearranged or reduced to a smaller set of factors. These factors can then be taken as a source of variability accounting for the observed interrelations in the data. Each set of data is composed of individual characteristics that tend to change in a parallel manner, and separate sets are composed of features that act independently of other sets. FA can be used as an exploratory, confirmatory, or measuring device (9). The exploratory uses are as a first step to detect a pattern of variables and to reduce the data by obtaining few descriptors without a loss of information. Furthermore, the confirmatory use can be performed to test the hypothesis of an expected number of significant factors and in the construction of indices to be used as new variables in later analysis. The purposes of this study were: (i) to verify the presence of good correlation coefficients not only among the several leads within each experimental condition but also among three different conditions (eyes closed, eyes open, and hyperventilation), comparing all the leads at different times; (ii) to extract from the pool of the EEG variables (in our case, 16 leads × 3 experimental conditions = 48 variables for each frequency band) some factors that should be able to give a concise but complete picture of the EEG pattern and of its changes; and (iii) to compare the results of the raw and transformed data obtained from the FA.

METHOD

Subjects

The sample consisted of 50 normal adults (mean age 35.16, SD 12.23), including 24 men (mean age 37.58, SD 12.48) and 26 women (mean age 32.92, SD 11.80). Before admission to the study, all subjects underwent an extensive screening to ensure that they were healthy. The subjects were selected on the basis of physical, neurologic, and psychiatric examinations to exclude any possible diseases. Additional exclusion criteria included current use of alcohol and prescription drugs and abnormal sleep patterns.

Experimental Procedures

Subjects were comfortably seated in a soundproofed and electrically shielded room and were instructed to relax as much as possible. If drowsiness or restlessness were noted, appropriate action was taken to either wake or relax the subject; this ensured maintenance of a relatively constant level of consciousness throughout the recording time. EEG was recorded under three experimental conditions: (i) resting, eyes closed, lasting 3 min; (ii) resting, eyes open, lasting 3 min; and (iii) hyperventilation with eyes closed (the subjects breathed deeply and regularly at a rate of about 20 respirations/min for a period of 4 min, with only the last 3 min being analyzed by computer. EEG measurements were taken with a conventional EEG examination, consisting of a 16-channel recording with 19 scalp electrodes placed according to the standard 10–20 system with reference to the two linked mastoids (F3, C3, P3, O1, F7, T3, T5, Fz, Pz, F4, C4, P4, O2, F8, T4, T6). The EEGs were recorded with a Nicolet 21-channel polygraph and the signal was analyzed by means of A-to-D conversion performed on-line by an IBM PC computer. The EEG signals were analogically filtered with a half-amplitude cutoff at 1 and 30 Hz; a 50-Hz notch filter was also on-line. Recordings were edited off-line on a second-by-second basis and then digitized at 250 Hz. Artifact-free 8-s epochs were FFT transformed: a mean number of 20 epochs for eyes closed, a mean number of 20 epochs for hyperventilation, and 18 epochs for eyes open were processed. For each of the 16 derivations, the values of absolute and relative power in the δ_1 (0–2 Hz), δ_2 (2–4 Hz), θ_1 (4–6 Hz), θ_2 (6–8 Hz), α_1 (8–10 Hz), α_2 (10–12 Hz), β_1 (12–18 Hz), and β_2 (18–30 Hz) frequency bands were computed and then the relative values were subjected to the above mentioned transformation (i.e., $Y = \log [X/(1 - X)]$).

Statistics

As a first step, the Kolmogorow–Smirnoff test was performed to check the distribution of absolute, relative, and log-transformed relative values of the 50 subjects for each derivation in each frequency band and condition (16 derivations, 8 frequency bands, and 3 conditions). Then the absolute and transformed values of the 50 subjects relative to each experimental session for each derivation in each frequency band were subjected to FA (9). FA as a first step involves constructing a correlation matrix R to determine a set of initial factors, often accomplished by the method of principal components. There is one option concerning the correlation matrix R, i.e., whether to replace the 1's on the diagonal of R with communalities (the variance of the linear combination C_j of the common factors for any variable X_j, i.e., the quantity measuring the information that the variable has in common with all the other variables through the common factors). Because this substitution, which alters the original R matrix in a not entirely satisfying theoretical way, is a part of the computer algorithm for FA, we first evaluated the correlations among variables (with Pearson produce–moment correlation). In our study the correlation matrix R consisted of the 16 leads for each one of the three different recording conditions (eyes closed, eyes open, hyperventilation), i.e., R 48 × 48, for each frequency band. In accordance with the results of correlation analysis, some options of FA procedure can be more firmly selected. In particular, because our data set was composed of variables that were all mutually related with highly significant correlation coefficients (see Results for details), we chose to use a mineigen value of at least 1.0, a principal component extraction method, and an oblique rotation of factors, performing FA separately for absolute and log-transformed values and for each frequency band (i.e., 8 frequency bands = 16 factor analyses). The initial factors, if constructed as principal components, are completely independent, thus satisfying one goal of FA analysis. Despite the fact that the initial factors provide a useful first impression, they are usually difficult to interpret directly without some further manipulation. Consequently another step, which entails rotation, is usually required to achieve conceptual meaningfulness. Therefore, we performed an oblique rotation because this can partially consider the high correlation among the initial set of variables, since the factors resulting from this method of rotation are also usually correlated to some extent (i.e., some or all of the factor cosines will be non-zero) (10). Finally, a factor loading score above 0.85 for one factor and below 0.15 for the others was considered satisfactory for each derivation.

RESULTS

According to the Kolmogorow–Smirnow statistic, raw values (i.e, absolute and relative EEG power values) did not show a normal distribution in any frequency band (statistically significant two-tailed $p = 0.05$). On the contrary, log-transformed values always showed distribution shapes very close to normal ones (two-tailed $p = $ not significant). As an example, Fig. 1 shows the distribution of absolute values, relative values, and log-transformed relative values for 01 derivation in the α_2 frequency band for each condition. Pearson produce–moment correlation coefficients among derivations for each frequency band have been calculated and for the most part, derivations were significantly correlated in each condition and across the three different experimental conditions.

The percentage of variance explained by each of three identified factors in each frequency band for absolute and transformed values are respectively shown in Figs. 2 and 3. The total percentage of variance explained by three factors was 68.2–89.3% for absolute and 71.7–89.2% for transformed values, depending on the frequency band. Factor 1 explained 34–77.1% of the

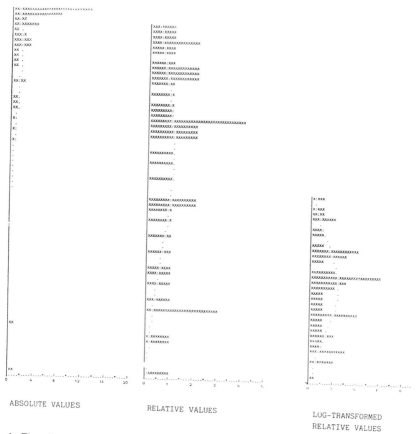

ABSOLUTE VALUES

RELATIVE VALUES

LOG-TRANSFORMED
RELATIVE VALUES

A

FIG. 1. The distributions of absolute, relative and log-transformed relative values are shown in each condition for left occipital derivation in α_2 frequency band; **A,** eyes closed; **B,** eyes open; **C,** hyperventilation.

total variance with absolute values and 48.6–75.4% after log-transformation, depending again on the different frequency bands. The second and third factors accounted for a reduced but nevertheless important percentage of the total variance. Figures 4 and 5 show the relationships between identified factors and experimental conditions in each frequency band on the basis of the factor loading scores of the 48 variables for absolute and transformed values, respectively. Before the transformation the variables corresponding to the leads during hyperventilation loaded completely in δ_1 and θ_2 and partially on Factor 1 in β_2 and on Factor 2 in δ_2, θ_1, θ_2, and β_1. The leads in eyes closed condition loaded completely in δ_2, θ_1, θ_2, and α_2, and partially in β_1 and β_2 on Factor 1 and on Factor 3 in δ_1, α_1, and β_1 frequency bands. The leads in eyes open condition loaded partially on Factor 1 in β_1 and completely on Factor 2 in δ_1, α_1, and α_2, and on Factor 3 in δ_2, θ_1, θ_2, and

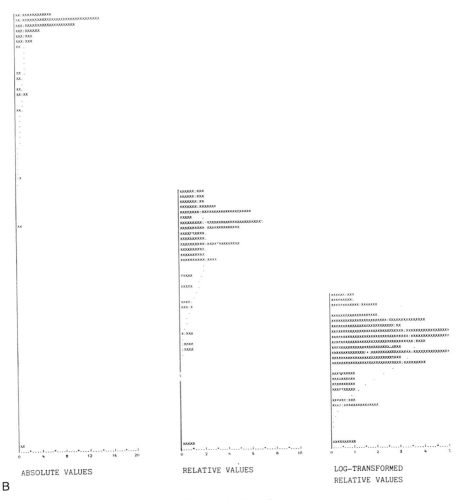

ABSOLUTE VALUES   RELATIVE VALUES   LOG–TRANSFORMED
                                                  RELATIVE VALUES

B

FIG. 1. *Continued*

β_2 frequency bands. After the log-transformation the eyes closed condition loaded completely in θ_1, θ_2, α_2, and β_1, and partially in α_1 and β_2 on Factor 1, and on Factor 3 in δ_1 and δ_2 frequency bands. Eyes open condition loaded on Factor 2 in all frequency bands except for θ_2 and on Factor 3 in the θ_2 band. Hyperventilation loaded completely in δ_1 and δ_2 and partially in α_1 and β_2 on Factor 1, on Factor 2 in θ_2, and on Factor 3 in θ_1, α_2, and β_1.

DISCUSSION

Absolute EEG values are not normally distributed, and to treat them by means of parametric statistics it is necessary to transform them. Our data

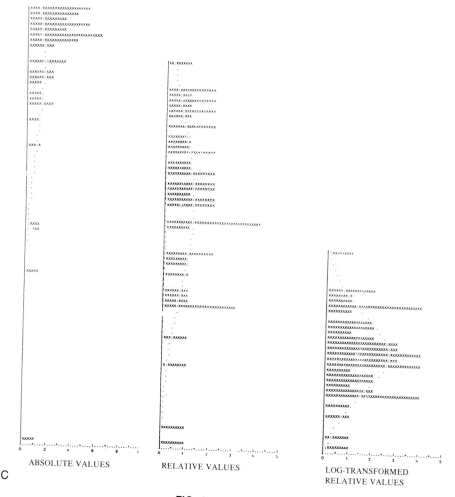

ABSOLUTE VALUES   RELATIVE VALUES   LOG-TRANSFORMED RELATIVE VALUES

C

FIG. 1. *Continued*

are consistent with previous recent findings (1,11,12) and call for a very cautious evaluation of the results of clinical neurophysiologic studies when parametric statistical tests are applied to absolute EEG values. Furthermore, the evidence of correlation among the different variables of EEG across three neurofunctionally different states makes it incorrect to consider the measurements from different electrodes on the same subject independently. It also confirms the soundness of FA as a statistical tool to reduce the massive amount of EEG data and to discover physiologically meaningful descriptors of the EEG changes. In our study, we submitted both absolute and log-transformed data to FA separately and found that the relationships between

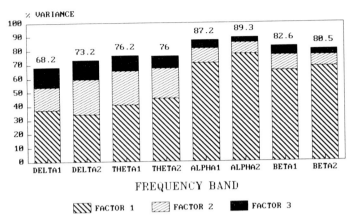

FIG. 2. Factor analysis: absolute values. Percentage of variance explained by factor for each frequency band.

identified factors and experimental conditions depend on transformation of the data. At present, many methods for multivariate analyses have been proposed, in some cases also relaxing the usual restrictive criteria such as for multinormal distribution of different variables. It is also known, however, that traditional FA is a highly efficient analytic method for both exploratory and confirmatory analysis of a set of variables, but that it requires multinormal distributions for continuous variables. When compared with the original non-transformed variables, the log-transformed variables showed a lower dispersion of data, thus hypothetically reducing some measurement bias in data description. Although a tendency toward distortion and artifacts has

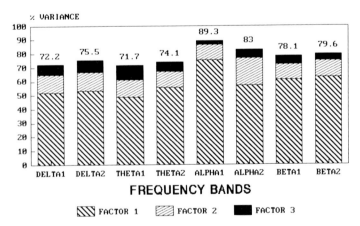

FIG. 3. Factor analysis: log-transformed relative values. Percentage of variance explained by factors for each frequency band.

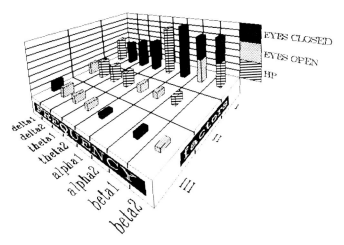

FIG. 4. EEG factor analysis: absolute values.

been reported for transformation that changes the characteristics of the original data (3) it is still unclear at this point whether these transformations have a negative effect on the final results. Following this reasoning, we chose to analyze log-transformed variables that fully satisfy the prerequisite assumption of normality for our preliminary analysis. Taking into account transformed values, Factor 1 explains at least 45% of the total variance in each EEG frequency band. It loads with hyperventilation on δ frequency band (δ_1 and δ_2). It therefore should be considered a good descriptor of the synchronization of the EEG activity related to the metabolic modifications induced

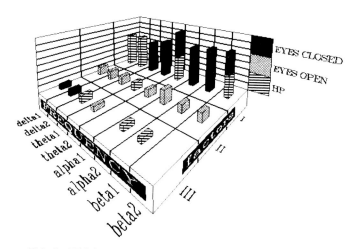

FIG. 5. EEG factor analysis: log-transformed relative values.

by hyperventilation. Factor 1 also explains a high variance in almost all the components of the EEG spectrum in eyes closed condition (i.e., θ_1 and θ_2 for slow frequencies, α_2 for central frequencies, and β_1 for fast frequencies). Therefore, it should be considered a good descriptor of the main electrical activity of the brain in the resting state. Factor 2 explains up to 19% of variance, therefore showing less importance in explaining the variance of EEG activity. Nevertheless, it loads in all frequency bands in the eyes open condition. Therefore, it should reflect the neurofunctional state of this condition, which is related to a certain level of desynchronization of EEG activity Factor 3 load with eyes closed in slow frequencies. It seems, therefore, that a certain amount of the EEG variance in the resting state is defined by slow activity, suggesting that a good definition of the EEG in the resting eyes closed state also depends on the slowest components on the EEG spectrum. Therefore, it could be considered a good additional descriptor of the main electrical activity of the brain in resting states. In conclusion, FA appears to be a useful statistical tool for reducing the large amount of data extracted by automated EEG analysis to fewer factors. Moreover, these factors appear to be related in a neurophysiologically meaningful way to the three basic conditions in which clinical neurophysiologists explore EEG-measured brain activity.

Repeated experimental work and additional evaluation of the influence of some demographic variables, such as age and sex, will be needed to confirm these very preliminary data.

REFERENCES

1. Oken BS, Chiappa KH. Statistical issues concerning computerized analysis of brainwave topography. *Ann Neurol* 1986;19:493–4.
2. John ER, Pricep LS, Easton P. Normative data banks and neurometrics: basic concepts, current status and clinical applications. In: Remond A, Lopes de Silva F, eds. *Computer analysis of EEG and other neurophysiological variables: clinical applications*. Amsterdam: Elsevier, 1987. (EEG handbook, vol 3).
3. Nuwer MR. Quantitative EEG: I. Techniques and problems of frequency analysis and topographic mapping. *J Clin Neurophysiol* 1988;5:1–43.
4. John ER, Pricep LS, Friedman J, Easton P. Neurometric topographic mapping of EEG and evoked potentials features: application to clinical diagnosis and cognitive evaluation. In: Maurer K, ed. *Topographic brain mapping of EEG and evoked potentials*. Berlin: Springer-Verlag, 1989:90–117.
5. John ER, Pricep LS, Chabot RJ. Quantitative electrophysiological maps of mental activity. In: Basar E, Bullock TH, eds. *Brain dynamics: progress and perspectives*. Berlin: Springer-Verlag, 1989:316–30.
6. Duffy FH. Brain electrical activity mapping: clinical applications. *Psychiatr Res* 1989;29:379–84.
7. Duffy FH, Maurer K. Establishment of guidelines for the use of topographic mapping in clinical neurophysiology: a philosophical approach. In: Maurer K, ed. *Topographic brain mapping of EEG and evoked potentials*. Berlin: Springer-Verlag, 1989:3–10.
8. Gasser T. Mocks J, Bacher P. Topographic factor analysis of the EEG with applications to development and to mental retardation. *Electroenceph Clin Neurophysiol* 1983;55:445–63.

9. Kim JO. Factor analysis. In: Bowman JH, Cahill J, eds. *SPSS*, 2nd ed. New York: McGraw–Hill, 1975:468–514.

10. Kleinbaum DG, Kupper LL, Muller KE. *Applied regression analysis and other multivariable methods*. Boston: PWS-KENT Publishing Company, 1988.

11. Van den Noort S, Conomy J, Davis E, et al. Special articles–assessment: EEG brain mapping. *Neurology* 1989;39:1100–01.

12. Gasser T, Bacher P, Macks J. Transformations towards the normal distribution of broad band spectral parameters of the EEG. *Electroenceph Clin Neurophysiol* 1982;53:119–24.

Psychiatry and Advanced Technologies, edited by L. Ravizza, F. Bogetto, and E. Zanalda. Raven Press, Ltd., New York © 1993.

8

A Statistical Approach to Computed Electroencephalography: Preliminary Data on Control Subjects and Epileptic Patients

M. Locatelli, O. Gambini, C. Colombo, F. Macciardi, and S. Scarone

Psychiatric Branch, Department of Biomedical and Technological Sciences, University of Milan Medical School, Scientific Institute San Raffaele, 20127 Milan, Italy

Despite the large number of statistical procedures available, it has been very difficult to compare computed electroencephalography (EEG) variables of clinically different groups, taking into account all statistical analysis requirements. Because of the redundancy and high correlation in multichannel EEG data sets (1), many efforts have been made to extract some summarizing feature with a neurophysiologic meaning. It is necessary to discover reliable descriptors of the brain's electric activity under different physiologic and pathologic functional conditions.

Recently, factor analysis (FA) has been suggested as a useful EEG data analysis technique for describing the entire EEG pattern under three experimental conditions (resting eyes closed, resting eyes open, and hyperventilation with eyes closed) by means of three extracted factors (2). Our findings in this study were that Factor 1 loaded under the hyperventilation condition in the δ range and in the eyes closed condition in all the other bands. Factor 2 loaded under the eyes open condition in all components of the EEG spectrum. Factor 3 loaded under the eyes closed condition in δ_1 and δ_2 frequency bands and during hyperventilation in the θ, α, and β ranges. This confirms the data reduction capability of FA. Furthermore, close relationships between factors and experimental conditions indicate a neurofunctional meaning of the three identified factors. The aim of the present study was to explore the confirmatory use of FA in comparing two groups with different neurofunctional pictures: 14 epileptic patients with generalized seizures and 50 normal subjects. Epilepsy is an example of central nervous system (CNS) functional pathology and, in addition to epileptoform discharges, is also characterized by abnormal interictal background activity, such as a slowing with a decrease of α power and an increase of θ and δ power. We tested the reliability of FA in assessing the functional impairment reflected by the interictal EEG of epileptic patients.

SUBJECTS

Fourteen epileptic patients (five men and nine women; mean age 27.5, SD 9.64), selected on the basis of a positive history of generalized seizures, were entered in the study. Ten had tonic–clonic seizures and four had absence seizures; all patients had been treated with such anticonvulsants as sodium valproate, phenobarbital, carbamazepine, or phenytoin at different dosages. A conventional visual inspection of interictal EEGs of these patients showed some irregularity in background activity without any epileptiform discharges. Fifty normal adults (24 men and 26 women; mean age 35.16, SD 12.23) acted as controls. The subjects were selected on the basis of normal physical, neurologic, and psychiatric examinations to exclude any possible disease. Additional exclusion criteria included current use of alcohol and prescription drugs and abnormal sleep patterns.

EXPERIMENTAL PROCEDURES

Subjects were comfortably seated in a soundproofed and electrically shielded room and were instructed to relax as much as possible. If drowsiness or restlessness were noted, appropriate action was taken to either wake or relax the subject. This ensured maintenance of a relatively constant level of consciousness throughout the recording time. EEG was recorded under three experimental conditions: resting (eyes closed, lasting 3 min); resting, eyes open (lasting 3 min); and hyperventilation with eyes closed (the subjects breathed deeply and regularly at a rate of about 20 respirations/min for a period of 4 min, with only the last 3 min being analyzed by computer. EEG measurements were taken in a conventional EEG examination consisting of a 16-channel recording with 19 scalp electrodes placed according to the standard 10–20 system with reference at the two linked mastoids (F3, C3, P3, O1, F7, T3, T5, Fz, Pz, F4, C4, P4, O2, F8, T4, T6). The EEGs were recorded with a Nicolet 21 channel polygraph and the signal was analyzed by an IBM PC computer. The EEG signals were analogically filtered with a half-amplitude cutoff at 1 and 30 Hz; a 50-Hz notch filter was also on-line. Twenty-two 8-s epochs for each experimental condition were submitted to the analogue-to-digital conversion and only the artifact-free ones were fast-Fourier transformed (FFT) (at least 15 for each experimental condition). For each of the 16 derivations, relative power in δ_1 (0–2 Hz), δ_2 (2–4 Hz), θ_1 (4–6 Hz), θ_2 (6–8 Hz), α_1 (8–10 Hz), α_2 (10–12 Hz), β_1 (12–18 Hz), and β_2 (18–30 Hz) frequency bands was computed and then the relative values were log-transformed according to the following formula: $Y = \log[X/(1 - X)]$ (2,3). Taking control subjects and epileptic patients together, FA was performed separately for each frequency band (i.e., 8 frequency bands = 8 factor analyses), considering three conditions together (eyes closed, eyes open, and hyperventilation) because the three conditions are mutually related to each other with highly significant correlation coefficients. A mineigen value of at least 1.0, the principal component extraction method, and oblique rotation of factors were chosen. The resulting factor scores of epileptic patients and healthy subjects were analyzed for each frequency band by analysis of variance (ANOVA) to check significant differences between the two groups.

RESULTS

Table 1 shows statistically significant results on factor scores of the two groups in different frequency bands. There are differences between epileptic patients and control subjects on Factor 3 in θ_1, Factor 1 in θ_2, and Factors 1 and 3 in α_1.

DISCUSSION

Epileptic patients show significant differences in the factor score means of the Factor 1 in θ_2 and α_1 EEG frequency bands. On the basis of normative data from our laboratory (4), this factor reflects the background electric activity in eyes closed condition. Therefore, our results suggest that background activity in the 6- to 10-Hz range is abnormally organized in epileptic patients in the resting, eyes closed condition, even in the absence of epileptic interictal abnormalities. Furthermore, significant differences between epileptic patients and controls were observed on factor score means of Factor 3 in θ_1 and α_1 EEG frequency bands; this factor reflects the background electrical activity under hyperventilatory conditions. Therefore, our results suggest that background activity in the 4- to 6- and 8- to 10-Hz ranges is abnormally organized in epileptic patients during hyperventilation, even in the absence of epileptic interictal abnormalities. This preliminary study confirms that computerized EEG results can be described by means of a statistical procedure that allows construction of factors with a neurofunctional meaning. Furthermore, this statistical method provides reduction of data without any

TABLE 1. *Epileptic patients vs. controls: ANOVA for factor scores*

Factor 3 score in θ_1 frequency band

	Mean	SD	Cases
Entire population	−5.551E-16	1.2908360	64
Normal subjects	0.1849229	1.3489376	50
Epileptic patients	−0.6604388	0.7842634	14

Source/between groups

Sum of squares/7.8163	D.F./1	Mean square/7.8163	F/4.9879	Sig./0.0291

Factor 1 score in θ_2 frequency band

	Mean	SD	Cases
Entire population	−2.776E-16	1.5959696	64
Normal subjects	−0.3584331	1.5032432	50
Epileptic patients	1.2801182	1.2519426	14

Source/between groups

Sum of squares/29.3656	D.F./1	Mean square/29.3656	F/13.8873	Sig./0.0004

Factor 1 score in α_1 frequency band

	Mean	SD	Cases
Entire population	−2.776E-16	1.3111743	64
Normal subjects	0.1832941	1.2979880	50
Epileptic patients	−0.6546217	0.1791485	14

Source/between groups

Sum of squares/7.6793	D.F./1	Mean square/7.6793	F/4.7314	Sig./0.0334

Factor 3 score in α_1 frequency band

	Mean	SD	Cases
Entire population	−2.498E-16	1.3112794	64
Normal subjects	−0.1874265	1.2603589	50
Epileptic patients	0.6693803	1.3144010	14

Source/between groups

Sum of squares/8.02943	D.F./1	Mean square/8.0294	F/4.9635	Sig./0.0295

D.F., degree of freedom; F, F values; Sig, significance.

loss of information and the opportunity of comparing different groups by means of a few components raised from FA. There has previously been interest in FA of spatial features of the multichannel EEG (5–7). Our study suggests the possibility of group comparisons by factor analysis not only of several electrodes at different times but also in different functional conditions, and could open new ways to deal with computed EEG data. Nevertheless, these data must be cautiously evaluated because of the small number of patients and their clinical and therapeutic heterogeneity. Undoubtedly, additional data need to be collected.

REFERENCES

1. Harner RN, Riggio S. Application of singular value decomposition to topographic analysis of flash-evoked potentials. *Brain Topogr* 1989;2:91–8.
2. John ER, Pricep LS, Chabot RJ. Quantitative electophysiological maps of mental activity. In: Basar E, Bullock TH, eds. *Brain dynamics: progress and perspectives*. Berlin: Springer-Verlag, 1989:316–30.
3. John ER, Pricep LS, Friedman J, Easton P. Neurometric topographic mapping of EEG and evoked potentials features: application to clinical diagnosis and cognitive evaluation. In: Maurer K, ed. *Topographic brain mapping of EEG and evoked potentials*. Berlin: Springer-Verlag, 1989;90:117.
4. Gambini O, Locatelli M, Colombo C, Macciardi F, Scarone S. The meaning of physiological computed electroencephalography: a statistical approach. In: Ravizza L, Bogetto F, Zanalda E, eds. *Psychiatry and advanced technologies*. New York: Raven Press, 1993:61–71 (this volume).
5. Skrandies W, Lehmann D. Spatial principal components of multichannel maps evoked by lateral visual half-field stimuli. *Electroenceph Clin Neurophysiol* 1982;54:662–7.
6. Gasser T, Mocks J, Bacher P. Topographic factor analysis of the EEG with applications to development and to mental retardation. *Electroenceph Clin Neurophysiol* 1983;55:445–463.
7. Harner RN. Topographic analysis of multichannel EEG data analysis. In: Samson–Dollfus D, Guieu JD, Gotman J, Etevenon P, eds. *Statistics and topography in quantitative EEG*. Paris: Elsevier, 1988:49–61.

Psychiatry and Advanced Technologies,
edited by L. Ravizza, F. Bogetto, and
E. Zanalda. Raven Press, Ltd.,
New York 1993.

9

Local Cerebral Glucose Metabolic Rates in Obsessive–Compulsive Disorder

Chawki Benkelfat, *Thomas E. Nordahl,
*William E. Semple, *A. Catherine King,
Dennis L. Murphy, and *Robert M. Cohen

*Section on Clinical Neuropharmacology, Laboratory of Clinical Science,
National Institute of Mental Health, NIH Clinical Center,
Bethesda, Maryland 20892; and *Section on Clinical Brain Imaging,
Laboratory of Cerebral Metabolism, National Institute of Mental Health,
NIH Clinical Center, Bethesda, Maryland 20892*

Obsessive–compulsive disorder (OCD), initially described by Esquirol (1) and Westphal (2), is a chronic anxiety disorder that generally begins during adolescence and has a fluctuating course throughout most of the patient's adult life. The disorder is characterized by repetitive and intrusive dysphoric thoughts and forceful ritualistic behaviors. Lifetime prevalence rates of OCD in the general population, originally estimated to be very low (0.05%) (1953), were recently found to be 25–60 times greater in a United States community sample of 18,500 individuals (1988). Understanding of the OCD symptom complex has been based primarily on psychodynamic interpretations and the theory of defense mechanisms (1937) that have evolved over the last 60 years. However, recent evidence collected over the past decade implicates neurobiologic abnormalities in patients with OCD.

Some of the evidence suggesting neural abnormalities in patients with OCD comes from many case report observations of comorbidity of obsessive–compulsive (OC) symptoms with various neurologic disorders (e.g., Von Economo encephalitis, epilepsy, Parkinson, Gilles de la Tourette syndrome, frontal and/or basal ganglion lesions) (for review, see ref. 3). In addition, increased "obsessiveness–compulsiveness" has been regularly observed in association with magnetic resonance imaging (MRI) identified frontal and/or basal ganglion lesions (4–7).

More recently, the established efficacy of selective serotonin-reuptake blockers (e.g., clomipramine) as potent antiobsessional medications, as well as the confirmed reports of successful treatment of refractory cases of OCD by stereotactic psychosurgery techniques, have rekindled interest in exploring further brain localization, mechanisms, and neurochemistry of OC symptoms.

Positron emission tomography (PET) is one of the few functional brain imaging techniques with the potential to address simultaneously issues of brain localization and neurochemistry in the living patient. Recently, using PET and the 2-deoxyglucose method, Baxter et al. (8) reported that symptomatic, nonmedicated OCD patients exhibit increased glucose metabolic consumption in the orbital frontal cortex and in the caudate nucleus. The full significance of these results is not yet known; however, the finding of metabolic hyperfunction in the orbital frontal cortex and the caudate nucleus in a significant percentage of OCD patients clearly distinguishes them from patients with other psychiatric illnesses, such as schizophrenia (9,10) and affective disorders (11).

In an attempt to replicate and extend these findings, we decided to examine regional glucose metabolic rates in symptomatic OCD patients before and during treatment with clomipramine, at various stages of the therapeutic response, and to compare them with those obtained in healthy volunteers. By carefully examining possible brain regional metabolic changes associated with clomipramine treatment, we hoped to obtain information to help delineate the functional anatomy of OCD and the mechanism of action of antiobsessional drugs. If we found that hyperfrontality and/or hypermetabolism in the caudate nucleus was specifically related to OC symptoms, then we could determine whether effective treatment with selective antiobsessional drugs, such as clomipramine, is associated with a return to more normal glucose metabolism in these brain areas.

SUBJECTS AND METHODS

Subjects

Thirteen drug-free OCD outpatients were selected as part of the National Institute of Mental Health (NIMH) fluorodeoxyglucose (FDG) PET study of OCD (12). Of this group, eight were considered nondepressed OCD patients and were scanned on two distinct occasions, before treatment and while taking the tricyclic antidepressant clomipramine. Selection criteria for these patients were as follows: (i) DSM-III-R primary diagnosis of OCD, according to two staff psychiatrists (C.B. and T.E.N.) (13). Clinical evaluations were carried out separately by each investigator, during a nonstructured screening interview; if there was any disagreement on diagnosis, the patient was dismissed from the study; (ii) minimal score of 7 for the NIMH Global OC Scale (ordinal scale of severity from 1 to 15); and (iii) normal results on physical examination, electrocardiogram, chest x-ray, and laboratory tests for renal, hepatic, hematologic, and thyroid functions. Subjects with either a current axis I diagnosis of major depression or a Hamilton Depression Rating Score (HDRS-17) of over 17 were excluded from the study. The patient sample (Table 1) consisted of four men (mean age ± 29.7, SD 7.1) and four women (mean age 34.5, SD 6.1), with a mean duration of illness at time of entry into the study of 19 ± 8 years, ranging from 8 to 30 years. For all patients, onset of illness occurred in late childhood or early adolescence. Four (three men and one woman) of the eight patients had a second axis I diagnosis as follows: generalized anxiety disorder ($n = 1$), chronic dysthymia ($n = 1$), atypical depression ($n = 1$), and adjustment disorder with depressed mood ($n = 1$). None of the patients reported a personal or family history of Gilles de la Tourette's syndrome. All patients were evaluated for severity of symptoms at the time of the first scan. Behavioral ratings obtained at this time reflected the patient's mental condition in the week before the first scan.

Clomipramine Treatment

The same eight OCD patients were treated with clomipramine alone in an open trial for a minimum of 12 weeks (mean 16.1 ± 3.2 weeks) at doses ranging from 125 to 300 mg/day. All patients but one were scanned after a minimum of 12 h after ingestion of the last clomipramine dose. At the time of the scan, mean plasma levels of clomipramine and its demethylated metabolite, desmethylclomipramine, were 103 ± 43 ng/ml and 419 ± 219 ng/ml, respectively.

Behavioral Task

The auditory continuous performance task (CPT) consisted of a random series of 500-Hz tones of 1-s duration and 2-s intertone intervals, with an intensity of 67, 75, or 86 decibels, measured at the earphone–ear interface. Subjects were instructed to press the handheld response button when the lowest tone was detected. The task was presented in successive 5-min blocks for 30 min after fluorodeoxyglucose (FDG) after injection. Almost all FDG–PET scans performed at NIMH use this CPT task. To minimize the effect of learning during the scanning procedure, we trained all patients to perform 18 of 20 correct identifications of this task in the hour preceding FDG injection.

PET Scan Procedure

All subjects remained in a supine position throughout the procedure, including the transmission scan. The total duration of scan was 90 min. Subjects, with eyes patched, began their auditory discrimination task several minutes before injection of the 5-mCi dose of FDG and completed the task

TABLE 1. *Clinical and demographic profile of the eight OCD patients treated with clomipramine*

Patient	Age	Sex	History of OCD (years)	Prior treatment	Axis I codiagnosis	Baseline CPRS-8	Baseline HDRS-17	CMI (weeks)	CMI/DCMI (ng/ml)	% Change CPRS-8	CMI response[a]
1	35	F	18	ALP-IMI	GAD	12	14	16	172/815	33	PR
2	24	M	11	—	—	10	8	15	96/227	50	GR
3	26	M	8	—	Dysthymia	13	10	18	108/314	38	PR
4	40	M	30	—	PD	11	9	15	60/215	56	GR
5	42	F	30	ALP	Atypical dep.	10	7	21	146/602	20	PR
6	29	M	16	—	—	9	5	20	81/265	67	GR
7	34	F	22	DMI	—	12	5	15	42/335	33	PR
8	27	F	17	—	ADDM	14	10	13	118/582	85	GR
Mean ± SD	32 ± 6.6	4F/4M	19 ± 8			11.4 ± 1.7	8.5 ± 3	16.6 ± 2.8	103 ± 43/419 ± 219	47 ± 21	4 GR/4 PR

ADDM, adjustment disorder with depressed mood; ALP, alprazolam; CMI, clomipramine; CPRS, Comprehensive Psychiatric Rating; DMI, desipramine; DCMI, desmethylclomipramine; GAD, generalized anxiety disorder; HDRS, Hamilton Depression Rating Score; IMI, imipramine; PD, panic disorder.

[a] GR, good responder; PR, partial or poor responder.

30–35 min after injection. Subjects were than scanned for the next 30 min. Scans were performed with a Scanditronix scanner with 5- to 6-mm full-width half-maximum in plane resolution and a transverse resolution of 11 mm. A transmission scan was used to calculate attenuation. Throughout the scanning procedure, the patient's head remained stationary with the use of hexalite plastic mask, which was heated, molded to the contours of the head, and then fixed to the scanner headrest. The tracer input curve was calculated from blood samples obtained from the radial artery (usually on the right side). The scanning procedure enabled us to obtain 28 slices (four sets of seven planes each) from each subject, starting at 5 mm above the plane parallel to the canthomeatal (CM) line. The interslice interval was approximately 3.5 mm. Each PET slice had at least 10^6 coincidence counts.

Region of Interest Analysis

Raw pixel values were converted to glucose metabolic rates in SI units of μmol glucose/100 g of tissue/min (14,15). To extract regional glucose metabolic rates, we measured 60 regions of interest in five standard planes (A, 94 mm above CM line; B, 81 mm above CM line; C, 67 mm above CM line; D, 53 mm above CM line; E, 40 mm above CM line) (Fig. 1) chosen from one of the four scans run, each containing seven slices. All the data presented here are extracted from planes D and E and consist of the following 11 regions of interest (ROI) reported by Baxter et al. (8) to be abnormal in OCD: left and right anterior orbital frontal gyri, left and right posterior orbital frontal gyri, inferior medial frontal cortex, left and right anterior putamen, left and right posterior putamen, and left and right caudate nuclei. The regions of

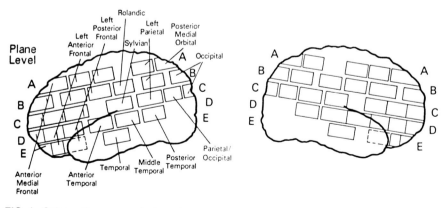

FIG. 1. Schematic representation of regions sampled in the left and right hemispheres is shown. Regions labeled as medial, although sampled from the medial portion of the cortex, are represented when possible as incomplete boxes on the lateral surface. The boxes outlined by dashed lines are sampled from the surface of the frontal cortex medial to the temporal cortex.

interest (rectangular box regions) were selected independently by two raters, blind to the identity and diagnosis of the patients they were evaluating; this was accomplished by placing the boxes through neuroanatomical matching to a standard template. This technique is similar to the ROI system analysis previously described (10,16). Anatomic structures were judged as contained within these regions according to the human brain atlas of Matsui and Hirano (17).

Metabolic rates are expressed as "global glucose metabolic rates" (estimates of the average value for glucose metabolism obtained from all the gray matter–rich areas of the brain sampled), "regional glucose metabolic rates" (average values for glucose metabolism obtained from the region of interest), and "normalized regional glucose metabolic rates" (regional metabolic rate/ global gray metabolism). The normalization procedure minimizes the effects of individual variation in global metabolism on regional metabolism and is similar in principle to the "reference ratio" or "landscape method" (18).

Statistics

All statistical comparisons of regional metabolic rates were made with normalized values. All normal controls/off-drug patient comparisons were performed with unpaired t tests. All off-drug/on-drug comparisons were performed with paired t tests. Two-tailed t tests were used exclusively except for comparisons of areas of the orbital frontal (E plane) and the basal ganglia, previously reported to be increased in untreated OCD patients. As we hypothesized that differences in glucose metabolism were state related, we expected that clomipramine would reduce glucose metabolic rates in these brain areas. Therefore, we performed one-tailed t tests for these regions of interest (left and right, anterior and posterior orbital frontal gyri; left and right caudate nuclei) in these two brain areas. We also elected to compare local cerebral glucose metabolism (LCGM) rates between normal controls ($n = 30$) and clomipramine-treated OCD patients, for the regions whose LCGM rates in untreated OCD patients differed from those of normal controls.

Correlations between scores obtained on the NIMH-OC and CPRS8-OC scales and LCGMR in the orbital frontal cortex and basal ganglia structures in unmedicated OCD patients were determined with the Spearman rank correlation, as these rating scales are not truly parametric. Correlations between clinical and metabolic changes during clomipramine treatment were also determined by nonparametric methods (Spearman rank correlation).

RESULTS

Clinical Severity Before and During Clomipramine Treatment

Most patients were rated in the moderate to moderately severe range for OC symptoms and did not exhibit signs of major depression. Before clomipramine treatment, mean behavioral rating scores were as follows (Table 1): total Maudsley inventory score 20.1 ± 5.0; NIMH Global OC score 8.9 ± 1.0; Comprehensive Psychiatric Rating Scale OC subscore (CPRS-OC 8) (19) 11.4 ± 1.7 HDRS-17 8.5 ± 3.0; Beck Depression Inventory (BDI) 9.7 ± 3.0; Spielberger Anxiety State Score (SASS) 45.9 ± 9.3.

As expected, paired comparisons of mean scores for all measures of OC symptoms showed that patient OC symptoms improved on clomipramine: CPRS-OC (off, 11.4 ± 1.7; on, 5.9 ± 2.5; $t = 5.31, p < 0.001$); NIMH-OC (off, 26.9 ± 3.7; on, 12.4 ± 5.8; $t = 7.48, p < 0.00001$); and NIMH-Global OC (off, 8.9 ± 1; on, 5 ± 1.5; $t = 6.67, p < 0.0003$).

The degree of clinical change in OC symptoms, based on a percentage change from baseline for the CPRS-OC and the NIMH-OC scores, varied from 20–85% (47.8 ± 21.1%) and 26–83% (54.1 ± 19.7%), respectively. Using a cutoff of 50% or greater improvement on CPRS-OC subscores, four patients were considered good responders, three patients considered partial responders (33–38% change), and one patient considered a poor responder (<30%). Comparisons between the plasma levels of clomipramine and desmethylclomipramine in these two subgroups (responders vs. partial or poor responders) did not yield significant differences, although poor or partial responders to clomipramine tended to have higher drug levels (clomipramine, 117 ± 56 vs. 89 ± 24; desmethylclomipramine, 516 ± 238 vs. 322 ± 174).

Comparisons of Normalized Local Cerebral Glucose Metabolism Between Unmedicated OCD Patients and Healthy Volunteers

Table 2 presents comparisons of normalized local glucose metabolic rates between unmedicated OCD patients ($n = 8$) and healthy volunteers ($n = 30$) of the orbital frontal cortex and some basal ganglion structures. Significantly higher metabolic rates in OCD patients were found at the level of the inferomedial frontal cortex ($p = 0.05$) and the right anterior ($p = 0.02$) and posterior orbital frontal cortex ($p = 0.04$). In addition, OCD patients exhibited significantly higher metabolic rates in the left caudate nucleus ($p = 0.03$) and the left anterior ($p = 0.04$) and posterior putamen ($p = 0.01$) than those obtained in normal controls.

Clinical–Metabolic Correlations in Untreated OCD Patients

We examined six correlations between scores of severity of OC symptoms (CPRS8-OC) and LCGMR collected in those brain regions which distinguished OCD patients from normal controls (inferomedial frontal cortex, right anterior and posterior orbital frontal cortex, left caudate nucleus, left anterior and posterior putamen): of the six correlations computed, only one

TABLE 2. Paired comparison of the means (± SD) for normalized local cerebral glucose metabolism in basal ganglia and orbital frontal cortex in eight OCD patients off and on clomipramine (one-tailed except for putamen)

	Normal controls (1) (n = 30)	OCD patients off CMI (2) (n = 8)	OCD patients on CMI (3) (n = 8)	% Change[a]	p value (1) vs. (2)	p value (2) vs. (3)
Frontal cortex						
Inferior medial	0.903 ± 0.06	0.953 ± 0.066	0.901 ± 0.063	−5.50	0.05*	0.045*
Left posterior	0.911 ± 0.08	0.945 ± 0.050	0.941 ± 0.058	0.00	0.24	NS
Right posterior	0.924 ± 0.105	1.011 ± 0.085	0.971 ± 0.046	−4.10	0.04*	0.15
Left anterior	0.867 ± 0.095	0.916 ± 0.085	0.906 ± 0.071	−1.00	0.20	NS
Right anterior	0.917 ± 0.086	1.007 ± 0.101	0.944 ± 0.088	−6.30	0.02*	0.057
Basal ganglia						
Left caudate nucleus	1.021 ± 0.107	1.123 ± 0.133	1.050 ± 0.104	−6.90	0.03*	0.01**
Right caudate nucleus	0.972 ± 0.110	1.048 ± 0.118	1.079 ± 0.165	3.30	0.10	NS
Left anterior putamen	1.060 ± 0.114	1.178 ± 0.223	1.182 ± 0.160	0.00	0.04*	NS
Right anterior putamen	1.005 ± 0.098	1.151 ± 0.185	1.202 ± 0.181	4.60	0.29	0.013**
Left posterior putamen	0.989 ± 0.100	1.123 ± 0.172	1.146 ± 0.191	2.10	0.01**	NS
Right posterior putamen	0.989 ± 0.079	1.073 ± 0.208	1.127 ± 0.105	7.10	0.08	NS

[a] Percent change and p values are for comparisons of OCD patients on vs. off clomipramine (CMI).
* $p < 0.05$; ** $p < 0.01$, NS, not significant.

was significant, at the level of the left posterior putamen ($n = 8$; ρ corrected for ties $= 0.779$, $p < 0.05$).

Effect of Clomipramine on Normalized Local Cerebral Glucose Metabolism

Changes in LCGM during treatment with clomipramine occurred predominantly in regions of the basal ganglia and the orbital frontal cortex (E plane) (Table 2). The LCGM decreased significantly in the left caudate (6.9%; $t = 2.99$, $p < 0.01$, one-tailed) and increased in the right anterior putamen (4.6%; $t = -1.65$, $p = 0.013$, two tailed). In addition, clomipramine decreased LCGM in three of the five orbital frontal areas (E plane): medial frontal cortex (5.5%; $t = 1.97$; $p = 0.045$), right posterior (4.1%; $t = 1.10$, $p < 0.16$, one-tailed, NS) and right anterior (6.3%; $t = 1.81$, $p < 0.06$, one-tailed) orbital frontal cortex.

Because OCD patients off medication had higher glucose metabolic rates in the orbital frontal cortex and parts of the basal ganglia as compared with normal controls, we decided to compare glucose metabolic rates of these patients on clomipramine again with the same set of normal volunteers. In this follow-up study, we found that none of the previously reported differences between untreated OCD patients and normal controls were present after clomipramine treatment.

Correlations With Clinical Change

Examination of the anatomic localization of drug effects included attempts to correlate changes in glucose metabolism and changes in OC symptoms. However, because type I and type II errors can occur with statistical evaluation of multiple correlations in small sample sizes, the correlation findings presented here should be interpreted with caution, despite our efforts to diminish these errors.

To reduce the risk of type II errors, we looked for possible correlations between the degree of clinical change in OC symptoms (% change CPRS8-OC) and changes in glucose metabolism only in the specific regions of interest where LCGM changes were found in patients on clomipramine (inferomedial frontal cortex, right anterior orbital frontal cortex, left caudate nucleus, right anterior putamen).

Clinical and metabolic changes correlated significantly only in one brain region, the left caudate nucleus, where a decrease in OC symptoms was associated with a reduction in glucose metabolic consumption ($n = 8$; $\rho = 0.776$, $p < 0.05$).

Glucose Metabolic Comparisons Between Clomipramine Responders and Partial or Poor Responders

As expected, OCD patients who responded well to clomipramine had significant differences in their mean percentage change in CPRS-OC scores as compared with partial or poor responders (63.7 ± 15 vs. 31 ± 7; $p < 0.01$). When both groups were compared (responders vs. partial or poor responders), we found that the percentage of change from baseline [(off-on/off)/100] in LCGM differed in certain brain regions. In particular, patients on clomipramine who responded well to the drug had a greater decrease in LCGM in the caudate nucleus as compared with partial or poor responders. This difference was significant on the left ($10.9 \pm 5\%$ vs. $2.1 \pm 3.6\%$; $p < 0.01$) with a similar trend on the right ($7.4 \pm 18.6\%$ vs. $-0.07 \pm 8.7\%$; NS).

DISCUSSION

Increased LCGMR in the OFC and Basal Ganglia in OCD

The results of this study are consistent with those obtained by Baxter et al. in two independent samples of depressed (8) and nondepressed OCD patients (20). We report here an increased rate of glucose metabolism in the right and medial orbital frontal cortex and in part of the basal ganglion in OCD patients, as compared with normal controls. Since publication of these findings, several other groups have reported brain structural and/or functional alterations in untreated OCD patients with MRI (21,22), single photon emission computed tomography (SPECT) (22) and PET (23), most of which point to the role of the orbital/prefrontal cortex and basal ganglion regions in mediating OC symptoms. Except for the report of Martinot et al. (24), all FDG-PET studies in OCD were associated with a hypermetabolic pattern in those areas.

Hypermetabolism in the Orbital Frontal Cortex: A Functional Representation in Brain of the Resistance to the Surge of Obsessional Ideation

Hypermetabolism in the orbital/prefrontal cortex and/or basal ganglion regions could represent either (i) a functional state or trait-dependent index of neural activation underlying the production of OC symptoms, (ii) a brain correlate of nonspecific behavioral events (e.g., fear, worries, ruminations), occurring during the uptake in brain of FDG, or (iii) a functional representation in the brain of the attempt made by patients to suppress/resist the overwhelming flow of OC symptoms.

Despite the small sample size of the study, the fact that neither the CPRS-OC nor the NIMH-OC scores correlated with the glucose metabolic rates in the orbital frontal cortex in our study, as in Baxter et al. (8) and Swedo et al. (23), argues against the interpretation that the OFC might represent a neural substrate for the production of obsessions. Rather, a careful examination suggests that active resistance best characterized most patients' subjective experience while lying under the PET camera: When successful, it enabled them to suppress the surge in obsessional concerns and keep their distress under control, ensuring smooth scanning. This was often the case for patients with fears of contamination (washers), who were more likely "concerned," tensed, and preoccupied by the various manipulations they were subjected to (e.g., insertion of venous and arterial catheters, touching of their face and hair for molding the head mask) to prepare them for scanning. Because of restraint, patients were prevented from carrying out their usual compulsive behaviors, resulting for some in increased distress. Although they appeared to tolerate the procedure well, they admitted later having to actively resist the urge of discontinuing scanning in order to complete their decontaminating rituals. A notable increase in the time spent in the bathroom at the end of the scan for performing these washing rituals reflected their past level of distress and resistance during scanning.

The interpretation that an overactive orbital frontal cortex might serve as the neural substrate for suppressing unwanted interference agrees well with the current theory that the prefrontal cortex plays a major role, through the display of inhibitory influences, on various limbic-based basic drives (e.g., aggression). For Fuster (25), a cardinal function of the prefrontal cortex consists of integrating motor acts in an orderly way, in accord with preestablished cognitive schemes; this is made operative under the control of three major subordinate functions, among them the ability of the prefrontal cortex to control interference. In carnivores and humans, but not in primates, this function seems to be based primarily in the orbital frontal cortex. In the cat, lesions of the orbital frontal cortex lower the threshold for aggressive behaviors elicited by the electrical stimulation of the hypothalamus (cited in 25, 26). Conversely, the electrical stimulation of the prefrontal cortex blocks attack behavior (cited in 25, 27). In humans, orbital frontal cortex lesions result in "the patient showing a failure to suppress a variety of internal representation, as well as impulses of motor and instinctual nature" (cited in 25–30). A hyperactive orbital frontal cortex could well represent a neural basis for the active resistance displayed by OCD patients when confronted with the surge of unwanted obsessional thoughts or motor compulsions encountered during the scanning situation.

Clomipramine Treatment Results in a Reduction of the OFC Glucose Metabolism

In this study, long-term clomipramine treatment of OCD patients resulted in various degrees of improvement in OCD symptoms, as well as regional changes in cerebral glucose metabolism. LCGM decreased in three of the five orbital frontal regions examined in our analysis [medial, right anterior and postorbital frontal cortex (E plane), and left caudate]. These changes, together with the findings that patients receiving clomipramine no longer differed from normal controls in their glucose metabolic rates in the orbital frontal cortex and the left caudate nucleus, support the hypothesis that the high glucose metabolic rates found in some untreated OCD patients may be partially reversible with drug treatment. Notably, some patients who responded well to clomipramine had more pronounced changes in the caudate nucleus than others who did not respond well to the drug, suggesting that changes in glucose metabolism in areas such as the caudate nucleus may be necessary for a positive drug response.

The clomipramine-induced reduction in the orbital frontal cortex metabolism, although of limited magnitude, may be directly related to the relative antiobsessional properties of the drug or may be a corollary of a less effortful, less distressful, more efficient "resistance." The latter interpretation would be in agreement with a broader view suggesting that an overactive orbital frontal cortex might not be specific for OCD per se but rather is a common feature of various stress-related conditions, all of which are characterized by the patient's inability to control/suppress unpleasant emotions, images, and/or cognitions, which could become rapidly overwhelming. This handicap is epitomized in true OCD patients but is also reported by other affective and anxiety disorder patients to a lesser degree. A recent report of a positive correlation in normal controls between an index of neuroticism (using the Eysenck personality inventory) and the orbital frontal cortex (OFC) metabolism (31) supports this view. At the other end of the clinical spectrum, it is notable that patients with personality disorders characterized by an inability to exercise impulse control tend to exhibit a lower OFC glucose metabolism (32).

A Neuroanatomic Model of OCD

"Ritualistic" behaviors include both a motor component and an associated ideational set. OCD patients are distinguished from patients with other anxiety disorders by their overwhelming and complex pattern of internal cognitive stimuli. Despite some elegant hypotheses, it is not yet known whether the ideation associated with OCD can help patients resist undesired motor impulses or intrusive thoughts, or whether these impulses are themselves recurrent "bursts" of intrusive thoughts.

To a large degree, investigators who evaluate PET data or the effects of anatomic lesions on behavior to identify anatomic loci associated with OCD are faced with similar ambiguities. These studies are unable to distinguish brain structures that are the sources(s) of the ideational and/or motor intrusions that prevent OCD patients from participating in a normal cognitive and behavioral life from brain structures that adapt in either fruitful or nonproductive manners in response to these intrusions.

Because considerable evidence already exists that the orbital frontal cortex and the basal ganglia (OFC–basal ganglia loop) (33,34) are involved in the expression of OCD (for review, see 35), one might postulate that affecting transmission through this neuroanatomic loop would also affect OC symptoms.

Indeed, the efficacy of psychosurgery in refractory OCD appears to be related to the lesioning of part of the orbital frontal cortex and/or disconnecting the orbital and medial frontal cortex from its limbic and/or subcortical connections (cingulotomy–stereotactic limbic leukotomy–bifrontal tractotomy) (for review see 36). In a preliminary study of LCGMRs measured with PET in refractory OCD patients undergoing capsulotomy, Mindus et al. (37) reported a postoperative reduction in the OFC metabolism in patients who responded well to surgery. Furthermore, as reviewed above, PET findings show an apparent abnormality in the orbital frontal cortex, and a change in the functioning of this region and the basal ganglia during treatment with clomipramine, perhaps the most effective and selective drug treatment for OCD. Although the role of clomipramine is not fully understood, it is conceivable that clomipramine merely resets the cortex–basal ganglia–thalamus loop which appears to be critical in determining OCD-related behaviors.

REFERENCES

1. Esquirol E. *Des maladies mentales considerées sous les rapports médicales, hygiénique et médico-légal.* Paris: Bailliere, 1838.
2. Westphal K. Ueber Zwangsvorstellungen. *Arch Psychiatr Nervenkr* 1878;8:734–50.
3. Kettl PA, Marks IM. Neurological factors in obsessive compulsive disorder: two case reports and a review of the literature. *Br J Psychiatry* 1986;149:315–9.
4. Laplane D, Widlocher D, Pillon B, Baulac M, Binoux F. Comportement compulsif d'allure obsessionnelle par nécrose circonscrite bilaterale pallido-striatale. *Rev Neurol* 1981;137: 269–76.
5. Laplane D, Dubois B, Pillon B, Baulac M. Perte d'autoactivation psychique et activite mentale stereotypée par lesion frontale: rapports avec le trouble obsessif compulsif. *Rev Neurol* 1988;144:564–70.
6. Tomkonogy J, Barreira P. Obsessive compulsive disorder and caudate-frontal lesions. *Neuropsychiatr Neuropsychol Behav Neurol* 1989;2:203–9.
7. Laplane D, Levasseur M, Pillon B, et al. Obsessive compulsive and other behavioral changes with bilateral basal ganglia lesions. *Brain* 1989;112:699–725.
8. Baxter LR, Phelps ME, Mazziotta JC, Guze BH, Schwartz JM, Selin CE. Local cerebral glucose metabolic rates in obsessive-compulsive disorder: a comparsion with rates in unipolar depression and normal controls. *Arch Gen Psychiatry* 1987;44:211–8.
9. Buchsbaum MS, De Lisi LE, Holcomb HH, et al. Anteroposterior gradients in cerebral glucose use in schizophrenia and affective disorders. *Arch Gen Psychiatry* 1984;41:1159–66.
10. Cohen RM, Semple WE, Gross M, et al. Dysfunction in a prefrontal substrate of sustained attention in schizophrenia. *Life Sci* 1987;40:2031–9.
11. Baxter LR, Schwartz JM, Phelps ME, et al. Reduction of prefrontal cortex glucose metabolism common to three types of depression. *Arch Gen Psychiatry* 1989;46:243–50.

12. Nordahl TE, Benkelfat C, Semple WE, Uhde TW, Cohen RM. *Metabolic rates in OCD: comparison with panic disorder*. Presented at the American Psychiatric Association, San Francisco, CA, May 6–11, 1989.
13. American Psychiatric Association. *Diagnostic and statistical manual of mental disorders, 3rd ed, revised*. Washington, DC: American Psychiatric Association, 1987.
14. Sokoloff L, Reivich M, Kennedy C, et al. The (14C) deoxyglucose method for the measurement of local cerebral glucose utilization: theory, procedure, and normal values in the conscious and anesthetized albino rat. *J Neurochem* 1977;28:897–916.
15. Brooks RA. Alternative formula for glucose utilization using labeled deoxy glucose. *J Nucl Med* 1982;23:538–9.
16. Clark C, Carson R, Kessler R, et al. Alternative statistical models for the examination of clinical positron emission tomography/fluorodeoxyglucose data. *J Cereb Blood Flow Metab* 1985;5:142–50.
17. Matsui T, Hirano A. *An atlas of the human brain for computerized tomography*. New York: Igaku-Shoin, 1978.
18. Phelps ME, Mazziotta JC, Kuhl DE, et al. Tomographic mapping of human cerebral metabolism: visual stimulation and deprivation. *Neurology* 1981;31:517–29.
19. Asberg M, Montgomery SA, Perris C, Schalling D, Sedvall G. A comprehensive psychopathological rating scale. *Acta Psychiatr Scand Suppl* 1978;271:5–27.
20. Baxter LR, Schwartz JM, Mazziotta JC, et al. Cerebral glucose metabolic rates in nondepressed patients with obsessive-compulsive disorder. *Am J Psychiatry* 1988;145:1560–3.
21. Garber HJ, Ananth JB, Chiu LC, Griswold VJ, Oldendorf WH. Nuclear magnetic resonsance study of obsessive-compulsive disorder. *Am J Psychiatry* 1989;146:1001–5.
22. Machlin SR, Harris GJ, Pearlson GD, Hoehn–Saric R, Camargo EE, Links JM. *SPECT and MRI in obsessive compulsive disorder*. 143rd APA Annual Meeting, New York: NR, 1990:173.
23. Swedo SE, Schapiro MB, Grady CL, et al. Cerebral glucose metabolism in childhood-onset obsessive compulsive disorder. *Arch Gen Psychiatry* 1989;46:518–23.
24. Martinot JL, Allilaire JF, Mazoyer BM, et al. Obsessive compulsive disorder: a clinical, neuropsychological and positron emission tomography study. *Acta Psychiatr Scand* 1990; 8:233–42.
25. Fuster JM. *The prefrontal cortex: anatomy, physiology, and neuropsychology of the frontal lobe*. New York: Raven Press, 1989.
26. Sato M, Onishi T, Otsuki S. Integrating functions of the prefrontal cortex on emotional behaviors. *Folia Psychiatr Neurol Jpn* 1971;25:283–93.
27. Siegel A, Edinger H, Koo A. Suppression of attack behavior in the cat by the prefrontal cortex: role of the mediodorsal thalamic nucleus. *Brain Res* 1977;127:185–90.
28. Meyer A, McLardy T. Posterior cuts in prefrontal leucotomy: a clinico-pathological study. *J Ment Sci* 1948;94:555–64.
29. Fulton JF. *Frontal lobotomy and affective behavior*. New York: Norton, 1951.
30. Stuss DT, Kaplan EF, Benson DF, Weir WS, Chiulli S, Sarazin FF. Evidence for the involvement of the orbito frontal cortex in memory function: an interference effect. *J Comp Physiol Psychol* 1982;96:913–25.
31. Semple WE, Cohen RM, Foer J, et al. Orbital frontal cortex metabolism and personality in normal results from two PET studies. *Biol Psychiatry* 1991;29:174.
32. Goyer PF, Andreassen PJ, Semple WE, et al. PET and personality disorders. *Biol Psychiatry* 1991;29:94.
33. Alexander GE, De Long MR, Strick PL. Parallel organization of functionally segregated circuits linking basal ganglia and cortex. *Annu Rev Neurosci* 1986;9:357–81.
34. Goldman–Rakic P, Selemon LD. Topography of corticostriatal projections in nonhuman primates and implications for functional parcellation of the neostriatum. In: Peters A, Jones EG, eds. *Cerebral cortex*. New York: Plenum Press, 1986;447:66.
35. Modell JG, Mountz JM, Curtis GC, Greden JF. Neurophysiologic dysfunction in basal ganglia/limbic striatal and thalamocortical circuits as a pathogenetic mechanism of obsessive compulsive disorder. *J Neuropsychiatry* 1989;1:27–36.
36. Marks IM. Obsessive compulsive disorder. In: Marks IM, ed. *Fears, phobias and rituals*. New York: Oxford University Press, 1987;423–53.
37. Mindus P, Nyman H, Mogard J, Meyerson BA, Ericson K. Frontal lobe and basal ganglia metabolism studied with PET in patients with incapacitating obsessive-compulsive disorder undergoing capsulotomy. *Nord Psykiatr Tidsskr* 1990;44:309–12.

Psychiatry and Advanced Technologies,
edited by L. Ravizza, F. Bogetto, and
E. Zanalda. Raven Press, Ltd.,
New York © 1993.

10

Spectroscopy: An Overview of Current and Future Applications in Neurology

Brian D. Ross

Huntington Medical Research Institutes, Pasadena, California 91105

Magnetic resonance (MR) techniques are now ubiquitous in medicine. Despite the great expense of the highly homogeneous magnets and the difficulty of operating them in a clinical environment, almost 3,000 whole-body imagers are installed in the United States. Possibly one-third of those are of a field strength of 1.5 tesla or more and potentially available for clinical spectroscopy, in addition to an ever-increasing array of magnetic resonance imaging (MRI) techniques. The temptation to apply MRI and MR spectroscopy (MRS) to the elucidation of intractable problems in neurology is overwhelming, and the capabilities of the technique are entirely appropriate.

MRI AND MRS IN NEUROLOGIC DISEASE

Figure 1 is a stylized "disease" as it might affect the brain. Etiology, progress, prognosis, and therapy might equally well be the subjects of study. In the category of etiology (the other components of the disease will not be discussed) are listed many of the suspected mechanisms of disease. On either side are the possible points of impact of MR technology at present available or under development. In the following discussion an illustration of each of these major points is presented, emphasizing spectroscopy methods.

Blood Flow and Substrate Delivery

MR angiography is now a well-established noninvasive technique, and together with diffusion/perfusion measurements, provides new insights into the flow of blood (and oxygen). However, metabolism, the key target of reduction in either method, can be detected only with MRS. Studies in neonates after hemorrhagic brain damage amply illustrate the point (1). ^{31}P-MRS

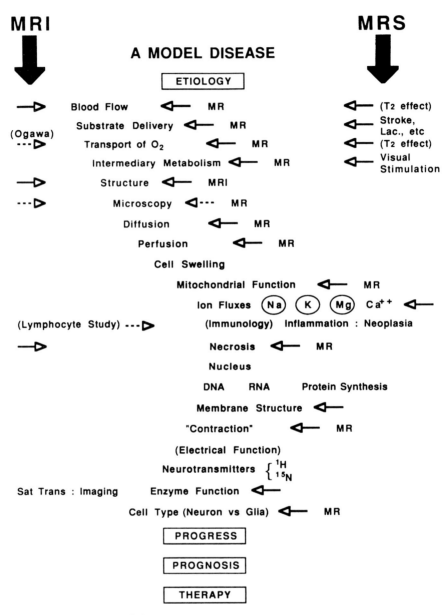

FIG. 1. A model of neurologic disease.

has proved equally interesting in adult stroke (this volume). However, it is probable that high resolution ^{1}H (proton)-MRS will prove even more valuable by virtue of its ability to monitor not only neuron loss (see below) but accumulation of lactate. Perfusion/metabolism disequilibrium might be a useful description of the recovering brain after stroke (Fig. 2).

Intermediary Metabolism

The range of metabolites, and hence the number of neurobiochemical pathways that can be directly observed by ^{31}P- or ^{1}H-MRS is strictly limited. Nevertheless, carefully planned clinical MRS studies can reveal disease processes by inference and may increasingly do so in the future. Thus, the amino acids alanine, phenylalanine, glutamate, and glutamine (2) can be directly observed in human brain by ^{1}H-MRS; accumulation of organic acids can be followed by pH determinations with ^{31}P-MRS.

Functional Stimulation

The ability of positron emission tomography (PET) to monitor and map significant metabolic responses to visual and other stimuli is fast being emulated by MRS techniques. In principle, the information is complementary but may be crucially different if PCr and ATP synthesis turn out to be equally or more relevant than glycolysis to neuronal function (Fig. 3). Associated with this approach is the ability of MRS to provide necessary spatial and temporal information about metabolism in a tissue as well organized as the brain. Thus, MR metabolite maps of the brain can now readily be generated in 30 min or less for each of the major metabolites of the spectrum: NAA, lactate, choline, creatine, phosphocreatine (see below), and creatine kinase flux.

Mitochondrial Function

Mitochondrial myopathy, in which one of the earliest successful ^{31}P-MRS studies was performed (3), has its counterpart in mitochondrial disorders of the brain (4). This is probably a rare hereditary disease, but mitochondrial dysfunction might also be acquired, for example, in hepatic encephalopathy (5) or Reye's syndrome. Either condition might usefully be examined by ^{31}P-MRS.

Ion Fluxes

MRS in vivo may have little to offer at present in this important area, although Na$^+$ imaging is well established. In in vitro and in functioning tissue

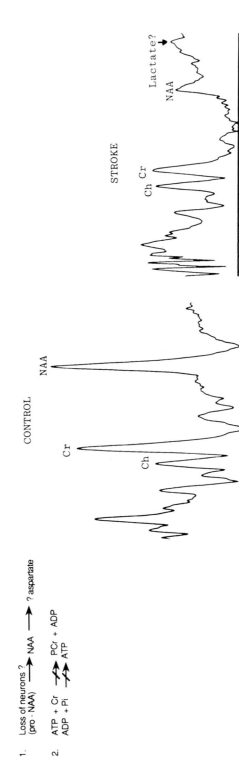

FIG. 2. Blood flow, oxygen and substrate delivery: Mechanism of "stroke." Proton spectra courtesy of Dr. Roland Kreis and Neil Farrow, Huntington Medical Research Institutes (HMRI). **Left:** Normal hemisphere; **right:** stroke region after 6 weeks, showing loss of NAA, Cr + PCr, and possibly minimal lactate accumulation.

Lactate: Glucose + ATP ⟶ G-6-P ⟶ Lactate | Rate

5

(ATP) ADP + Pi ⟶ ATP | 1

PCr Cr + ATP ⟶ PCr | 10

Creatine kinase

~ 10 x ox phos;

~ 2 x glycolysis

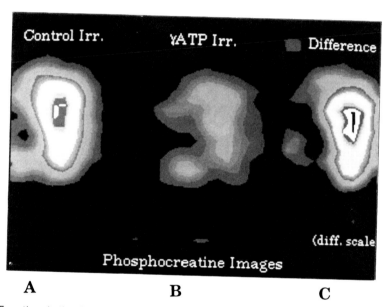

A   **B**   **C**

FIG. 3. Functional stimulation: the three sources of energy from metabolism. Images acquired by ^{31}P MRS in macaque brain. **A:** PCr map. **B:** Residual PCr mapped during γ-ATP irradiation. Result is suppression of PCr in proportion to CPK flux. (Reproduced courtesy of Dr. Bassem Mora and P.T. Narasimhan, HMRI.)

preparations, ^{19}F-MR is a valuable tool for Ca^{2+} determination, and Rb^+-MR has been developed to clarify potassium fluxes.

Immune Disease

MRS in AIDS dementia is extensively discussed in this volume. Direct monitoring of lymphocyte metabolism within the brain has thus far proved beyond the capability of MRS, but in in vitro cultures of lymphocytes their response to interleukin-2 and PHA can readily be assayed by ^{31}P- or ^{1}H-MRS (Fig. 4) (6).

Neurotransmitters

The key to success of a novel technique in neurochemistry might reside in its ability to detect and measure even a few of the myriad neurotransmitter substances under discussion in disease states. This is a difficult task for MRS, for which the lower limit of sensitivity may be 10^{-4} M. Nevertheless, some progress can be anticipated in determining the components listed in Fig. 5 with ^{1}H- or ^{15}N-MRS (7).

Enzyme Function

This broad area of disease is well within the scope of modern methods of in vivo ^{31}P- and ^{1}H-MRS. A particularly valuable technique is magnetization transfer, in which flux through an enzyme (in contrast to the more usual output of MRS, which is steady-state concentration of the substrate or product of the enzyme) is determined. Changes in creatine kinase flux, for example, may prove to be important in neurophysiology (Fig. 3) or neuropathology. Saturation transfer imaging is now feasible for ^{31}P and for water protons (i.e., standard MRI!).

Cell Type

Whether MRS can resolve cell type in the brain is very doubtful, but at least one metabolite in the ^{1}H-MRS spectrum, i.e., N-acetyl aspartate (NAA), is almost certainly confined to neurons. It may therefore be a "neuronal marker."

Conversely, ^{15}N-MRS shows that $^{15}NH_4^+$ rapidly enters $^{15}\gamma$-N-glutamine in intact brain (8). Because the sole enzyme capable of performing this synthesis (glutamine synthetase) is confined to the astrocyte, ^{15}N-MRS may also be capable of defining cell type in an indirect assay.

CONCLUSIONS

MR is a relatively new tool in medicine. Like chemistry before it, there is almost no aspect of disease to which MR cannot be applied. MRI and MRS techniques are evolving rapidly. Some are very demanding of equipment and expertise, whereas others (e.g., ^{15}N) are currently effective only in vitro. In neurology, noninvasive diagnosis with MRS (^{31}P or ^{1}H) is well advanced,

Lymphocyte — cell interaction		31P	1H		
Biological response modifiers					
interleukins		31P	1H		
INFLAMMATION	31P				
NEOPLASIA	31P	1H	13C	15N	

HUMAN LYMPHOCYTES

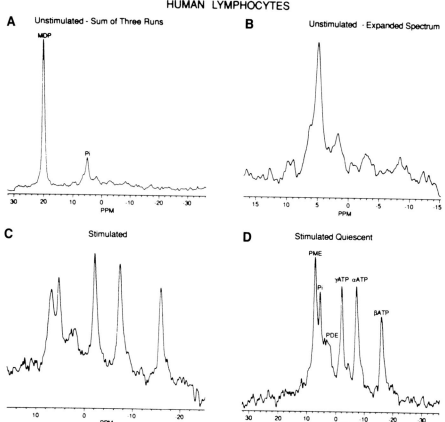

FIG. 4. Immune disease. ^{31}P-MR spectra of human peripheral blood lymphocytes encapsulated in alginate gels and perfused with phosphate-free medium containing IL-2 (50° flip angle; 300 ms interpulse delay). **A:** Nonstimulated lymphocytes: spectrum is a total of 448,000 acquisitions obtained by addition of three preparations. Methylene diphosphonate (MDP) capillary was used as a chemical shift standard and for quantitation. Total number of lymphocytes was 774 × 10⁶. **B:** Expanded spectrum of nonstimulated lymphocytes: additional resonances for ATP, PDE, and PME can be observed. **C:** Stimulated lymphocytes: spectrum is sum of 160,000 acquisitions for 32 × 10⁶ lymphocytes. The spectrum shows AJP, PME, and PDE in much increased concentration. **D:** Stimulated "quiescent" lymphocytes. Cells (1,050 × 10⁶) were allowed to divide in culture until they achieved a quiescent state. Spectrum is the addition of 64,000 acquisitions. Reproduced from ref. 6.

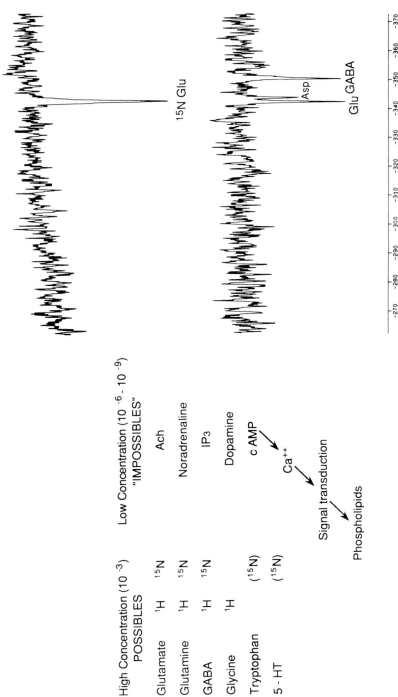

FIG. 5. Neurotransmitters that might be assayed: ^{15}N spectra of rat brain enriched with α-^{15}N-glutamate. After intraventricular injection, ^{15}N label appeared in aspartate and GABA. The ^{15}N spectra were acquired from ex vivo brain tissue by Dr. Keiko Kanamori, HMRI.

and ^{13}C-MRS and sodium imaging are established as research techniques. Application of MRS to psychiatric diagnosis and therapeutic monitoring has thus far utilized only a fraction of the available techniques.

Note added in proof: A novel diagnosis in Alzheimer's disease demonstrates application of ^{1}H MRS. Patients show significantly elevated *myo*-inositol and reduced *N*-acetyl asparate compared to matched controls. Together, these changes appear to be specific for early Alzheimer's disease (9).

ACKNOWLEDGMENT

Work cited in this brief review was performed in collaboration with colleagues in Oxford, Hammersmith, South San Francisco, Huntington Medical Research Institutes, and the California Institute of Technology, Pasadena. Clinical MRS was supported by a grant from the Whittier Foundation of California and ^{15}N-MRS studies by the Norris Foundation. The ^{1}H spectra for Fig. 2 were obtained by Dr. Roland Kreis and Neil Farrow.

REFERENCES

1. Cady E, Dawson M, Hope P, et al. Non-invasive investigation of cerebral metabolism in newborn infants by phosphorus nuclear magnetic resonance spectroscopy. *Lancet* 1983;1: 1059–62.
2. Ross BD, ed. Proton spectroscopy in clinical medicine (mini-categorical course proceedings of the Society of Magnetic Resonance in Medicine, 1990). *NMR Biomed* 1991;4:47–116.
3. Radda GK, Bore PJ, Gadian DG, et al. ^{31}P NMR examination of two patients with NADH-CoQ reductase deficiency. *Nature* 1982;295:608–9.
4. Eleff S, Barker P, Blackband S, et al. Phosphorus magnetic resonance spectroscopy of patients with mitochondrial encephalomyopathies. *Soc Magnet Reson Med* 1989;1:451.
5. Ross B, Tropp J, Roberts J, Bass N, Hawryszko C, Derby K. [31]P spectroscopic imaging of the brain shows energy deficit of thalamus in chronic hepatic encephalopathy [Abstract]. *Soc Magnet Reson Med* 1989;1:465.
6. Shankar Narayan K, Freeman D, Moress E, Ingram M, Ross B. Lymphocyte metabolism and cytotoxic activity monitored with ^{31}P magnetic resonance spectroscopy. *J Biol Response Mod* 1990;9:241–246.
7. Farrow NA, Kanamori K, Ross BD, Parivar F. An N-15 NMR study of cerebral, hepatic and renal nitrogen metabolism in hyperammonemic rats. *Biochem J* 1990;270:473–81.
8. Kanamori K, Ross BD, Farrow NA, Parivar F. An N-15 NMR study of isolated brain in portacaval shunted rats after acute hyperammonemia. *Biochim Biophys Acta* 1991;1096: 270–6.
9. Miller BL, Moats R, Shonk T, Ernst T, Woolley S, Ross BD. *In vivo* abnormalities of cerebral *myo*-inositol and N-acetyl residues in Alzheimer disease [Abstract]. *Soc Magn Reson Med* 1992;WIP:760.

Psychiatry and Advanced Technologies,
edited by L. Ravizza, F. Bogetto, and
E. Zanalda. Raven Press, Ltd.,
New York © 1993.

11

Recent Progress in Spectroscopic Imaging

M. Paley, D. Lampman, J. Murdoch, J. McNally, and *B. Miller

*NMR Advanced Technology Group, Picker International, Inc., Cleveland, Ohio 44143; and *MRI Center, Harbor-UCLA Medical Center, Torrance, California 90509*

Magnetic resonance (MR) imaging has become a powerful tool for the investigation of a wide range of pathological conditions in many parts of the human body. Most of the MR signal from the body is from water molecules, which are relatively free to move. However, much weaker signals also can be detected from other molecular constituents, such as methyl and methine groups. The signals received are at characteristic frequencies dispersed from the water signal, which allows identification with particular molecules through spectral analysis.

The strength of the signal received is related (in a somewhat complicated way) to the concentration of the molecular species present. By comparison with in vitro assays and animal studies, the major MR-observable biochemical species in the human brain have been identified and published, together with their approximate concentrations. These include *N*-acetyl aspartate (a neuronal marker), choline- and creatine-containing compounds and, in certain cases, lactate.

Recently, studies have been extended to investigation of a range of disease processes including tumors, response to therapies, and neurologic disorders. Technical problems that have been overcome to allow these advances include suppression of the abundant water signal, which is four orders of magnitude stronger than the metabolites of interest, and improvements in system sensitivity to allow relatively high spatial resolution (typically 10 mm in plane) to be achieved. The ability to acquire data from multiple locations in a single study has also improved the efficiency of in vivo studies and allowed the spatial distribution of metabolites to be examined (1–10).

THE MESA-3D TECHNIQUE

The specific technique used in the present study is the MESA-3D spectro-scopic imaging sequence. This is a multiple spin–echo method in which magnetic field gradients are applied along three orthogonal axes for successive echoes. This localizes the signal to a region of the brain, previously identified on a normal proton image, located to exclude lipid signal from the scalp. The initial radio frequency excitation pulse is specially designed to stimulate only the frequencies corresponding to the molecules of interest and not water.

To generate spatial maps, multiple repetitions of the pulse sequence are applied with incremental magnetic field gradients, known as phase-encoding gradients. Typically 8×8 or 16×16 voxels are acquired over a time ranging from 15 to 40 min. The maps are reconstructed by applying three successive Fourier transformations, the first being a time-frequency transform and the second pair being spatial transforms. Filtering of the data allows the signal-to-noise ratio to be optimized.

It is possible to form multiple metabolite maps from one acquisition. The height, area or ratios of the different biochemical species can be used to form metabolic images.

Each of the lines in the acquired spectra has unique time constants for signal decay (T2) and recovery to equilibrium (T1) after initial excitation by the radio frequency pulse. This knowledge can be used to generate spectral "contrast" by adjustment of the delay time before data is acquired and the time between repetitions.

METHODS

All spectra were acquired on a Picker 1.5T whole-body imager fitted with the SpectroVista research package. Data were acquired with a conventional quadrature head receiver coil.

These studies used a repetition time of 1,500 ms, an echo time of 270 ms, and 12 signal repetitions on each of the 64 phase encodes. The voxel size before subdivision into 64 subvoxels measured $8 \times 8 \times 3$ cm, resulting in a subvoxel size of 3 cm^3.

Patients and volunteers all gave informed consent for the examinations. The patient was laid supine with the head located in a holder and positioned centrally within the radiofrequency coils and magnet. Patient movement must be avoided to obtain successful data collection.

The MR signal was optimized by calibration of the radiofrequency pulses, and the spectral linewidth was minimized by careful adjustment of the magnet homogeneity. The magnet was adjusted to one part in 10 million accuracy, which is essential for acquiring high-quality data.

MR images were acquired to localize the voxel of interest, which was placed centrally in the brain above the ventricles.

RESULTS

Figure 1 illustrates the central 12 voxels of a MESA-3D acquisition from a normal volunteer. The peaks from left to right represent choline-containing compounds, creatine-containing compounds, and *N*-acetyl aspartate.

Spectra acquired from a tumor patient after radiation therapy are illustrated in Fig. 2. The spectra are numbered 1–4. Spectrum 1 is in the region of the tumor in which four peaks are observed. The first three are as described above and the fourth peak on the right represents lactate. The decrease in *N*-acetyl aspartate, the initial increase in choline, and the increase in lactate in the tumor are clearly visualized in moving from region 4 to region 1. The patient is being followed to track outcome.

Quantitative analysis of spectra from patients with Alzheimer's disease has been performed by fitting theoretical curves, consisting of Lorentzian lines, to the data, as shown in Fig. 3. The spectra acquired in a small number of patients indicate that the ratio of *N*-acetyl aspartate to choline concentration may be increased in comparison with normal volunteers. However, further work is required to establish this trend (11–16).

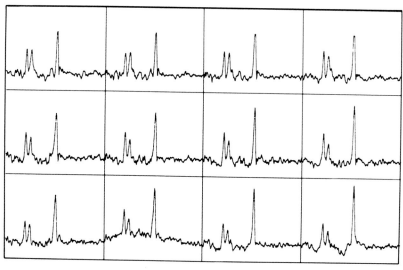

FIG. 1. Central 12 voxels from a MESA-3D data set acquired from a healthy volunteer, illustrating high spectral and spatial resolution.

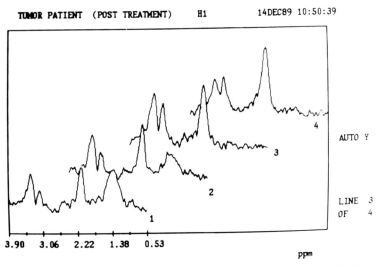

FIG. 2. A set of MESA-3D spectra obtained from adjacent voxels in a patient with a tumor (courtesy of MetroHealth Medical Center, Cleveland, OH, U.S.A.). Parameters are the same as for Fig. 1. Spectrum 4 corresponds to a normal region on the proton image; spectrum 1 corresponds to a region located inside the tumor. The reduction in NAA and increase in lactate in the tumor region are evident.

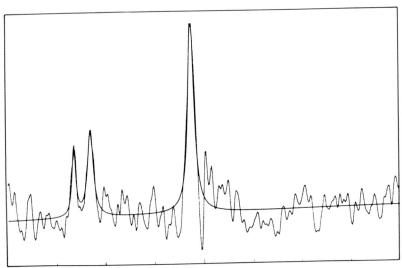

FIG. 3. Fit of a model function consisting of three Lorentzian lines to a proton spectrum acquired with MESA-3D. The relative areas and widths of all the lines can be obtained from the fitting procedure.

DISCUSSION

These studies indicate the potential of MR proton spectroscopy in conjunction with MR imaging to provide a detailed in vivo analysis of some important brain biochemicals, together with morphologic data on their distribution. The potential for monitoring the effects of therapy, including those of psychoactive drugs exists and will probably be extended over the next decade as MR moves beyond its conventional role in radiology to further support biochemistry, pharmacology, and psychiatry. The potential for collaborative efforts with pharmaceutical manufacturers also offers the potential for development of new strategies for effective drug treatments.

REFERENCES

1. Luyten PR, van Rijen PC, Berkelbach JW, Sprenkel VD, Tulleken CAF, Den Hollander JA. Society of Magnetic Resonance in Medicine, Seventh Annual Meeting, August 20–26, 1988, San Francisco: p. 753.
2. Lampman DA, Paley M, McNally J. SMRI Seventh Annual Meeting. *Magnet Reson Imaging* 1989;1(suppl):189.
3. Bottomley PA. Human in vivo NMR spectroscopy in diagnostic medicine: clinical tool or research probe? *Radiology* 1989;170:1.
4. Frahm J, Bruhn H, Gyngell ML, Merboldt K, Hanicke W, Sauter R. *Magnet Reson Med* 1989;11:49.
5. Lampman DA, Hurst G, McNally J, Paley M. Volume selective proton spectroscopy with solvent suppression, SMRI Fourth Annual Meeting. *Magnet Reson Imaging* 1986;4:115.
6. Lampman et al. In-vivo spatially encoded magnetic resonance with solvent suppression. File No. PKR 2 024, 1988 (U.S. Patent No. 4,771,242).
7. Haase A. Localisation of unaffected spins in NMR imaging and spectroscopy (LOCUS Spectroscopy). *Magnet Reson Med* 1986;3:963–969.
8. Paley M et al. Continuation PKR 2 161. 1988. (U.S. Patent Application Serial no. 392,480).
9. Lampman DA, Murdoch J, Paley M. In vivo metabolite maps using the MESA 3D technique. *Magnet Reson Med* 1991;18:169–80.
10. Hore PJ, Solvent suppression in Fourier transform magnetic resonance. *J Magnet Reson* 1983;4:539.
11. Miller B, Jenden DJ, Cummings JL, et al. Abnormal erythrocyte choline and influx in Alzheimer's disease. *Life Sci* 1986;38:485–490.
12. McGeer PL, McGeer EG, Suzuki J, et al. Aging, Alzheimer's disease, and the cholinergic system of the basal forebrain. *Neurology* 1984;34:741–745.
13. Blusztajn JK, Wurtzman RJ. Choline and cholinergic neurons. *Science* 1983;221:614–620.
14. Jenden DJ, Rice KM, Roch M, Booth RA. Effects of nicotinamide on choline and acetylcholine levels in rats. In: Wurtman RJ, Corkin S, Growdon J, Ritter–Walker E, eds. *Advances in neurology, Alzheimer's disease*. New York: Raven Press, 1990;51:65–71.
15. Freeman JJ, Jenden DJ. The source of choline for acetylcholine synthesis in brain. *Life Sci* 1976;19:949–962.
16. Dross K, Kewitz H. Concentration and origin of choline in the rat brain. *Naunyn Schmiedebergs Arch Pharmacol* 1972;274:91–106.

Psychiatry and Advanced Technologies,
edited by L. Ravizza, F. Bogetto, and
E. Zanalda. Raven Press, Ltd.,
New York 1993.

12

Positron Emission Tomography as a Tool to Investigate Cerebral Glucose Metabolism in Neurologic and Psychiatric Diseases: Studies in Alzheimer's Disease and in Obsessive–Compulsive Disorder

*†Pietro Pietrini, †Mario Guazzelli, †Pietro Sarteschi,
*Cheryl L. Grady, *James V. Haxby, ‡Susan E. Swedo,
‡Judith L. Rapoport, *and Mark B. Schapiro

*Laboratory of Neurosciences, National Institute on Aging, National Institutes of
Health, Bethesda, Maryland 20892; †Clinical Psychiatry I, University of Pisa,
56100 Pisa Italy; and ‡Child Psychiatry Branch, National Institute of Mental
Health, National Institutes of Health, Bethesda, Maryland 20892*

Positron emission tomography (PET) is a new noninvasive technique that allows the study of brain metabolism and blood flow in living human subjects. Since its appearance, PET has been widely used to investigate cerebral metabolic correlates of physiologic and cognitive processes (1–3), of aging (4,5), and of neurologic and psychiatric disorders (6–10). We summarize here the results of "resting state" cerebral glucose metabolism from PET studies of two diseases, obsessive–compulsive disorder (OCD) and Alzheimer's disease (AD), which, besides differing from each other in terms of age of onset, clinical picture, natural history, and neuropathology, have been recently suggested to be related to two phylogenetically distinct neural systems (11–14). We conclude that PET is a useful and powerful tool to investigate brain metabolism in neurologic disorders whose neuropathologic correlates are well known, as well as in psychiatric disorders whose biological roots, despite a growing body of evidence, remain controversial. New experimental procedures and methodological developments may overcome current limitations of PET, and lead to a great expansion of its potential in exploring brain function and dysfunction.

INTRODUCTION

Noninvasive measurements of brain function have been sought since the beginning of modern medicine. Because most psychiatric disorders are not associated with definable structural abnormalities, one approach to the understanding of these diseases has been the in vivo study of brain function in human subjects. One of the earliest functions investigated was cerebral blood flow, whose coupling to brain metabolism had been postulated since the last century (15). In 1948, Kety and Schmidt (16) applied the Fick principle, which governs the relation between the arterial delivery of a chemically inert substance, its brain uptake, and its clearance into the venous system, to develop a technique to measure cerebral blood flow. Their original method used nitrous oxide, a freely diffusible and nonmetabolizable substance, as an indicator of blood flow. However, this technique was invasive, requiring carotid artery injection and internal jugular sampling, and could only provide measurements of the average rates of whole-brain blood flow with no regional information. Subsequent modifications of the original method led to the 133-Xenon technique (17–19), which uses the γ-emitting compound ^{133}Xe and multiple scintillation probes. With this method it was possible to measure regional cerebral blood flow with either inhalation or intracarotid artery injection of ^{133}Xe with extracranial radiation detection and no internal jugular sampling. Its use, however, is limited to the investigation of large cortical areas, owing to limited spatial resolution and inability to examine subcortical regions.

During the last decade, with the introduction of PET, it has become possible to investigate brain functional activity in awake human subjects in a noninvasive way. With the increasing availability of positron-emitting compounds, the number of brain functions that can be studied has increased. Using [^{18}F]-2-fluoro-2-deoxy-D-glucose (18FDG), rates of glucose utilization can be determined within regions of the human brain smaller than 3 mm in diameter, on the cortical surface as well as subcortically (20). Because glucose is the major substrate for brain oxidative metabolism, its rate of consumption is a direct measure of regional brain functional activity (21). Moreover, PET scans can be repeated, thus allowing brain metabolic patterns to be evaluated in the same subject under different clinical conditions, such as before and after pharmacologic treatment or during longitudinal follow-up of a degenerative disorder. By identifying brain regions affected at the early stages of progressive neurodegenerative disorders such as AD, it may be possible to better understand their pathogenesis and the roles played by genetic, biologic, and environmental factors, as well as by the different central neurotransmitters involved. Furthermore, PET studies performed during life can be compared with postmortem neuropathology and neurochemistry, to help determine which brain regions are initially affected in a given disorder and which degenerate in a secondary manner (14).

In an attempt to show some of the applications of PET in neuropsychiatric research, we chose two diseases, AD and OCD, that differ from each other in terms of age of onset, clinical features, natural history, and neuropathology. Moreover, several pieces of evidence, including results from PET studies, suggest that each disease involves a distinct network of brain regions. As suggested by Rapoport (11–14), several groups of brain regions that are anatomically and functionally connected within a system by a process of "vertical evolution" underwent selective expansion or differentiation ("integrative phylogeny") during recent evolution of primates, particularly hominids. System I regions include the association neocortices as well as the nucleus basalis of Meynert, the entorhinal cortex, and subdivisions of the septum, hippocampal formation, and amygdaloid complex. Alzheimer's disease and two other dementing processes, Pick's disease and the dementia of Down's syndrome, have been shown to affect preferentially System I regions with relative sparing of System II structures. System II regions include the segregated circuits involving parts of the frontal cortex, basal ganglia, thalamus, and substantia nigra (13,14). Obsessive–compulsive disorder appears to result from dysfunction of this system (13,14). System II regions also appear to be involved in Huntington's disease, Parkinson's disease, progressive supranuclear palsy, and striatonigral degeneration (see Table 1).

Obsessive–compulsive disorder is a psychiatric disorder that frequently appears in childhood and persists for life. According to DSM-III-R (22), OCD is characterized by recurrent obsessions or compulsions sufficiently severe to cause marked distress, to be time consuming, or to interfere significantly

TABLE 1. *Principal features distinguishing AD from OCD*

Disease	AD (neurologic)	OCD (psychiatric)
Phylogenic system involved	I	II
Neurotransmitter(s) deficient	Multiple	Serotonin (?)
Dementia	+	−
Heritable	+	±
Demonstrable neuropathology	+	−
Animal model	−	+
Age of onset	Late (adult)	Early (childhood)
CT scan	Ventricular enlargement Cortical atrophy	Normal ventricles Caudate nuclear atrophy
PET scan	Decreased rCMRglc in association neocortices	Increased rCMRglc in frontal association, cingulate gyrus, and caudate nucleus
Therapy	−	+ (serotonin reuptake inhibitors)

As discussed in the text, differences between AD and OCD are not only limited to pathophysiologic, clinical, and therapeutic aspects. According to the theory of integrative phylogeny, AD and OCD involve two distinct neural systems (I and II), which underwent separate vertical evolutionary processes during recent evolution of primate (adapted from ref. 13).

with the person's normal routine, occupational functioning, or usual social activities or relationships with others.

Previously thought to be rare, recent epidemiologic studies suggest that OCD may affect as much as 2% of the population in the United States (23). Freud (24) attributed the origin of the obsessive neuroses and states to repressed memories of sexual guilt and, especially in the United States, OCD had been considered predominantly a domain of psychoanalysis for a long time. However, "organic" features in OCD have been reported since the last century (25) and, in recent years, a growing body of evidence has led to an increasing interest in the neurobiology of OCD. The association of OCD with certain neurologic disorders, such as Sydenham's chorea (26), postencephalitic Parkinson's disease (27), and Gilles de la Tourette's syndrome (28), as well as the presence of soft neurologic signs in about two thirds of OCD patients (29,30), strongly supports a neurobiologic basis for OCD. Further support for neurobiologic mechanisms has come from psychopharmacologic studies, which showed a selective clinical response to serotonin reuptake inhibitors, such as clomipramine and fluoxetine, in OCD patients (31). Serotoninergic neurons are widely distributed in the brain and are particularly concentrated in the basal ganglia (32,33). As discussed later, structures such as the basal ganglia that act as important "relay stations" between sensory input and motor and cognitive output seem to be dysfunctional in OCD.

Alzheimer's disease is a degenerative brain disease characterized by progressive impairment of memory, cognitive functions, and adaptive behavior. It affects approximately 5–10% of the population over the age of 65 years and 47% of those over the age of 85 years (34,35). The rate of cognitive decline can vary among patients, but death occurs on average 8 years after diagnosis (36). The accuracy of diagnosing AD during life is about 90% (37); cerebral biopsy or postmortem brain examination is required for confirmation of diagnosis. The neuropathologic features of AD include extensive neuron loss, neurofibrillary tangles, and senile plaques in specific regional and laminar patterns of distribution (38). This pathology is found mainly in the phylogenetically new association neocortex and in noncortical brain regions functionally and anatomically connected with the neocortex, such as the medial septal nucleus, nucleus basalis of Meynert, CA1 and subicular subfields of hippocampal formation, layers II and IV of entorhinal cortex, and parts of the amygdaloid complex. As discussed earlier, these brain regions belong to a system (System I) and share a common evolutionary profile as well as vulnerability to certain neurodegenerative diseases (13,14).

METHODS

Subjects

With regard to OCD and AD, patient groups and methodology have been reported in detail elsewhere (39,40). For the OCD group, 18 patients (9 men

TABLE 2. *Clinical data from the 18 OCD patients*

Clinical variable (ref.)	Mean ± SD	Range	Maximum possible score
Age (years)	27.8 ± 7.4	20–46	—
Age of onset (years)	8.9 ± 2.6	4–13	—
Ward (71)	13.5 ± 3.3	4–18	20
CPRS OCD[a] (42)	10.4 ± 4.1	2–17	24
NIMH OCD[b] (43)	27.2 ± 10.4	0–44	56
Global function (72)	5.8 ± 1.7	1–9	15
Global OCD (72)	6.7 ± 1.9	1–9	15
Global anxiety (72)	5.8 ± 1.9	2–9	15
Global depression (72)	4.3 ± 2.0	1–8	15
Hamilton Depression[c] (73)	8.6 ± 7.9	2–30	40
Spielberger Anxiety State[d] (53)	48.3 ± 11.7	28–68	80

Modified from ref. 39.
[a] Comprehensive Psychopathological Rating Scale.
[b] National Institute of Mental Health OCD Rating Scale.
[c] Hamilton Depression Rating Scale.
[d] Spielberger Anxiety State Questionnaire.

and 9 women; mean age 28 years, SD ± 7 years, age range 20–46 years), meeting the DSM-III (41) criteria for primary OCD, were studied. Potential subjects with physical, neurologic, or other concomitant psychiatric disorders were excluded. Severity of OCD symptomatology was assessed with specific rating scales, including the Comprehensive Psychopathological Rating Scale-OCD Subscale (42) and the National Institute of Mental Health-OCD Scale (43) (Table 2). All patients refrained from taking psychotropic drugs for at least 4 weeks and any medication at all for at least 2 weeks before the PET scan. The control group for the OCD patients consisted of 18 healthy volunteers (9 men and 9 women; mean age 32 years, SD ± 7 years) who were carefully screened to exclude medical, neurologic, or psychiatric disorders (4).

For the AD group, 47 patients with probable AD according to the NIN-CDS–ADRDA criteria (44) and otherwise in good health, were divided into three subgroups of dementia severity with the Folstein Mini-Mental State Examination (45): severe (score 0–9; $n = 11$; mean age 68 ± 11 years); moderate (score 10–19; $n = 19$; mean age 68 ± 9 years); and mild (score 20–30; $n = 17$; mean age 66 ± 11 years). They were compared to 30 age- and sex-matched healthy controls. Concomitant physical illness or history of major psychiatric disorder, stroke, epilepsy, significant head trauma, and transient ischemic attacks were among the exclusion criteria for both groups. All subjects were drug-free (as described above).

PET Scan

PET scans for both patients and controls were performed in a similar manner, on a Scanditronix PC1024-7B tomograph (Uppsala, Sweden). This is a seven-slice machine with a transverse resolution of 6 mm (FWHM) and an axial resolution of 10 mm. Subjects fasted for at least 2 h and refrained from alcohol, caffeine, and smoking for at least 24 h before the PET scan. Catheters were placed in a radial artery for drawing blood samples and in the antecubital vein of the opposite arm for injecting the isotope. Subjects were placed in the scanner in a quiet, dimly lit room with minimal background noise, with their eyes covered and ears occluded, and their heads held in place by a thermoplastic mask. After transmission scans were performed for attenuation correction, a bolus of 5 mCi of 18FDG was injected through the intravenous line. The emission scans were begun after a 45-min uptake period. Two interleaved scans were obtained parallel to and 10–100 mm above the inferior orbitomeatal (IOM) line, resulting in a total of 14 slices. In all subjects, arterial blood samples were drawn throughout the procedure at fixed intervals for measurement of plasma radioactivity and glucose concentration. Regional cerebral metabolic rates for glucose (rCMRglc) were calculated in mg glucose/100 g tissue/min by a modification (46) of the operational equation of Sokoloff et al. (47) and a lumped constant of 0.418. Patient and control scans were intermixed to avoid machine drift and bias.

Data Analysis

PET data were analyzed with a template composed of circular regions of interest (ROIs) which were 8 mm in diameter (48 mm^2). The ROIs were spaced evenly throughout the cortical ribbon and centered in subcortical regions. The template for each slice was placed over the matching slice for each subject and manually adjusted to fit (see Fig. 1a in ref. 40 for an illustration of the template). Regional metabolic rates were obtained by averaging values in the circular regions that were included in the larger anatomic areas, such as the superior parietal or superior temporal areas. These anatomic areas were identified by comparing the PET images to a standard atlas (48). Because the image analysis was performed by three individuals, inter-rater reliability coefficients (49) were calculated on all the regions; these ranged from 0.87 (left orbitofrontal) to 0.99 (left inferior parietal).

In addition to the absolute rCMRglc values, ratios of rCMRglc to the mean cortical gray matter were calculated to normalize the regional metabolic values and reduce variance. Right–left rCMRglc asymmetry indices were calculated for homologous right and left brain regions with the following formula: Asymmetry = $100 \times 2[\text{rCMRglc, right} - \text{rCMRglc, left}]/[\text{rCMRglc, right} + \text{rCMRglc, left}]$ (50).

RESULTS

OCD Patients

The main clinical features of the OCD patients are summarized in Table 2. As a group, the patients showed moderately severe OCD symptomatology but were neither depressed nor anxious, as concomitance of other psychiatric disorders, such as depression or anxiety, was an exclusionary criterion. Compared with the age-matched healthy controls, the 18 OCD patients showed increased rCMRglc in the left orbitofrontal, right sensorimotor, left premotor, right thalamus, and bilateral prefrontal and anterior cingulate regions ($p < 0.05$). Figure 1 clearly shows hypermetabolism in several brain regions in a patient with OCD as compared with a matched healthy control. Increased rCMRglc was also found in the right inferior temporal, right cerebellar and left paracentral regions (Table 3). No difference in whole-brain or mean cortical gray matter rCMRglc, nor any abnormal right–left asymmetry, was seen.

In contrast with previous reports (51,52), mean caudate nuclei rCMRglc did not differ significantly between the OCD patients and controls (Table 3). The left anterior cingulate/mean cortical gray matter ratio and the right prefrontal/mean cortical gray matter ratio were significantly higher in the

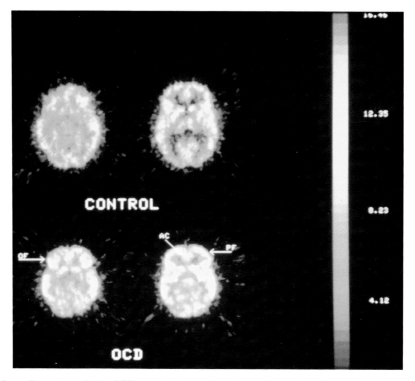

FIG. 1. Transverse brain PET scan images at two levels from a healthy control (**top**) and a sex- and age-matched OCD patient (**bottom**). rCMRglc values reported on the colorimetric scale are in units of mg/100 g/min. In the OCD patient, significantly higher rCMRglc values are shown in the orbitofrontal (OF), prefrontal (PF), and anterior cingulate (AC) regions in comparison with a matched control.

TABLE 3. *Absolute rCMRglc values (mean ± SD)*

Regions	rCMRglc (mg/100 g/min)	
	Controls ($n = 18$)	OCD ($n = 18$)
Prefrontal		
Right	8.45 ± 1.25	9.55 ± 1.28*
Left	8.48 ± 1.28	9.40 ± 1.38**
Orbitofrontal		
Right	7.67 ± 1.28	8.47 ± 1.44
Left	7.77 ± 1.31	8.65 ± 1.12**
Premotor		
Right	9.39 ± 1.42	10.23 ± 1.70
Left	9.52 ± 1.58	10.57 ± 1.50**
Sensorimotor		
Right	8.71 ± 1.27	9.72 ± 1.53**
Left	9.00 ± 1.48	9.72 ± 1.51
Medial parietal		
Right	9.13 ± 1.13	9.45 ± 1.88
Left	9.32 ± 1.54	9.65 ± 1.87
Inferior temporal		
Right	6.54 ± 0.94	7.33 ± 1.09**
Left	6.66 ± 1.11	7.18 ± 1.03
Medial temporal		
Right	8.20 ± 1.08	9.04 ± 1.53
Left	8.58 ± 1.16	8.97 ± 1.39
Paracentral		
Right	8.57 ± 1.03	9.44 ± 1.56
Left	8.88 ± 1.18	9.99 ± 1.62**
Cerebellum		
Right	6.86 ± 1.10	7.73 ± 1.36**
Left	6.84 ± 1.16	7.54 ± 1.34
Insula		
Right	8.97 ± 1.07	9.65 ± 1.81
Left	9.05 ± 1.18	9.56 ± 1.74
Lenticular nucleus		
Right	9.80 ± 1.70	10.47 ± 1.75
Left	9.95 ± 1.34	10.61 ± 1.71
Caudate nucleus		
Right	9.13 ± 1.73	10.25 ± 1.77
Left	10.06 ± 1.21	10.47 ± 1.54
Thalamus		
Right	8.61 ± 1.37	9.89 ± 1.99**
Left	9.13 ± 1.57	9.85 ± 1.74
Anterior cingulate		
Right	8.46 ± 1.29	9.37 ± 1.28**
Left	8.55 ± 1.26	9.78 ± 1.53*
Posterior cingulate	9.82 ± 1.59	10.81 ± 2.30
White matter		
Right	2.21 ± 0.52	2.39 ± 0.70
Left	2.26 ± 0.68	2.35 ± 0.61
Global gray matter	8.59 ± 1.14	9.37 ± 1.48
Whole brain	6.57 ± 0.91	7.22 ± 1.09

Modified from ref. 39.

[a] Metabolic rates are expressed as mg of glucose/100 g of brain tissue/min.

* $p \leq 0.01$.

** $p < 0.05$.

TABLE 4. *Correlations between rCMRglc and baseline OCD severity, state measures, and response to drug treatment[a]*

rCMRglc	Clinical variable	r^b	p
R orbitofrontal	Rank order severity	+0.52	0.03
R orbitofrontal/mean cortical gray matter	Rank order severity	+0.53	0.03
R prefrontal/mean cortical gray matter	Spielberger Anxiety[c]	+0.72	0.008
L prefrontal/mean cortical gray matter	Spielberger Anxiety[c]	+0.63	0.005
R orbitofrontal/mean cortical gray matter	Spielberger Anxiety[c]	+0.50	0.03
R prefrontal/mean cortical gray matter	Mean for 8 patients with panic > 10 without		
L premotor	Mean for 8 patients with panic < 10 without		
R prefrontal/mean cortical gray matter	Mean for patients with resistance > patients without		
R anterior cingulate			
R orbitofrontal	6 Nonresponders ≫ 11 responders > NC		

[a] See text for details.
[b] Spearman's correlation coefficient.
[c] Spielberger Anxiety State Questionnaire (53).

OCD group compared with controls ($p < 0.05$). Correlations between rCMRglc and clinical measurements (Table 4) showed that right orbitofrontal rCMRglc and the right orbitofrontal/mean cortical gray matter metabolism ratio were positively correlated with clinical OCD severity rank (the 18 OCD patients were rank-ordered in terms of clinically-rated OCD symptom severity from the least ill, No. 1, to the most severely ill, No. 18). However, no correlation was found between rCMRglc and any individual rating scale or duration of illness. Positive correlations were present between right prefrontal, left prefrontal, and right orbitofrontal ratios to mean cortical gray matter rCMRglc and anxiety during the PET scan, as assessed by the Spielberger State Anxiety Questionnaire (53). Moreover, a lower left premotor rCMRglc and a higher right prefrontal/mean cortical gray matter ratio were found in 8 OCD patients who admitted feelings of panic during the scan compared with the other 10 OCD patients who did not (Table 4). No statistically significant difference in rCMRglc was shown between patients with and without obsessive thoughts or compulsive urges during the PET scanning. The right prefrontal/mean cortical gray matter ratio, however, was higher in a subgroup of OCD patients reporting resistance against obsessions and compulsions during the scan ($p < 0.03$).

Right anterior cingulate and right orbitofrontal rCMRglc were significantly higher in 6 OCD patients who later did not respond to clomipramine treatment compared with the 11 who did respond (Table 4).

AD Patients

As a group, the AD patients showed significantly reduced rCMRglc in most neocortical gray matter regions compared with the normal volunteers.

Such reductions were present even in the mildly demented patients, and were most severe in the neocortical association areas, with the parietal, medial and lateral temporal, and premotor regions being the most impaired. Primary neocortical areas and subcortical regions appeared to be relatively spared, even in the severely demented AD patients (Fig. 2).

Whole-brain and mean cortical gray matter rCMRglc values were significantly lower than normal in all three groups. Because calcarine regions (primary visual) were the most spared neocortical areas, calcarine rCMRglc was used to normalize rCMRglc values and to calculate ratios. rCMRglc/calcarine rCMRglc ratios were significantly decreased bilaterally in the parietal lobes in the mildly demented AD patients, in the parietal, lateral temporal, and premotor regions bilaterally in the moderately demented AD group, and in the prefrontal, premotor, parietal, lateral temporal, sensorimotor, posterior medial temporal, occipital association, and orbitofrontal regions bilaterally

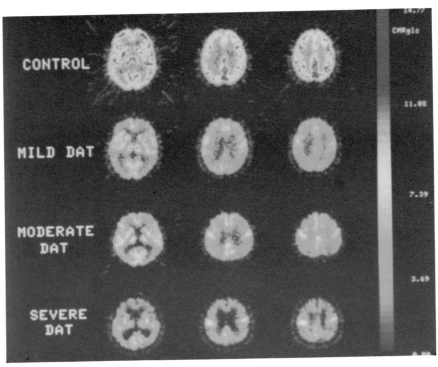

FIG. 2. Transverse images at three different levels of brain PET scans in a normal control and in patients with mild, moderate, and severe AD, respectively (from **top** to **bottom**). rCMRglc values reported on the colorimetric scale are in mg/100 g/min. rCMRglc reductions are present mostly in the association areas and become more severe as AD progresses. Primary neocortical areas are relatively spared, even in the latest stages of the disease.

in the severely demented AD patients. Significantly larger variances of right–left asymmetry were shown, as compared with healthy controls, in the frontal, parietal, and temporal association regions, but not in the sensorimotor or calcarine neocortex, of mildly and moderately demented AD patients. In addition, severely affected AD patients had statistically significant rCMRglc asymmetries in the caudate nucleus and the thalamus.

DISCUSSION

OCD Patients

The most relevant differences between OCD patients and normal controls were increased rCMRglc values in frontal neocortical regions and in the anterior cingulate gyrus bilaterally. These results are consistent with previous PET findings (51,52,54) and with several pieces of evidence suggesting a role of frontal cortex in OCD (55). Neuropsychologic studies in OCD patients, for instance, reveal striking spatial–perceptual abnormalities suggestive of frontal lobe and/or caudate dysfunction (56,57). Data from psychosurgery in OCD also implicate the frontal cortex in this disease. Anterior capsulotomy, a lesion of the anterior limb of the internal capsule, and cingulotomy, a lesion of the anterior portion of the cingulate gyrus, have successfully reduced obsessive–compulsive symptomatology in patients resistant to other treatments (58,59). Both procedures interrupt connections between the frontal lobe and the cingulate gyrus. Moreover, a PET study with 18FDG conducted in five patients with severe anxiety disorders including OCD, before and after cingulotomy, showed a significantly increased frontal cortex rCMRglc value at baseline in the patients compared with matched healthy controls; this higher frontal rCMRglc was lowered significantly after cingulotomy (60).

Further support for the involvement of frontal regions in OCD comes from the results of posttreatment PET scans. To evaluate the effects of drug treatment on rCMRglc, 13 of the 18 OCD patients underwent a second PET exam with 18FDG after at least 1 year of therapy. As a group, the OCD patients had significantly improved on all OCD and anxiety rating scales, and showed a significant decrease in the orbitofrontal rCMRglc (61). Therefore, our results and other reports (51,62) strongly suggest an involvement of the frontal lobes, the cingulate gyrus, the basal ganglia, and their interconnections in OCD.

Recently, it has been proposed that obsessive–compulsive behavior might be due to a disinhibition of striatum caused by a dysfunction of the corticostriatal circuit that normally suppresses obsessive behavior in humans (63). According to the "integrative phylogeny" hypothesis, this circuit involves regions that belong to segregated circuits in System II (11–14).

AD Patients

Our results in patients with probable AD demonstrate that rCMRglc is impaired predominantly in the association neocortical areas throughout the course of the disease. The primary sensorimotor cortex, primary visual cortex, cerebellum, thalamus, and caudate and lenticular nuclei are relatively spared, although they are affected to a lesser extent in all stages of the disease. Although the parietal association cortex, especially in the earlier stages of AD, is usually the most severely impaired region, the pattern of metabolic impairment may differ widely among patients. Moreover, in the same patient, homologous right and left hemispheric regions may be affected at different rates (right–left asymmetries). Equivalent numbers of patients have left-sided and right-sided asymmetries, and about one third of AD patients have symmetric rCMRglc values in all the association neocortices (64). As one would expect, in contrast to the significantly increased asymmetry in the association areas at all stages of AD, primary sensorimotor and occipital cortex rCMRglc values are not more asymmetric in AD patients than in controls ($p > 0.05$), further confirming their relative sparing.

The topographical localization of rCMRglc impairment in AD patients in life is consistent with the distribution of postmortem neuropathology, which is greatest in association neocortical regions and in subcortical regions that are functionally and anatomically connected with the association neocortex. Furthermore, metabolic and neuropathologic abnormalities are distributed mainly in the brain regions that belong to System I, a network of regions that underwent vertical evolution through the process of integrated phylogeny (11–14).

Other studies in our laboratory have shown that in moderately demented AD patients, different patterns of nonmemory neuropsychological impairment were significantly and appropriately related to different patterns of reduced rCMRglc in the association neocortices (50,66,67). Studies of patients with focal brain damage show that syntax comprehension, mental arithmetic, and immediate verbal memory are related to left parietal and temporal functions, whereas visuospatial construction is related to right parietal function (64,65,67). Accordingly, PET studies in moderately demented AD patients demonstrate disproportionate left-sided hypometabolism associated with disproportionate language impairment, whereas disproportionate right-sided hypometabolism is associated with visuospatial impairment. These observations demonstrate that different topographical localizations of alterations in regional brain function may be responsible for the interindividual differences in the pattern of nonmemory language and cognitive impairments seen in patients with moderate AD. Of more interest is the observation that patients with mild AD did not show any statistically significant impairment in the above-mentioned nonmemory neuropsychologic functions, but did present the same variability in rCMRglc reductions in the association neocortex. Although no correlations were found between their nonmemory neuro-psychologic test scores and right–left rCMRglc asymmetries at the initial evaluation (65), after a mean follow-up period of 24 months these same patients had developed significant impairments of nonmemory language and visuospatial functions, which then were significantly and consistently correlated with the earlier right–left metabolic asymmetries (66). Over this same period of time, the direction and magnitude of right–left metabolic asymmetries were remarkably stable (68). These results strongly suggest that rCMRglc abnormalities detected by PET in the association neocortical areas appear before any impairments, and predict later reductions in neocortically mediated visuospatial and language functions.

CONCLUSION

The studies of resting state glucose metabolism described here illustrate the usefulness of PET for investigating the cerebral metabolic dysfunction related to the pathophysiology of a neurologic and a psychiatric disorder.

Of course, one must recognize that PET with 18FDG in the resting state still presents some limitations. For instance, it has not allowed a preclinical diagnosis of AD (69) and is unable to examine cerebral function in connection with obsessive behavior, e.g., compulsive rituals. Use of PET scanners with increased resolution, along with new technical developments such as MRI–PET superimposition, may allow a more precise anatomic definition of even the smallest subcortical brain regions. Therefore, PET might provide useful information about structures known to be among the first affected in AD, such as the amygdaloid complex, hippocampal formation, and entorhinal cortex. Furthermore, the study of rCMRglc patterns in these regions, not simply limited to the singular regions per se but extended to the analysis of the interregional functional correlations, may be able to detect abnormalities even in the preclinical stages of AD, as well as in individual subjects "at risk" for disease (70).

The metabolic correlates of the clinical and behavioral features of OCD and AD can be further examined by using PET with [^{15}O]-water, a radionuclide that allows measurements of regional cerebral blood flow (rCBF). Because rCBF is coupled to cerebral metabolism, different rCBF patterns reflect different patterns of brain activation. Given the very short half-life of [^{15}O]-water, rCBF can be measured several times in the same subjects during the same PET scanning. In this way, rCBF during the resting state can be compared to rCBF during "activation," e.g., while the subject is performing a neuropsychologic task or is confronting a "trigger" condition (for example, application of dirt on the hand of a washer, a patient with an obsession about contamination and a compulsion to wash). Finally, new experimental paradigms, such as cognitive stimulation studies or pharmacologic probes, will certainly expand the application of PET in neuropsychiatry and lead to a deeper understanding of brain function in health and disease.

ACKNOWLEDGMENT

We thank E. Wagner for her technical assistance in acquiring the data reported here.

REFERENCES

1. Fox PT, Raichle ME, Thach WT. Functional mapping of human cerebellum with positron emission tomography. *Proc Natl Acad Sci USA* 1985;82:7462–6.
2. Fox PT, Mintun MA, Raichle ME, Miezin FM, Allman JM, Van Essen DC. Mapping human visual cortex with positron emission tomography. *Nature* 1986;323:806–9.
3. Pardo JV, Fox PT, Raichle ME. Localization of a human system for sustained attention by positron emission tomography. *Nature* 1991;349:61–4.
4. Duara R, Margolin RA, Robertson–Tchabo EA, et al. Cerebral glucose utilization as measured with positron emission tomography in 21 resting healthy men between the ages of 21 and 83 years. *Brain* 1983;106:761–75.
5. Frackowiak RSJ, Wise RSJ, Gibbs JM, Jones T. Positron emission tomographic studies in aging and cerebrovascular disease at Hammersmith Hospital. *Ann Neurol* 1984;15(suppl): S112–8.
6. Kuhl DE, Phelps ME, Markham CH, Metter JE, Riege WH, Winter J. Cerebral metabolism and atrophy in Huntington's disease by 18 FDG and computed tomographic scan. *Ann Neurol* 1982;12:425–34.
7. Duara R, Grady CL, Haxby JV, et al. Positron emission tomography in Alzheimer's disease. *Neurology* 1986;36:879–87.
8. Mazziotta JC, Phelps ME. Positron emission tomography studies of the brain. In: Phelps ME, Mazziotta JC, Schelbert HR, eds. *Positron emission tomography. Principles and applications for the brain and heart.* New York: Raven Press, 1986;493–579.
9. Dolan RJ, Friston MA. Positron emission tomography in psychiatric and neuropsychiatric disorders. *Semin Neurol* 1989;9:330–7.
10. Holcomb HH, Links J, Smith C, Wong D. Positron emission tomography: measuring the metabolic and neurochemical characteristics of the living human nervous system. In: Andreasen NC, ed. *Brain imaging: application in psychiatry.* Washington, DC: American Psychiatric Press, 1989;235–370.
11. Rapoport SI. Brain evolution and Alzheimer's disease. *Rev Neurol* 1988;144:79–90.
12. Rapoport SI. Hypothesis: Alzheimer's disease is a phylogenic disease. *Med Hypoth* 1989; 29:147–50.
13. Rapoport SI. Integrated phylogeny of the primate brain, with special reference to humans and their diseases. *Brain Res Rev* 1990;15:267–94.
14. Rapoport SI. Topography of Alzheimer's disease: involvement of association neocortices and connected regions; pathological, metabolic and cognitive correlations; relation to evolution. In: Rapoport SI, Petit H, Leys D, Christen Y, eds. *Imaging, cerebral topography and Alzheimer's disease.* Berlin: Springer-Verlag, 1990;1–17.
15. Roy CS, Sherrington CS. On the regulation of the blood supply to the brain. *J Physiol* 1890; 11:85–108.
16. Kety SS, Schmidt CF. The nitrous oxide method for quantitative determination of cerebral blood flow in man: theory, procedure and normal values. *J Clin Invest* 1948;27:475–83.
17. Obrist WD, Thompson HK Jr, King CH, Wang HS. Determination of regional cerebral blood flow by inhalation of 133-Xenon. *Circ Res* 1967;20:124–35.
18. Obrist WD, Thompson HK Jr, Wang HS, Wilkinson WE. Regional cerebral blood flow estimated by 133-Xenon inhalation. *Stroke* 1975;6:245–56.

19. Risberg J. Regional cerebral blood flow measurements by 133-Xe-inhalation methodology and applications in neuropsychology and psychiatry. *Brain Lang* 1980;9:9–34.
20. Jagust WJ, Eberling JL, Baker MG, et al. Hippocampal glucose metabolism in Alzheimer's disease. *Abst Soc Neurosci* 1990;1:283.
21. Raichle ME, Grubb RL Jr, Gado MH, Eichling JO, Ter-Pogossian MM. Correlation between regional cerebral blood flow and oxidative metabolism. In vivo studies in man. *Arch Neurol* 1976;33:523–6.
22. American Psychiatric Association, Committee on nomenclature and statistics: *Diagnostic and statistical manual of mental disorders*, 3rd ed., revised. Washington, DC: American Psychiatric Association, 1987.
23. Karno M, Golding J, Sorenson S, Burnham M. The epidemiology of obsessive compulsive disorder in five US communities. *Arch Gen Psychiatry* 1988;45:1094–9.
24. Freud S. The neuropsychoses of defence (1894). In: Freud S, ed. *The standard edition of the complete psychological works of Sigmund Freud*, vol 3. London: Hogarth, 1962:45–61.
25. Kettl PA, Marks IM. Neurological factors in obsessive compulsive disorder. Two case reports and a review of the literature. *Br J Psychiatry* 1986;149:315–9.
26. Swedo SE, Rapoport JL, Cheslow DL, et al. High prevalence of obsessive compulsive symptoms in patients with Sydenham's chorea. *Am J Psychiatry* 1989;146:246–9.
27. Von Economo C. *Die Enceptalitis lethargica*. Vienna: Deutcke; 1917.
28. Pauls DL, Towbin KE, Leckman JF, Zahner GEP, Cohen DJ. Gilles de la Tourette's syndrome and obsessive compulsive disorder. *Arch Gen Psychiatry* 1986;43:1180–2.
29. Denckla MB. Neurological examination. In: Rapoport JL, ed. *Obsessive compulsive disorder in children and adolescents*. Washington DC: American Psychiatric Press, 1989:107–15.
30. Hollander E, Schiffman E, Cohen B, et al. Signs of central nervous system dysfunction in obsessive compulsive disorder. *Arch Gen Psychiatr* 1990;47:27–32.
31. Leonard HL. Drug treatment of obsessive compulsive disorder. In: Rapoport JL, ed. *Obsessive compulsive disorder in children and adolescents*. Washington DC: American Psychiatric Press, 1989:237–49.
32. Pazos A, Palacios J. Quantitative autoradiographic mapping of serotonin in rat brain: I: Serotonin I receptors. *Brain Res* 1985;356:205–31.
33. Pazos A, Cortes R, Palacios J. Quantitative autoradiographic mapping of serotonin in rat brain: II: Serotonin II receptors. *Brain Res* 1985;356:231–49.
34. Katzman R. Alzheimer's disease. *N Engl J Med* 1986;314:964–73.
35. Evans DA, Funkenstein HH, Albert MS, et al. Prevalence of Alzheimer's disease in a community population of older persons. *JAMA* 1989;262:2551–6.
36. Heston LL, Mastri AR, Anderson VE, White J. Dementia of the Alzheimer type. Clinical genetics, natural history, and associated conditions. *Arch Gen Psychiatry* 1981;38:1085–90.
37. Ron MA, Toone BK, Garralda ME, Lishman WA. Diagnostic accuracy in presenile dementia. *Br J Psychiatry* 1979;134:161–8.
38. Morrison JH, Hof PR, Campbell MJ, et al. Cellular pathology in Alzheimer's disease: implications for cortical disconnection and differential vulnerability. In: Rapoport SI, Petit H, Leys D, Christen Y, eds. *Imaging, cerebral topography and Alzheimer's disease*. Berlin: Springer-Verlag, 1990:19–40.
39. Swedo SE, Schapiro MB, Grady CL, et al. Cerebral glucose metabolism in childhood-onset obsessive compulsive disorder. *Arch Gen Psychiatry* 1989;45:518–23.
40. Kumar A, Schapiro MB, Grady CL, et al. High-resolution PET studies in Alzheimer's disease. *Neuropsychopharmacology* 1991;4:35–46.
41. American Psychiatric Association, Committee on Nomenclature and Statistics. *Diagnostic and statistical manual of mental disorders*, 3rd ed. Washington, DC: American Psychiatric Association, 1980.
42. Thoren P, Asberg M, Cronholm B, Jornestedt L, Traskman L. Clomipramine treatment of obsessive compulsive disorder, I: A controlled clinical trial. *Arch Gen Psychiatry* 1980;37:1281–5.
43. Insel TR, Murphy DL, Cohen RM, Alterman I, Kilts C, Linnoila M. Obsessive compulsive disorder: a double-blind trial of clomipramine and clorgyline. *Arch Gen Psychiatry* 1983;40:605–12.
44. McKhann G, Drachman D, Follstein M, Katzman R, Price D, Stadlan EM. Clinical diagnosis of Alzheimer's disease: report of the NINCDS-ADRDA work group under the auspices

of the Department of Health and Human Services Task Force on Alzheimer's disease. *Neurology* 1984;34:939–44.

45. Folstein MF, Folstein SE, McHugh PR. "Mini Mental State" a practical method for grading the cognitive state of patients for the clinician. *J Psychiatr Res* 1975;12:189–98.

46. Brooks RA. Alternative formula for glucose utilization using labeled deoxyglucose. *J Nucl Med* 1982;23:538–9.

47. Sokoloff L, Reivich M, Kennedy C, et al. The (14C)-deoxyglucose method for the measurement of local cerebral glucose utilization: theory, procedure and normal values in the conscious and anesthetized albino rat. *J Neurochem* 1977;28:897–916.

48. Eycleshymer AC, Shoemaker DM. *A cross-section anatomy.* New York: Appleton and Co., 1911.

49. Bartko JJ, Carpenter WT. On the methods and theory of reliability. *J Nerv Ment Dis* 1976; 163:307–17.

50. Haxby JV, Duara R, Grady CL, Cutler NR, Rapoport SI. Relation between neuropsychological and cerebral metabolic asymmetries in early Alzheimer's disease. *J Cereb Blood Flow Metab* 1985;5:193–200.

51. Baxter LR, Phelps ME, Mazziotta JC, Guze BH, Schwartz JM, Selin CE. Local cerebral glucose metabolic rates in obsessive compulsive disorder. *Arch Gen Psychiatry* 1987;44: 211–8.

52. Baxter LR, Schwartz JM, Mazziotta JC, Phelps ME, Pahl JJ, Guze BH. Cerebral glucose metabolic rates in nondepressed patients with obsessive compulsive disorder. *Am J Psychiatry* 1989;145:1560–3.

53. *Spielberger 20-item State Anxiety Questionnaire-Manual.* Palo Alto, CA: Consulting Psychologist Press, 1968.

54. Nordahl TE, Benkelfat C, Semple WE, Gross M, King AC, Cohen RM. Cerebral glucose metabolic rates in obsessive compulsive disorder. *Neuropsychopharmacology* 1989;2:23–8.

55. Khanna S. Obsessive compulsive disorder: is there a frontal lobe dysfunction? *Biol Psychiatry* 1988;24:602–13.

56. Behar D, Rapoport JL, Berg CJ, et al. Computerized tomography and neuropsychological test measures in adolescents with obsessive compulsive disorder. *Am J Psychiatry* 1984; 141:363–9.

57. Cox CS, Fedio P, Rapoport JL. Neuropsychological testing of obsessive compulsive adolescents. In: Rapoport JL, ed. *Obsessive compulsive disorder in children and adolescents.* Washington, DC: American Psychiatric Press, 1989:73–86.

58. Mindus P. Capsulotomy, a psychosurgical intervention considered in cases of anxiety disorders unresponsive to conventional therapy. In: *Workshop on anxiety disorders.* Stockholm: Committee on Drug Information, the Swedish National Board of Health and Welfare, 1986.

59. Ballantine HT, Boucksoms AJ, Thomas EK, Giriunas IE. Treatment of psychiatric illness by stereotactic cingulotomy. *Biol Psychiatry* 1987;22:807–19.

60. Mindus P, Ericson K, Greitz B, Meyerson A, Nyman H, Sjogren I. Regional cerebral glucose metabolism in anxiety disorders studied with positron emission tomography before and after psychosurgical intervention. *Acta Radiol* 1986;369(suppl):444–8.

61. Pietrini P, Swedo SE, Grady CL, Rapoport JL, Rapoport SI, Schapiro MB. Post-treatment cerebral glucose metabolism (CMRglc) in obsessive compulsive disorder (OCD) assessed by PET. *Biol Psychiatry* 1991;29:311S.

62. Luxenberg JS, Swedo SE, Flament MF, Friedland RP, Rapoport J, Rapoport SI. Neuroanatomic abnormalities in obsessive-compulsive disorder detected with quantitative X-ray computed tomography. *Am J Psychiatry* 1988;145:1089–93.

63. Wise SP, Rapoport JL. Obsessive-compulsive disorder: is it basal ganglia dysfunction? In: Rapoport JL, ed. *Obsessive compulsive disorder in children and adolescents.* Washington, DC: American Psychiatric Press, 1988:327–46.

64. Haxby JV. Cognitive deficits and local metabolic changes in dementia of the Alzheimer type. In: Rapoport SI, Petit H, Leys D, Christen Y, eds. *Imaging, cerebral topography and Alzheimer's disease.* Berlin: Springer-Verlag, 1990:109–19.

65. Haxby JV, Grady CL, Duara R, Schlageter NL, Berg G, Rapoport SI. Neocortical metabolic abnormalities precede non-memory cognitive deficits in early Alzheimer-type dementia. *Arch Neurol* 1986;43:882–5.

66. Haxby JV, Grady CL, Friedland RP, Rapoport SI. Neocortical metabolic abnormalities

precede non-memory cognitive impairments in early dementia of the Alzheimer type: longitudinal confirmation. *J Neural Transm* 1987;24(suppl):49–51.
67. Benton A. Visuoperceptual, visuospatial and visuoconstructive disorders. In: Heilman KM, Valenstein E, eds. *Clinical neuropsychology*, 2nd ed. Oxford: Oxford University Press, 1985.
68. Grady CL, Haxby JV, Schlageter NL, Berg G, Rapoport SI. Stability of metabolic and neuropsychological asymmetries in dementia of the Alzheimer type. *Neurology* 1986;36: 1390–2.
69. Pietrini P, Grady CI, Haxby JV, et al. Resting cerebral glucose metabolism does not identify subjects "at-risk" for familial Alzheimer disease. *Ann Neurol* 1991;2:287–8.
70. Clark CM, Amman W, Martin WRW, Ty P, Hayden MR. The PET/FDG methodology for early detection of disease onset: a statistical model. *J Cereb Blood Flow Metab* 1991;19: 663–78.
71. Flament MF, Rapoport JL, Berg CJ, et al. Clomipramine treatment of childhood obsessive-compulsive disorder: a double-blind controlled study. *Arch Gen Psychiatry* 1985;42:977–83.
72. Murphy DL, Pickar D, Alterman IS. Methods for the quantitative assessment of depressive and manic behavior. In: Burdock EL, Sudilovsky A, Gershon S, eds. *The behavior of psychiatric patients*. New York: Marcel Dekker, 1982:355–92.
73. Hamilton M. Development of a rating scale for primary depressive illness. *Br J Soc Psychol* 1967;6:278–96.

Psychiatry and Advanced Technologies,
edited by L. Ravizza, F. Bogetto, and
E. Zanalda. Raven Press, Ltd.,
New York © 1993.

13

Microcomputer-Assisted Assessment of DSM-III-R Diagnoses

Michael B. First

*Department of Clinical Psychiatry, Columbia University, New York, New York;
and New York State Psychiatric Institute, New York, New York, 10032*

The benefits achieved by the use of a standardized psychiatric classification system depend on its accurate and nonidiosyncratic application. The complexity of the DSM-III-R classification, coupled with studies suggesting that the criteria are not always applied correctly, suggests that the introduction of computer technology into the diagnostic process may be useful. Two basic approaches to computer-assisted assessment have been generally adopted: the development of a diagnostic expert system that interacts with the clinician, and computerized interviewing. Caution should be taken in trusting the results of computerized interviews when no clinician has played an active role in the elicitation and interpretation of the diagnostic criteria. Two software packages (DTREE and Mini-SCID) that conform to certain basic design principles are discussed here.

INTRODUCTION

The introduction of computer technology into the field of mental health has proceeded relatively slowly as compared with its widespread adoption in the business, scientific, and educational arenas. The most common use of computers in the field of mental health has been for the processing of financial and demographic information about patients (e.g., office and hospital management) (1). The use of computers in clinical practice settings has thus far been extremely limited. This chapter discusses the potential application of computer technology to the field of diagnostic assessment, specifically to the making of DSM-III-R diagnoses (2).

WHY COMPUTERIZED ASSESSMENT?

A psychiatric classification system utilizing diagnostic criteria serves several critical functions in facilitating research and clinical practice. First, it functions as a language for communication among researchers and clinicians working in widely different settings by providing a concise shorthand for use in discussing phenomenology. For example, by saying that a patient's symptoms "meet diagnostic criteria for panic disorder," clinicians can instantly indicate to their colleagues information about the expected pattern of symptomatology and the minimum limits on the frequency of the attacks. Communication is also facilitated by providing standardization of terminology so that clinicians and researchers who are not in close geographic proximity can be assured of understanding one another. Finally, another important function of a classification system is to serve as a basis for including subjects in research studies. Replication of research findings and interpretation of the clinical significance of results is facilitated by clarifying the phenomenologic characteristics of the research sample.

The *Diagnostic and Statistical Manual of Mental Disorders*, Third Edition (DSM-III) (3), the official psychiatric classification system of the American Psychiatric Association, was the first complete psychiatric nomenclature to use diagnostic criteria; for each diagnostic category, necessary and sufficient criteria are prescribed. In terms of utilization, DSM-III and its successor, DSM-III-R, have been overwhelmingly successful. Since its introduction in 1980, DSM-III has been adopted as the official nomenclature in virtually all mental health facilities in the United States, and is used as the basis for psychiatric diagnosis by mental health professionals from all disciplines. It has also been translated into at least 14 different languages, spurred by widespread international interest, especially among researchers.

In view of this widespread dissemination, the true value of DSM-III in enhancing communication is critically dependent on correct application of the diagnostic criteria. Idiosyncratic interpretation of the diagnostic criteria or haphazard application of the diagnostic algorithms can undermine the value of the system as a diagnostic standard. For example, if the criteria for diagnosing major depression are applied in a way that is at variance with the specified diagnostic algorithm (for instance, making the diagnosis if only three items are present, rather than the required five items), then the use of the term "major depression" in association with a particular patient or group of patients will be at the very least misleading and may lead to adoption of an incorrect treatment plan.

Although very little research has investigated clinician's accuracy in applying the DSM-III diagnostic classification, several studies suggest that the criteria are not being applied correctly. A study by Skodol and colleagues (4) investigated the accuracy of intake diagnosis by psychiatric residents under supervision by faculty who had played a major role in the development of DSM-III. Taking the supervisors' DSM-III diagnoses as a standard, they found that 37% of the residents' diagnoses were incorrect, with 75% of these incorrect diagnoses being due to the misapplication of criteria or DSM-III conventions. Another study (5) examined the effect of the introduction of the DSM-III classification on chart diagnoses in a state hospital chronic care facility and found significant rates of apparent misdiagnosis, although the majority of charts (80%) lacked sufficient documentation of relevant psychopathology for a confident DSM-III diagnosis to be made. Finally, a third study (6), which tested knowledge of the diagnostic criteria for major depression among the clinical staff at an outpatient university-affiliated mental health facility, found incorrect responses on a questionnaire at a rate ranging from 13–48% (for example, 48% incorrectly thought that insomnia was *required* for a diagnosis of major depression). These findings suggest both that the diagnostic classification system is being used suboptimally and that proper documentation of the symptomatology underlying diagnostic decision making is typically lacking.

One solution to these problems is to apply the capabilities of a computer to assist the clinician in making a DSM-III diagnosis. Potential problems that may contribute to making an inaccurate or incomplete diagnostic assessment include the following: (i) incorrect application of DSM-III diagnostic algorithms: this may be due to lack of diligence on the part of the clinician or to difficulty in using the manual (which is a likely possibility owing to its length and complexity; DSM-III-R lists over 250 disorders in 360 pages); (ii) idiosyncratic interpretation of the meaning of diagnostic criteria; (iii) clinically significant conditions being missed because of premature closure of the diagnostic process (i.e., the tendency of the clinician to inquire only about symptoms directly related to the patient's chief complaint). Another problem in diagnostic assessment alluded to by the chart review study is the often poor state of medical records with regard to documentation of the relevant psychopathology; this may make it impossible to verify whether or not the assigned diagnosis is justifiable, in turn making chart review difficult.

Computer technology can be of assistance in dealing with each of these problems. A major strength of computers is that they apply rules and procedures with exact precision. By encoding the DSM-III-R diagnostic algorithms into a computer program, a procedurally accurate diagnostic assessment can be ensured. By providing definitions of diagnostic terms in "help" screens that are displayed at relevant points in the diagnostic process, the computer can guide the clinician as to the intended meaning of the diagnostic criteria. By having the computer collect data directly from the patient or by having the computer force the clinician to consider all diagnostic possibilities, premature closure can be curtailed. Finally, computers are excellent record keepers and can therefore provide a complete record of the symptomatology considered during the diagnostic process, thus instantly furnishing chart documentation.

DESIGN AXIOMS

Before specific methods of computers used in diagnostic assessment are discussed, two basic axioms relevant to the design of such systems should be mentioned. A common concern in the potential introduction of computer technology into the diagnostic process is whether the clinical interview (and, by extension, the clinician) will be rendered obsolete. The first proposed design axiom is that, given the current state of computer technology, a human clinician must remain a necessary component of the diagnostic process to ensure a certain level of diagnostic validity. This axiom is important for several reasons. First, a computer is unable to adequately collect and evaluate nonverbal data from the patient that may be relevant to the diagnostic process. The computer–human interface depends entirely on communication through verbal or symbolic language. Although in theory some nonverbal behaviors could be input by physiologic monitoring, many potentially critical nonverbal cues (e.g., facial expressions, speech pattern, vocal tone and inflections) are not amenable to computer analysis, given the current limitations of technology. Second, verbal communication between the patient and the computer is usually limited to having the patient make a selection from a set of fixed choices (e.g., YES/NO, MILD/MODERATE/SEVERE, multiple-choice items). The full range of verbal communication characteristic of a clinical interview is simply not possible because computers are unable to comprehend unrestricted English. This technologically necessary reductionistic approach can be somewhat mitigated by having the experienced clinician use his or her judgment in making these categorical determinations (as opposed to leaving this judgment to the patient). Third, computers are notoriously poor at representing and processing such information as the time course of illness and the temporal relationships of clusters of symptoms, both of which are often a crucial part of the definition of a particular disorder. The computer's shortcomings in dealing with such issues can be compensated to some extent by relying on the clinician's natural ability to do temporal reasoning. Finally, the computer cannot assess the clinical significance of a patient's report of a symptom because it cannot apply clinical judgment to the assessment process. Therefore, any scheme that proposes to use the computer as a clinical assessment tool must be designed in such a way that the clinician provides clinical judgment both in data gathering and in the interpretation of the clinical significance of symptomatology.

The second design axiom is that a necessary condition for the ultimate success of the computer program is that the clinician must thoroughly understand the strengths and limitations of the computer-assisted assessment procedure. In clinical practice, the clinician is ultimately responsible for the accuracy of the diagnostic assessment. Therefore, for a computer program to be truly useful, the clinician must completely understand the process by which the computer arrives at its diagnostic conclusions. It should not merely operate as a "black box" into which clinical data are input and a diagnosis (or a list of possible diagnoses) is output. Historically, developers of computer programs designed to aid in diagnosis have focused almost exclusively on improving the accuracy and comprehensiveness of the program's diagnostic capabilities, and have paid relatively little attention to its explanatory capabilities. Not surprisingly, such programs have been little used in clinical settings.

APPROACHES TO COMPUTER-ASSISTED ASSESSMENT

Two basic approaches for computer-assisted diagnosis have been generally adopted: using the computer as an "expert system," and using it to collect data directly from the patient by administering a diagnostic interview or questionnaire. With the expert system approach, the computer functions as would a diagnostic expert: the clinician consults the computer after initially collecting the diagnostic data from the patient, chart records, and/or family members or other informants. In this situation, the clinician judges the diagnostic significance of the raw data collected from the patient and other sources. In the second approach, the computer interviews the patient, with the patient responding directly to the computer's questions on a display screen or typewriter using either a keyboard, touch screen, joystick, or other simple input device.

Both approaches have the potential advantage of increased accuracy of application of the diagnostic criteria (since the diagnostic algorithms can be embedded into the flow of the computer program) and increased diagnostic coverage (since the computer program can ensure that all areas of potential psychopathology are considered). The main purported advantage of computer interviewing programs is their potential to reduce the amount of time the clinician must devote to the diagnostic process, since these programs have been designed to take over the time-consuming task of clinical interviewing. However, as mentioned above, this possible advantage is counterbalanced by the potentially great reduction in diagnostic validity that would result from eliminating the clinician's role in the data-gathering process. The major drawback of the expert system approach is that it may actually make the diagnostic process *more* time consuming for the clinician. No matter what other benefits may accrue, it clearly takes more time to consult an expert system program than to make a diagnostic assessment without consulting anything but one's memory of the diagnostic criteria. Ultimately, for an expert system program to be accepted by clinicians, the amount of time required must be relatively short, and the potential benefits of increasing diagnostic accuracy, coverage, and providing documentation must be perceived as relatively important.

DTREE AND MINI-SCID: TWO SOFTWARE EXAMPLES

"DTREE: The Electronic DSM-III-R" (7,9) is a computer-assisted diagnostic software package that adopts the expert system approach. DTREE guides the clinician through the process of making DSM-III-R diagnoses by offering a series of YES/NO questions for the clinician to answer. A decision tree model is used to determine the order of the questions (i.e., the selection of which question is asked next is determined by the answers to previous questions). Using DTREE, the clinician specifies the basic areas of disturbance (e.g., psychotic symptoms, mood symptoms, anxiety symptoms) that require further investigation. To ensure completeness of the evaluation, the clinician can choose to start with a series of 20 basic questions designed to inquire about all relevant areas of psychopathology, thus providing complete diagnostic coverage from the outset. For each symptom area selected, DTREE presents the complete differential diagnosis for that symptom and then attempts to narrow the list by presenting additional questions that check for the presence or absence of the relevant diagnostic criteria. For example, if the presenting symptomatology is paranoid delusions, the clinician selects the "psychotic tree" and DTREE starts by indicating the complete differential diagnosis (e.g., organic delusional disorder, dementia, delirium, brief reactive psychosis, schizophrenia, schizophreniform disorder, delusional disorder, psychotic mood disorder, schizoaffective disorder, psychotic disorder not otherwise specified). DTREE then tries to verify whether or not there are any etiologic organic factors in order to rule out organic delusional disorder and remove it from the differential diagnosis list.

Critical to the design and implementation of DTREE is its emphasis on informing the clinician about each aspect of the diagnostic process. Two design features have been added for this purpose: DTREE displays its reason for asking each question along with the question, and the clinician has a "help" key available for each question, which displays one or two pages of additional explanatory text, such as the diagnostic significance of the criterion being asked about, suggestions on how to assess the item, and other differential diagnostic issues (e.g., how a symptom may present differently in the context of different disorders). Therefore, by the time the DTREE evaluation is concluded, the clinician should have a complete understanding of the reasoning behind DTREE's final diagnosis. In addition, DTREE documents the process by producing a diagnostic summary report that includes two lists of diagnoses: those DSM-III-R diagnoses present (along with the criteria that justified giving the diagnosis), and a list of those diagnoses that were ruled out (along with the criteria whose absence justified ruling the diagnoses out).

The Mini-SCID software (8) is an example of the second approach, i.e., using the computer to collect diagnostic information directly from the patient. However, unlike many other programs that may produce diagnoses of questionable validity, Mini-SCID does not specify a particular DSM-III-R diagnosis. It is not intended to stand alone but is to be used in conjunction with an expert system program (such as DTREE), as follows. The diagnostic evaluation starts by having Mini-SCID ask questions that cover many different areas of psychopathology, thus ensuring a broad range of diagnostic coverage from the outset. The program then produces a summary of its findings, which is followed up by a clinical interview. After the confirmatory interview, the clinician then refers to the expert system (i.e., DTREE) to arrive at the final diagnosis. This hybrid process is intended to provide the best of both worlds: the potentially time-saving aspects and broad diagnostic coverage of computerized interviewing coupled with the diagnostic accuracy of an expert system, with the clinical interview acting as the cornerstone of the diagnostic process.

CONCLUSIONS AND FUTURE DIRECTIONS

The true value of using a standardized diagnostic classification system depends to a large degree on how accurately and consistently it is applied in the clinical setting. The desire to improve diagnostic accuracy in clinical practice has led to the application of computer technology to the diagnostic process; specifically, in this case, the DTREE and Mini-SCID software packages. These have been designed with the goals of providing the clinician with a complete understanding of the diagnostic process so as to allow the clinician to be confident in how the computer arrived at the results, a necessary feature for its acceptability in an actual clinical setting. Although the use of these software packages takes more time and effort than not using them, they offer the potential of improving diagnostic accuracy and documentation. Although pilot work examining the use of these programs in an inpatient setting (9) suggests both their acceptability to clinicians and their reliability in agreeing with expert clinical diagnoses, a more extensive field trial is needed to determine whether the potential benefits (i.e., improved diagnoses, complete documentation) outweigh the disadvantages (lengthening the evaluation process).

REFERENCES

1. Lieff JD. *Computer applications in psychiatry.* Washington, DC: American Psychiatric Press, 1987.
2. American Psychiatric Association. *Diagnostic and statistical manual of mental disorders,* 3rd ed. Washington, DC: American Psychiatric Press, 1980.
3. American Psychiatric Association. *Diagnostic and statistical manual of mental disorders,* 3rd ed. revised. Washington, DC: American Psychiatric Press, 1987.
4. Skodol AE, Williams JBW, Spritzer RL, Gibbon M, Kass F. Identifying common errors in the use of DSM-III through supervision. *Hosp Community Psychiatry* 1984;35:251–5.
5. Lipton AA, Simon FS. Psychiatric diagnosis in a state hospital: Manhattan State revisited. *Hosp Community Psychiatry* 1985;36:368–73.
6. Rubinson EP, Asnis GM, Harkavy Friedman JM. Knowledge of the criteria for major depression: a survey of mental health professionals. *J Nerv Ment Dis* 1988;176:480–4.

7. First MB, Williams JBW, Spitzer RL. *DTREE: The electronic DSM-III-R* (computer software, User's Guide, Case Workbook). Washington DC: American Psychiatric Press; Toronto, Canada: Multi-Health System, 1990.
8. First MB, Gibbon M, Williams JBW, Spitzer RL. *Mini-SCID: Computer-administered DMS-III-R screener based on the structured clinical interview for DMS-III-R*, (computer software, User's Guide), Washington, DC: American Psychiatric Press; Toronto, Canada: Multi-Health System, 1990.
9. First MB, Opler LA, Hamilton RM, et al. Utility of computer-assisted DSM-III-R diagnosis. *Compr Psychiatry* (in press).

Psychiatry and Advanced Technologies,
edited by L. Ravizza, F. Bogetto, and
E. Zanalda. Raven Press, Ltd.,
New York © 1993.

14

Applications of Computer and Laser-Disk Technology in Assessing Cognitive Abilities

Anastasia Zadeik–Hipkins, Gary Simson, and Thomas Crook

Advanced Psychometrics Corporation, Bethesda, Maryland 20814-3126

Recent technological advances have provided clinicians and scientists with increasingly precise tools for examining brain structures and neurophysiologic functions thought to underlie cognitive abilities. However, the direct behavioral assessment of these abilities is often a decidedly "low-tech" undertaking. Cognitive abilities are usually assessed by paper-and-pencil performance tests developed decades ago (1,2) or by standardized interviews in which the patient is asked to perform simple cognitive tasks such as identifying the date and place of the interview (3). Both behavioral assessment techniques are designed to measure the ability of individuals to perform critical cognitive tasks of daily life. Unfortunately, interviews tap only abilities on the most basic of tasks, and performance tests usually bear little or no resemblance to everyday cognitive tasks (4). For example, subjects may be asked to remember abstract geometric drawings (5), to arrange blocks in a prescribed pattern (2), or to remember pairings of words that bear no logical relationship to one another (1).

With computer and laser-disk technologies, some of the principal limitations of existing cognitive assessment techniques can be overcome. These technologies enable refined tests to be developed that simulate the actual cognitive tasks of interest to the clinician. In this regard, it may be considered paradoxical that electronic technologies can be used to provide increased clinical relevance and, indeed, to simulate tasks of daily life in a controlled manner within a clinical setting. Of course, aside from the issue of clinical relevance, electronic technologies allow precise control of stimulus and response conditions, construction of complex algorithms and methods of stimulus presentation, exact recording of response time, and automatic scoring and data storage. These factors can be expected to result in greatly improved test reliability and validity.

In 1985 we initiated an effort to develop a battery of tests for cognitive assessment using what was then state-of-the-art computer and laser-disk technology. Our objectives were as follows:

1. To develop measures that relate closely to critical behavioral tasks of daily life dependent on learning and memory.
2. To employ advanced theoretical paradigms of human cognitive processes.
3. To develop measures sensitive both to normal age-related memory loss and to cognitive symptoms seen early in the course of adult-onset cognitive disorders.
4. To develop measures that meet the highest standards of inter-rater and test–retest reliability.
5. To develop tests appropriate for different languages and cultures and therefore appropriate for use in multinational studies.
6. To develop measures available in at least five alternate forms for repeated use in drug trials or longitudinal studies.
7. To develop extensive normative data in different cultures and extensive data on the patterns of deficits seen in different neurologic disorders.
8. To develop measures sensitive to drug effects, including measures based on paradigms of learning and memory found sensitive to drug effects in experimental animals.
9. To develop a battery that would measure empirically and theoretically distinct parameters of cognitive function.

In an effort to meet these objectives, research aimed at test development and refinement was begun in 1985 and is now under way in multiple clinics, universities, and community settings in Belgium, Denmark, England, Finland, France, Holland, Italy, Sweden, and the United States.

Early in our research we became acquainted with the advantages and limitations of laser-disk technology. The first system we used was developed by Panasonic and employed individually programmable laser disks. This meant that each disk was unique. Because our computer programs call live video from the laser disk using reference frames, and because the reference frames were unique on each laser disk, we were forced to rewrite and compile the programs for each new test site. This became a significant problem as our research effort grew.

In 1986 we moved to our current system, in which we employ Pioneer laser disks that are pressed from a master and are therefore identical. This system uses a Pioneer LDV6010A laser-disk player interfaced with an AT&T 6300 personal computer (PC), a SONY monitor with a touch-sensitive membrane, a Panasonic KXP1080i printer, and peripheral devices such as a telephone connected through a DTMF decoder. All of these peripheral devices are controlled by PC programming and many graphic stimuli are stored on the PC as well. All live audio and video are stored on the laser disk.

In testing, the patient is seated in front of the SONY monitor and asked to respond to test stimuli in one of three ways: by touching a designated space or stimuli on the monitor; by responding verbally to the test administrator; or by using familiar manipulanda such as a telephone. Although advanced technology is used, the patient is not asked to utilize manipulanda such as joysticks or keyboards, which might be alien. This is of particular importance in assessing cognition in the elderly or neurologically impaired and, of course, in cultures where such devices are unfamiliar. We believe that although advanced technology offers clear advantages in testing, it is equally important to create a comfortable, nonthreatening testing environment.

The technology is employed at several levels to create clinically useful tests. At the most basic level, we have taken tests that can be administered with low-tech methods and simply used the computer to facilitate test administration and scoring. For example, we employ the classic Bushcke Selective Reminding paradigm (6) but we require subjects to recall a grocery list rather than unrelated common words (7). Similarly, we employ tests based on a classic paired associate learning paradigm. However, instead of the abstract associations such as "Pen-Dark" used in the Wechsler Memory Test (1), we ask subjects to make associations between first and last names "John-Harris," or "Susan-Peterson" (1,7). These two tests illustrate our effort to translate existing paradigms into concrete, common behavioral tasks.

At the next level of technological advancement, we have developed tests that can be administered without our technology but in which the technology greatly enhances the clinical relevance of the measure. For example, in a reaction-time test we measure the time taken by the subject to move a finger from a simulated brake pedal to a simulated gas pedal on the monitor screen as a traffic light on the screen changes between red and green (8). Other noncomputerized manipulanda are available to measure reaction time, but we believe this is a more realistic task than the typical test in which a telegraph key device is employed. Similarly, a realistic digit-recall task can be implemented with a telephone rather than by simply asking a patient to repeat a series of digits verbally (9).

At a third level of test development are those measures that *require* computer technology, e.g., assessing the ability to discriminate between faces seen for the first time and those seen previously. To assess this behavioral phenomenon we have developed two unique paradigms (10,11). In the first test of facial recognition we utilize a model from experimental psychology, delayed nonmatching to sample, in which the subject is presented with a group of facial photographs: first one, then two, then three, up to 25. With each presentation a novel facial photograph is added to the array. The subject's task is to identify the new face by touching it on the screen. In a second facial recognition test a signal detection model is used (8). In this case, the subject is presented with more than 150 facial photographs over 12 min. As each face appears, the subject is asked to identify whether or not the face has been presented before by simply touching an illuminated YES or NO box on the screen. Both of these facial recognition tests would be difficult to administer by hand with any precision. In each case, the computer program executes a complex algorithm for timing and order of facial presentation. For example, the signal detection paradigm requires an equal number of faces to be repeated at various delay intervals and requires that during any given minute of test administration an equal number of repeats for each delay interval must be presented.

At the next level, the computer can no longer handle the presentation of stimuli and laser-disk technology must be employed as well. Live audio and video stimuli, for example, necessitate a laser disk. In one task of topographic memory, the subject is driven through the city of San Diego, California and asked to recall the path taken (12). Live audio and video are also used as stimuli in a realistic test of name–face association (13). This is the most common memory problem across many cultures and, of course, is greatly exaggerated in neurologic disorders such as Alzheimer's disease in which a patient is simply unable to recall the name of a single individual, despite many reintroductions. In measuring this ability, we believe that live video is critical. In fact, in producing the test for each nationality, we re-film natives of the country so that the expressional and acoustic cues common to the culture are available in addition to facial distinctiveness.

Although the tests in our battery are unique because of their design, they would have little utility if they could not discriminate among clinical populations. In fact, they discriminate remarkably well among clinical populations (8,14,15) and among healthy persons of different ages across the adult life span (8,13). The battery also enables us to identify dimensions of cognition (16,17) and different cognitive subtypes of patients (18).

Of course, technology is changing rapidly, and we are applying new interactive digital video technology, using a compact disk in place of the laser disk. Digital Video Interactive ("DVI") technology, developed by Intel, represents the most recent advance in multimedia technology. Rather than combining digital with analog signals, as is done in our current laser-disk system, the DVI system is entirely digital. All live visual or audio stimuli and graphic images are stored in digital format, either on the hard disk of the PC or on compact disk. The implementation of DVI will enable us to overcome some of the difficulties we have noted in the current laser-disk system, particularly the lack of portability and problems related to customized hardware. The new system is much more compact and easily transportable. Finally, the flexibility of the hardware and software will enable future development of much more robust tests and simulations.

The hardware needed for the multimedia DVI environment is as follows:

1. Pro750 Application Development Platform (ADP) 386-25 MHz CPU
2. Sony CDU-520 Half Height Internal CD-ROM player

3. CDC Wren IV 306 MB hard drive
4. Samsung Monochrome 12″ monitor
5. Sony CPD-1390 color monitor for graphics and video display
6. Microsoft serial mouse
7. SS-X6A stereo speakers
8. 1 DVI ActionMedia Delivery Board

Requisite software is DVI software version 2.12 and 386MAX memory manager for 386 systems.

In summary, we believe that recent technological advances have greatly increased the ability of the clinician and scientist to examine not only the structure and neurophysiologic function of the human brain but also the cognitive behavioral abilities of ultimate interest.

REFERENCES

1. Wechsler D. A standardized memory scale for clinical use. *J Psychol* 1945;19:87–95.
2. Wechsler D. *Wechsler adult intelligence scale. Manual.* New York: Psychological Corporation, 1955.
3. Follstein MF, Follstein SE, McHugh PR. Mini-mental state: a practical method for grading the cognitive state of patients for the clinician. *J Psychiatr Res* 1975;12:189–98.
4. Crook T. Cognitive assessment in the year 2000. In: Gaitz C, Niederehe G, Wilson N, eds. *Aging 2000 our health care destiny: psychosocial issues*, New York: Springer-Verlag, 1985: 119–25.
5. Benton AL. *The revised visual retention test*, 4th ed. New York: Psychological Corporation, 1974.
6. Buschke H. Selective reminding for analysis of memory and learning. *J Verb Learn Verb Behav* 1973;12:543–549.
7. Youngjohn JR, Larrabee GJ, Crook TH. First-last names and the grocery list selective reminding test: two computerized measures of everyday verbal learning. *Arch Clin Neuropsychol* 1991;6:287–300.
8. Crook TH, Johnson BA, Larrabee GJ. Evaluation of drugs in Alzheimer's disease and age-associated memory impairment. In: Benkert O, Maier W, Rickles K, eds. *Methodology of the evaluation of psychotropic drugs*. Berlin: Springer-Verlag, 1990:37–55.
9. West RL, Crook TH. Age differences in everyday memory: laboratory analogues of telephone number recall. *Psychol Aging* 1990;5:520–9.
10. Crook TH, Larrabee GJ. Changes in facial recognition memory across the adult life span. *J Gerontol* 1992;47:138–41.
11. Flicker C, Ferris SH, Crook T, Bartus RT. Impaired facial recognition memory in aging and dementia. *Alzheimer's Dis Assoc Disorders* 1990;4:43–54.
12. Zappala G, Martini E, Crook T, Amaducci L. Ecological memory assessment in normal aging. *New Dev Neuropsychol Evaluat* 1989;5:583–94.
13. Crook TH, West RL. Name recall performance across the adult life span. *Br J Psychol* 1990;81:335–349.
14. Ivnik RJ, Malec JF, Sharbrough FW, Cascino GD, Hirschorn KA, Crook TH. Traditional and computerized assessment procedures applied to the evaluation of memory change after temporal lobectomy. *Arch Clin Neuropsychol* 1993;8:69–81.
15. Youngjohn JR, Larrabee GJ, Crook TH. Discriminating age-associated memory impairment and Alzheimer's disease. *Psychol Assessment* 1992;4:54–9.
16. Larrabee GJ, Crook TH. Dimensions of everyday memory in age-associated memory impairment. *Psychol Assessment* 1989;1:92–7.
17. Crook TH, Larrabee GJ. Interrelationships among everyday memory tests: stability of factor structure with age. *Neuropsychology* 1988;2:1–12.
18. Larrabee GJ, Crook TH. Performance subtypes of everyday memory function. *Dev Neuropsychol* 1989;5:267–83.

Psychiatry and Advanced Technologies,
edited by L. Ravizza, F. Bogetto, and
E. Zanalda. Raven Press, Ltd.,
New York © 1993.

15

Design and Implementation of an Integrated Image and Patient Record Database System to Support Schizophrenia Research

*†‡Harry Loats, *Teresa Rippeon, †‡Henry Holcomb, and †Carol Tamminga

Loats Associates Inc., Westminster, Maryland 21157; †University of Maryland Psychiatric Research Center, Baltimore, Maryland 20201; and ‡Johns Hopkins Medical Institution, Bethesda, Maryland

A rapid access database system that incorporates large image data sets is a rapidly growing requirement for both research and clinical medicine. The integration of image data with numerical and descriptive patient and experimental data greatly increases the potential for analysis and understanding of both experiment-derived and clinically derived information. Rapid, interactive review and analysis of large image data sets are required to support scientific experiments and clinical evaluations related to the brain. Current extension of research techniques to the volume analysis of combining functional and structural images gives rise to extremely large image data sets.

A Macintosh-based image database has been developed to accommodate the wide variety of image and support information characterized by combined experiment and clinical protocols. It integrates descriptive and quantitative experiment and numerical results. The system incorporates an object-oriented relational database and is structured to capture sequential and ad libitum nonsequential events. Imaging data sessions and nonimaging protocols, such as physical or psychologic examinations, are included. Information derived from the database analysis is easily exported to standard spreadsheet and statistical programs and to other database systems.

Data storage is implemented on either read–write or WORM optical disks. Large volumes of data are accommodated with a multiple-disk "jukebox." Image data sets are stored in a sequential fashion on WORM optical disks. The capability to automatically accommodate and characterize the wide variety of images derived from various acquisition systems and exhibiting various formats is included. The system data storage is implemented with read–write or write-only optical disks. A large-capacity (6.5 gigabyte), low-cost optical disk jukebox is used for database management.

The system has been designed to provide rapid recall and display of corre-lated sets of magnetic resonance imaging/positron emission tomography/sin-gle-photon emission tomography (MRI/PET/SPECT) images and image-de-rived data for human studies and various tissue section images for primates and other animals, by keying the images to appropriate anatomic atlases. The system can perform user-guided and atlas-aided image sampling and stores the image information in a database which contains pertinent subject and patient information. Specific user input that results in relational informa-tion is standardized by customized pull-down and tear-off lists.

The system concept is currently being used with a 20,000 + image brain-bank, which includes multiple MRI and PET data sets for patients exhibiting multiple diseases and conditions including schizophrenia, stroke, head trauma, epilepsy, Alzheimer's disease (AD), and Huntington's disease (HD). The image databasing concept has also been successfully applied to applica-tions including a pharmacology-oriented multiexperiment database and anal-ysis system and a (endoscopy) clinical trial multiple-user system for a large (400) marmoset colony with record lengths up to 20 years.

INTRODUCTION

Modern psychiatric research and practice are just beginning to reap the benefits of automated computer databases and behaviorally related clinical imaging. The rapid decrease in the cost of computer systems, accompanied by the accelerating increase in computing power, gives rise to capabilities for understanding patient behavior and for coupling image-derived psychiat-ric test data and observational data into meaningful information bases for patient diagnosis.

Specific behavioral paradigms have been developed to contrast the meta-bolic activity of normal and affected subjects. These paradigms rely on the relative stability of cortical metabolic patterns for individuals and classes of individuals. Previously it was impossible to develop an in vivo picture of the metabolic activity of normal subjects or affected individuals. The advent of modern PET technology, coupled with continuous-performance behavioral tasks, provides a new way to assess the condition and state of the brains of schizophrenic patients on and off neuroleptics.

Imaging research programs at the Maryland Psychiatric Research Center (MPRC), specifically aimed at understanding the effects of neuroleptic drugs on low-effective-state schizophrenics, have generated the need for a compre-hensive data analysis system combining patient visit information, psychiatric test data, and image test results in an interactive and user-friendly way. To serve this need, we have developed an integrated image and conventional data analysis system capable of acquisition, analysis, and storage of large data sets derived from multipatient imaging trials. The following describes the makeup and functioning of an integrated image data management system to support schizophrenia research.

PSYCHIATRIC RESEARCH INFORMATION SYSTEM

The Psychiatric Research Information System was designed to support the large patient database in the current outpatient schizophrenia project operated by the MPRC under the direction of Carol Tamminga, M.D. The project incorporates the capability to accommodate longterm patient populations.

The key feature of this program is the combination of MRI and PET images for brain volume and surface analysis with patient-oriented test and descriptive data. For the schizophrenia research projects, the diagnosis of condition and state of patients with psychiatric disease or conditions is implemented by the employment of behavioral pattern vector analysis coupled with computerized visit-oriented information on patient status, condition, and history. The behavioral patterns are analyzed in a computer utility designed to measure volumetric and surface metabolic brain patterns derived from specifically constructed behavioral paradigms using in vivo PET. The behavioral paradigms are constructed to include specific anatomic regions and circuits for which differences between normal subjects and schizophrenic patients have been identified or hypothesized.

BRAIN VOLUME AND SURFACE ANALYSIS

Volume data sets and surface projections are created from multiple-registered serial data sets that span the brain in at least a single axis. Our results to date have used MRI as the primary data set for structural anatomy. PET is the primary data set used to provide functional (metabolic activity) information (Fig. 1). The MRI data set serves as the baseline owing to inherently higher spatial resolution. The new Brain Volume and Surface Mapper is capable of using data from various registered modalities and from various species, from rats to humans.

Axial serial data sets are transformed into three-dimensional volume data sets by spatial resampling (Figs. 2 and 3). A local contrast filter is used to compensate for variable spacing of the different data sets and is particularly useful for landmark recognition enhancement on the primarily structural MRI images. The co-registered volume data sets are then used to derive registered cortical MAPs, co-planar images at different locations and orientations than

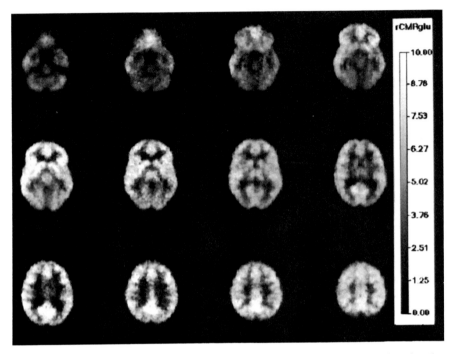

FIG. 1. Images collected for an individual experiment for a normal subject performing the auditory CPT.

would be provided in the primary acquisition plane, and volume region of interests (ROIs) or volume ROI displays (Figs. 4 and 5).

The program that is implemented on a high-resolution Mac II computer provides the following options: cortical surface MAPs centered on user-selected gyri and defining user-selected depth; planar images at any angle centered on arbitrary user-selected locations; volume region of interest; subcortical volume measures with activity centroids; wireframes and shaded surface display of subcortical objects; and location of planar and volume regions of interest in a stereotaxic coordinate system.

The sources of data for the cortical surface image can be: human PET, CT, MRI, and histologic; monkey PET and MRI and histologic; and rat metabolic and histologic.

BRAIN VOLUME/SURFACE ANALYSIS PROGRAM

The Brain Volume/Surface Analysis Program (BVSAP) is a quantitative image analysis program which has developed out of research performed by Loats and Holcomb over the past 4 years and particularly the latter 2 years.

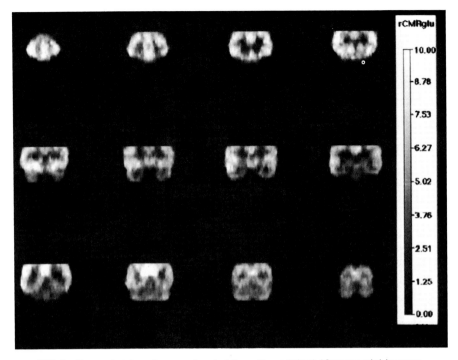

FIG. 2. Coronal data set reconstructed from the original 12 transaxial images.

It is based on co-registered multimodality images, particularly PET, MRI and computed tomography (CT). These capabilities were developed to allow the quantitative analysis of the relatively low-resolution metabolic PET images using the higher-resolution MRI images from the same subjects as ROI templates. This technique was facilitated by the development at Loats Associates of the multi-image quantitative image capabilities for the analysis of PET and other images which is currently in wide general use (MPRC, Johns Hopkins Medical Institution). This capability pioneered the redirected sampling of multi-modality co-planar images.

Specialized Analysis Features

Planar Images

The program allows the user to select image planes from the data set oriented to different axes than those supplied in the original acquisition data set. This enables the user to readjust single planes of data or complete serial data sets to accommodate the detailed analysis of anatomic features not

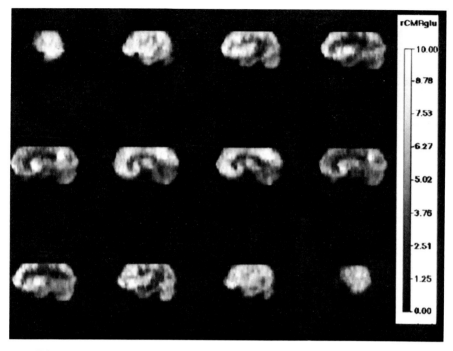

FIG. 3. Sagittal data set reconstructed from the original 12 transaxial images.

coincident with the original acquisition, or to adjust two data sets acquired with different axial alignments.

Volume Region of Interest

The program is designed to facilitate the selection of three-dimensional (volume) ROIs. For specific anatomic targets, this is accomplished under user guidance from the identification of the boundaries of the anatomic feature on serial planar images. Boundary identification can be done with the polygon or edge-detection modes. For the general case of severely unsymmetrical shapes (i.e., ventricles), this identification must be repeated in an orthogonal plane. The other method involves user-adjustable, regular-shaped ROIs (e.g., rectangular parallelepipeds or ellipsoids).

Subcortical Volume

The capability for identifying volume ROIs, as well as the capability of defining volumes in both relative and physical units and the capability to

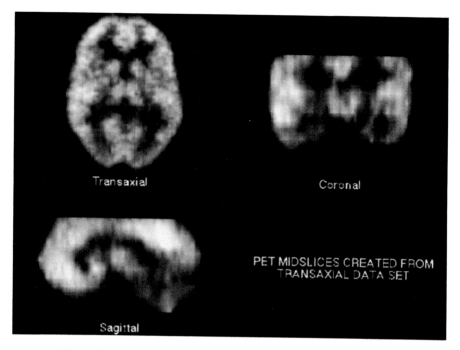

FIG. 4. PET midslices created from the original 12 transaxial images.

redirect the volume sample to other modalities, is included. In addition, the capability to determine both volumetric and activity centroids for the primary and redirected data is included.

Stereotaxic Coordinate System

Stereotaxic coordinate reference is important for comparison with data from other research agencies and studies. It is becoming conventional to reference ROI data to a common stereotaxic reference frame (1). The program provides the capability to express all spatial units relative to a stereotaxic coordinate system selected by the user. To facilitate this, the user specifies both the center of the system and its planar alignment relative to the axes selected in the acquisition data set.

Cortical Surface MAP

Cortical surface MAPs depict the metabolic patterns for carefully con- structed behavioral paradigms. To derive the map, cortical gyral regions are identified from the co-registered MRI images. Because the regions are

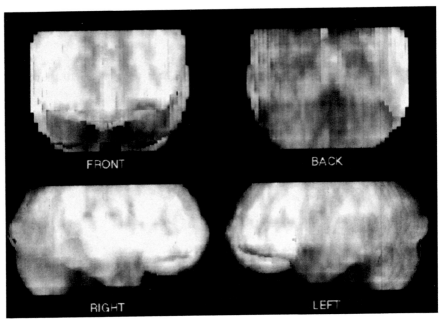

FIG. 5. Equivalent surface images for the PET data set.

registered in a volume sense to the corresponding behaviorally driven PET images, the mean and standard deviations of the metabolic activity of each region can easily be acquired.

VISIT-ORIENTED PATIENT INFORMATION

A Psychiatric Research Information System (PRIS) was developed to provide the features of an integrated database in both a research and a clinical setting. The system integrates pertinent image analysis capabilities with the ability to store both quantitative image data (e.g., metabolic activity parameters) and qualitative descriptive data (e.g., psychiatric test evaluations). The system provides the ability to manage the capture, storage, and analysis of large image data sets. Features are included to easily identify and measure areas of interest on an image and extract the appropriate measurement parameters from the region of interest. In addition, the system allows for easy entry of all descriptive test data. The system manages the collection of all pertinent data into a comprehensive data set, linking all quantitative data with the appropriate descriptive data. In a research setting, the system allows for experiment management of image and de-

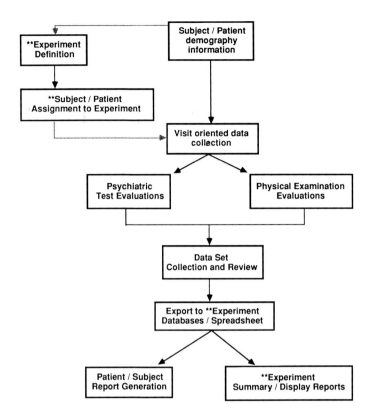

FIG. 6. The main modules of the Psychiatry Information System. The system collects and manages descriptive data as well as quantitative data in such a way as to provide a comprehensive data set for a subject or experiment.

scriptive data collected over various research sites. The database information is easily exportable to standard spreadsheet and statistical programs for additional user-defined analysis. Figure 6 illustrates the main modules of the PRIS.

All information stored in the database is keyed to particular subject events. Experiment data sets can be extracted from the database by making an appropriate subject assignment to an experiment protocol. Subject information stored in the database includes subject identification, date of birth, sex, among other data.

Event-oriented information is collected for both psychiatric tests, physical examination imaging sessions, and specific behavioral paradigms (Fig. 7). Qualitative psychiatric test results are recorded in such a way to constrain

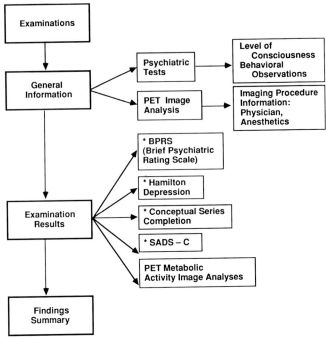

FIG. 7. Visit information; all information is saved in an event-oriented fashion. Various types of events can be stored in the database and are accounted for in a similar manner; therefore, similar functions are used in a collection of all events.

the results to be as uniform as possible and easy to use in statistical analysis by a commercial spreadsheet. For every testing session, the following information is recorded: general information concerning level of consciousness and behavior, examination test results for all standard test classes, and examination summary and diagnosis information.

Figure 8 illustrates entry of a psychiatric test evaluation of higher cognitive functions of a schizophrenic. Data entry of appropriate response levels is accomplished via selection from pop-up lists. All data are translated to a quantitative level, if possible, for use in plotting and comparing results.

Evaluation of higher cognitive functions often shows the early effects of cortical damage. Unsatisfactory completion of these tests may arise before more basic processes of attention, language, and memory are impaired. Subsequent physical evaluation of cortical damage via an imaging session can be related to this psychiatric test evaluation in the database to show the progression of cortical damage.

Patient image analysis, including measurements of metabolic activity pat-

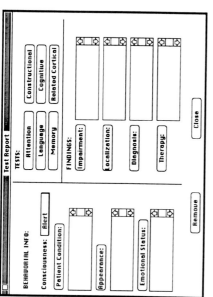

FIG. 8. The Psychiatric Information System provides ease of use in data entry for descriptive data. Data are entered via pop-up lists, pull-down menus, and buttons. In addition, qualitative data are translated to quantitative levels, if possible, for use in comparison of results.

terns, can be completed after the appropriate cortical surfaces have been created from the image data sets (see previous section). A custom "atlas" is created for each subject so that the computer will automatically measure the appropriate brain region over various imaging sessions. This is accomplished by "registering" co-planar stereotaxic atlases of a human brain region to a subject MRI image slice region; the user must outline each brain region for the subject and store this atlas in the database. Subsequent PET functional images can be displayed, and by choosing a particular region on the subject MRI atlas, the corresponding region on the PET image is measured. Various parameters stored in the database include transmission, optical density, area, perimeter, and texture characteristics. Figures 9 and 10 show cortical surface maps that would be used in the evaluation of activity in a region of the brain based on the selection of the region from the subject's cortical surface atlas.

A summary review can be made of all physical evaluations that are recorded in the database. A composite view of all events, with the associated images used in analysis for the appropriate event, are displayed. Various measurement parameters can then be plotted to follow activity patterns over time. In addition, visit/event information can be reviewed quickly within the composite review.

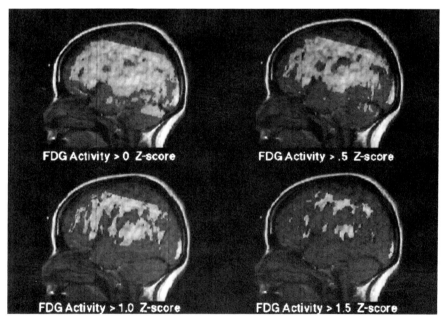

FIG. 9. A series of overlays depicting the spatial distribution of z-scored hyperactivity for the on-neuroleptics condition for a schizophrenic subject performing the continuous-attention visual task.

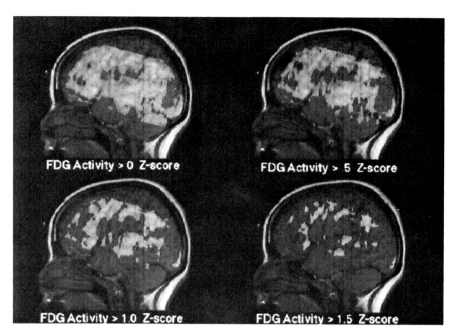

FIG. 10. PET–MRI cortical overlay for Study 2, the off-neuroleptics condition for a schizophrenic subject performing the continuous-attention visual task.

Test reports are completed for the various types of events recorded in the database. Behavioral test and psychiatric test report hardcopy output can be obtained from the system. In addition, blood curves can be generated for blood tests, and summary reviews of physical evaluations can be made.

Full image analysis capabilities are included in the program. These include annotation and measurement of regions of interest, calibration of the region of interest to a known area, resampling of an ROI and image/feature enhancement (e.g., application of various filters to images for smoothing, edging, etc. and application of various palettes to the image). Various tools have been developed for the annotation of a region of interest, including polygon and freehand drawing.

All visit information can be exported to an external database manager or spreadsheet package. Further subject or experiment analysis can be completed in these commercial packages. Hamilton Anxiety and MPRC test results are shown in Fig. 11. These results were exported to and plotted in a commercial statistics/graphing package. The MPRC Involuntary Movement results show the clustering of high levels of impairment in the facial and upper limb regions. These results are consistent with the disease demonstrated by this particular patient.

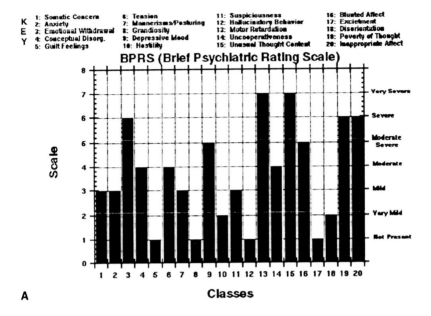

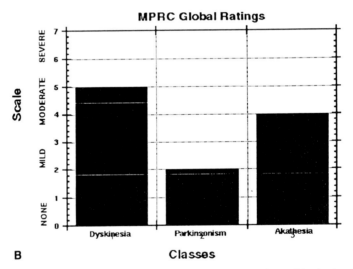

FIG. 11. Qualitative data are translated to quantitative levels, if possible, in the database. Test results are exported from the database to spreadsheets/grafting packages and plotted.

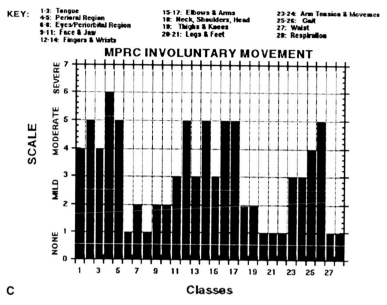

KEY:
1-3: Tongue
4-5: Perioral Region
6-8: Eyes/Periorbital Region
9-11: Face & Jaw
12-14: Fingers & Wrists

15-17: Elbows & Arms
18: Neck, Shoulders, Head
19: Thighs & Knees
20-21: Legs & Feet

23-24: Arm Tension & Movemes
25-26: Gait
27: Waist
28: Respiration

FIG. 11. *Continued.*

CONCLUSIONS

An interactive information system has been developed to support both clinical evaluation and research programs for a large, patient-oriented schizophrenia project. Descriptive, psychiatric test, and imaging data are combined in a patient/visit-oriented, computerized database and information system. The system is built around an automated visit-oriented database which combines the imaging data with all event-oriented information related to the patient population. This system also allows the incorporation of data and images from corollary animal research programs.

REFERENCE

1. Fox, PT, Purlmutter JS, Raichle ME. A stereotactic method of anatomical localization for positron emission tomography. *J Comput Assist Tomography* 1985;9:141–153.

Psychiatry and Advanced Technologies,
edited by L. Ravizza, F. Bogetto, and
E. Zanalda. Raven Press, Ltd.,
New York © 1993.

16

Expert Systems as Decisional Support in Psychiatry

P. Pancheri and P. L. Marconi

III Psychiatric Clinic, University of Rome "La Sapienza," 00185 Rome, Italy

The introduction of neuroleptic drugs during the early 1950s enabled us to face the problem of treatment of schizophrenia with alternatives to physical restriction or electroconvulsive therapy.

Study of the pharmacodynamic activity of neuroleptic drugs, the marked analogy between schizophrenic delusions and hallucinations on the one hand and those induced by the administration of amphetamine on the other (1), and studies on cerebral dopamine receptor density, both postmortem (2) and in vivo, with positron-emission tomography (PET) technique (3) support the hypothesis that at the basis of schizophrenic symptomatology is a pathogenetic mechanism related to dopaminergic hyperactivity. The dopamine hypothesis of schizophrenia is presently receiving general consensus but does not explain some features associated with this disease.

Neuroleptic drugs, all of which have some degree of antidopaminergic activity, are only partially effective in relieving the symptoms of schizophrenia. Furthermore, their side effects may iatrogenically induce and/or maintain negative schizophrenic symptoms. Regarding this partial ineffectiveness, it should be observed that such drugs appear to be effective mainly in Crow's type I schizophrenic syndrome, which is characterized by the so-called "positive" schizophrenic symptoms, such as delusions, hallucinations, and formal thought disorder. Neuroleptic therapy does not appear to influence the symptomatic core of Crow's type II schizophrenic syndrome, which typically involves "negative" symptoms such as affective flattening and blunting, impoverished speech, apathy, anhedonia, and social and emotional withdrawal. Such considerations, as well as critical re-examination of the facts in favor of the dopamine hypothesis of schizophrenia, promoted the search for more integrated approaches to the biochemistry and treatment of schizophrenia.

In an attempt to understand better the biochemistry of schizophrenia, interest has been directed towards neurotransmitter systems other than that of dopamine. Furthermore, overall "transmitter–receptor" system functioning was considered to be responsible for both physiologic and pathologic behavior instead of merely synaptic neurotransmitter concentration. The importance of the receptor mechanism has been increasingly recognized in recent years. Therefore, the original dopamine hypothesis of schizophrenia is now described in terms of pre- and postsynaptic receptor activity. Because such receptor activity is under the influence of nondopaminergic factors, the receptor-centered approach permits the introduction and integration into the dopaminergic model of other factors that exert a modulatory action on dopamine receptor activity.

This is the case of the neuropeptides, which exert their action over longer time intervals as compared with classic neurotransmitter activity. In the context of the pathogenetic hypotheses of schizophrenia, peptides such as cholecystokinin (in particular its C-terminal octapeptide fragment) (4) and gamma-endorphin (its des-Tyr_1 or desenkephalin fragments) (5) have found a place in the pathogenetic chain of this disorder. However, the low intensity or short duration of their clinical effects in schizophrenia, the relatively high cost of peptide products, and their unpredictability and/or their difficulty in crossing the blood–brain barrier do not currently support their widespread clinical use.

Studies on classic neurotransmitters have yielded no clear-cut results regarding the GABAergic (6) and cholinergic systems (7); a greater, albeit apparently secondary involvement, has been advocated for the noradrenergic system (8).

A greater interest has focused on the serotonergic system. On the basis of the symptoms induced by lysergic acid diethylamide (LSD), a drug once thought to be a pure serotonergic agonist, pathogenetic hypotheses were proposed during the 1960s which implicated serotonin in the onset of schizophrenic symptoms. At that time, however, overall neurotransmitter activity and not area-specific transmitter–receptor interactions were considered, a fact that may partially explain the uncertain results obtained by measuring total post-mortem brain serotonin in schizophrenics (9). An abnormality in the serotonergic system, at least in one subpopulation of schizophrenic patients, is suggested by the reduction of 5-hydroxyindoleacetic acid (5-HIAA) levels in the cerebrospinal fluid of schizophrenics with prevalent negative symptomatology and cerebral ventricular enlargement, found in one study (10).

Perhaps the most interesting data are those deriving from recent studies of clinical pharmacology, because they enable us to consider the final clinical effect of pharmacologic perturbations on serotonergic systems.

Pipamperone has been commercially available for more than 20 years. It is characterized by significant anti-D_2 and anti–5-HT_2 activity. Clinically, it possesses "anti-autistic and resocializing" properties, but such properties have yet to be adequately assessed. Therefore, the eventual correlation between antiserotoninergic activity and its efficacy in treatment of negative schizophrenic symptomatology is purely speculative (11).

Clozapine is an atypical antipsychotic drug, already marketed in some countries, which possesses significant anti–5-HT$_2$ and anti-D$_1$, -D$_2$ and -D$_3$ activity preferentially exerted on mesocorticolimbic tracts. In various clinical studies, clozapine was shown to be effective in improving schizophrenic patients resistant to other treatments. Furthermore, it is devoid of the typical side effects of neuroleptics, such as extrapyramidal and neuroendocrine (hyperprolactinemia) effects. However, the pharmacodynamic profile of clozapine is not limited to the dopaminergic and serotonergic systems; this renders the drug an inadequate probe for investigating the role of serotonin in schizophrenic conditions (11).

Ritanserin, on the other hand, is a molecule shown to possess prominent antiserotoninergic activity, especially on 5-HT$_2$ receptors, antagonizing the action of LSD (a partial 5-HT$_{1c}$/5-HT$_2$ agonist). Clinical studies of this drug showed not only anxiolytic activity on some components of anxiety but an antidepressant action as well (the latter led some authors to propose the term "thymosthenic" for this drug). For the purposes of the present report, it should be noted that this drug, coadministered to schizophrenic patients with neuroleptics, improved "negative" symptomatology significantly more than neuroleptics alone (11).

Risperidone has been shown to possess high anti–5-HT$_2$ activity as well as lower but significant antidopaminergic activity in basic pharmacologic studies. Its clinical use in open and double-blind controlled studies revealed significant antipsychotic activity also, parallel to a positive effect on negative symptomatology and an absence of extrapyramidal side effects (11).

These data led to postulation of a role for serotonergic systems in negative symptomatology of schizophrenia, probably exerted through modulation of cortical dopaminergic activity, although the importance of complex interactions between the two systems in other brain areas cannot be excluded. At present, an interpretive model has been proposed that hypothesizes the existence of frontal dopaminergic hypoactivity associated with mesolimbic dopaminergic hyperactivity in the pathogenesis of schizophrenia. The former would be related to elevated 5-HT$_2$/D$_2$ activity ratio and negative symptomatology (11).

In this perspective, therefore the principal clinical activity of a neuroleptic drug is as an antipsychotic, which correlates with its anti-D$_2$ activity and may be related to some aspect of its anti-D$_1$ activity. The further discrimination of therapeutic activity against mainly positive versus negative symptomatology requires a thorough evaluation of such drugs regarding their anti–5-HT$_2$ and anti-D$_2$/anti-D$_3$ activity (11).

The pharmacodynamic activity of neuroleptics is not confined to the dopaminergic and serotoninergic systems but also extends to the cholinergic, noradrenergic, and histaminergic systems. Such collateral activities differ among the various neuroleptic drugs; therefore, their clinical effect is related not only to the intensity of such activities but also to the dose regimen, which is correlated to anti-D_2 activity (12). Incorrect administration of such drugs bears the risk of transforming the acute clinical picture in chronic, neuroleptic-induced situations, characterized by motor retardation, weakness, sleepiness and, at times, mental confusion, symptoms that are likely to trigger dangerous vicious circles in which neuroleptic-induced symptomatology, misinterpreted as drug inefficacy, may prompt dose increases with consequent worsening of collateral symptomatology (12). Hence, it is necessary to consider the entire clinical picture in the choice of a neuroleptic, not only to minimize the emergence of side effects but eventually to therapeutically exploit its collateral activities, e.g., to diminish agitation, insomnia, or extrapyramidal symptoms (12).

With regard to the collateral activities of administered neuroleptics, clinical practice already tends to consider them heuristically. However, the descriptions of the various neuroleptic drugs are largely undefined, whereas the number of options presently considered constitute only a small part of those actually available. In Italy, more than 20 molecules are presently available that possess neuroleptic activity. Their diverse pharmacodynamic profiles are distributed throughout such a wide range of activities that they can be used for almost individually targeted therapy. Unfortunately, the average psychiatrist usually considers only five or six of these agents in treating schizophrenic patients.

Furthermore, the previously described interpretive model offers the possibility to define a further criterion for the choice of neuroleptic drugs, based on the 5-HT_2/D_2 activity ratio and aiming at optimizing the effect on negative symptomatology.

It is therefore clear that the clinical problem of drug treatment in schizophrenia is complex. As a consequence, the adoption of decisional support instruments based on artificial intelligence (AI) techniques may help to better resolve problems posed by complex clinical cases, thus enhancing the index of efficacy of drug treatment. In fact, through the construction of expert systems (ES), such techniques permit reproduction of the complexity of some aspects of human reasoning on a computer, maintaining its heuristic characteristics but at the same time ensuring the completeness of the assessment, a coherent respect of the protocols, and the possibility of a "natural" access to the rationale at the base of every choice.

AIMS OF THE STUDY

The Beta Project continues our experience begun with the Alpha Project in the context of applications of AI in psychiatry. The preceding experience focused on pharmacologic treatment of panic attacks and stressed the importance of correct formalization of preknowledge to achieve a prototype with adequate flexibility. As was the case with the Alpha Project, the interest in such tools stemmed from the possibility to formalize heuristic clinical knowledge according to modalities that permit immediate operative use. The choice of a syndromic-type knowledge is strictly connected to these considerations, first because it derives from empirical clinical experience and second because psychiatry generally lacks widely accepted interpretive models (13).

The first aim of the Beta Project is to define a logical connection (preknowledge) that allows operationalization of the heuristic rules for assessing the different therapeutic options. The structure thus created has been utilized to achieve the second aim of the project, i.e., the choice of the most adequate neuroleptic therapy, based on the clinical picture and pharmacodynamic drug profile, in the framework of the 5-HT/DA hypothesis of the pathogenesis of schizophrenic conditions.

Regarding this last point, the system may also constitute a useful tool for the evaluation of decisional consequences deriving from the application of a group of heuristic rules that constitutes a clinical operative translation compatible with a syndromic approach to an interpretive model of schizophrenia (in our case, the model based on the $5\text{-HT}_2/\text{D}_2$ activity ratio).

THE INSTRUMENTS: NEXPERT OBJECT

The commercially developed environment NEXPERT Object, produced by Neuron Data, Palo Alto, CA was used for realization of the project (16). This shell permits the realization of ES, whose knowledge structure has been conceived for the symbolic creation, manipulation, and destruction of abstract entities called "objects." Objects can correspond to real entities of the external world or to abstract conceptual entities. Knowledge Bases (KBs) created with NEXPERT Object contain the knowledge to work with objects; this knowledge is formalized in two different modalities.

The first modality is realized on a descriptive level and structures knowledge through a classification system in which objects can be identified by their properties. The classification system therefore permits collections of objects that share properties of the same type in homogeneous sets (classes). Furthermore, objects can be related to other objects that constitute one of their own components (e.g., a tissue as related to an organ) or to the whole to which they belong (e.g., example, the organism as related to a single organ). In turn, classes can be grouped according to similar criteria into higher-order classes (e.g., the butyrophenone class, identified on the basis of chemical structure, belongs to the class of neuroleptics, which is identified on the basis of clinical activity). Through this descriptive level, properties and property values of objects can be deduced as a function of their own definition.

The second modality consists of the representation of knowledge through a set of rules that are hierarchically organized at the level of reasoning. Such hierarchical organization permits the solution of a problem (goal) to be broken down into the solution of subproblems (subgoals). From an operative viewpoint, the atom of knowledge at this level is not the object but the "fact." The latter is defined as the value of a property of an object belonging to one or more sets of objects (classes). The conceptual hinge of the entire KB, however, remains the object. The rules on the level of reasoning are constituted from relations between facts of the type:

IF a certain antecedent is true

THEN a certain consequent is true

(structure according to production rule format).

Production rules are composed of two parts: the antecedent and the consequent. The antecedent is the set of facts that render the conclusions of the rule likely. The consequent is constituted from the set of facts which can be deduced as probable if the conditions of the antecedent are true. In NEXPERT Object, the consequent of rules is further broken down into the logical consequence (the hypothesis or the subgoal under consideration) and operative consequences. For the purpose of the reasoning process, the practical difference between the two types of consequents is that hypotheses that may also be present in the antecedent allow backward chaining of different rules to break the problem down into various subproblems, whereas the operative consequences propagate forward the effect of their own actions, thereby activating the antecedents of other rules until an exhaustive assessment of all derivable consequences is obtained. NEXPERT Object presents a remarkable facilitation of the complete procedure of knowledge formalization, supplying an advanced interface that frees the user from the most difficult aspects of syntax and grammar constraints required by the Inferential Engine (IE). However, it does not present a management of certainty factors, which instead should be managed with ad hoc procedures defined by the user. It is possible to manage incomplete information by undefined credibilities of the "I do not know" type. NEXPERT Object is capable of distinguishing "I do not know" because it was "not investigated" (UNKNOWN) from "I do not know" because of "lack of available information" (NOT KNOWN).

The system is written in C language and is widely open to integration with external systems, for example, the principal Data Management Systems, by which known facts are retrievable and conclusions can be stored.

NEXPERT Object can operate both in Apple Macintosh and in IBM-compatible personal computers.

RESULTS

The Logical–Conceptual Structure of Beta Knowledge Base

Beta reaches its conclusions by evaluating available drugs through a heuristic comparison between their pharmacodynamic profile and the facts of the clinical context. Such comparison uses the knowledge contained in KB and formalized in its descriptive structures and its production rules. This knowledge can be conceptually broken down into blocks hierarchically ordered according to the subproblems faced. As in the organigram of any operative organization, we have a *strategic, apical level*, in which the general objectives of the intervention are defined, a *tactic, intermediate level*, in which strategic indications are translated into specific operative choices, and an *executive peripheral level*, in which decisions of superior levels are translated into the concrete performance of actions.

The hierarchically most elevated knowledge block defines therapy in its strategic aspects, i.e., how many interventions to perform, with which objectives, and with which instruments. These decisions are made on the basis of heuristic rules that take into account the general characteristics of the problem (general operative context). First, diagnosis is considered, which per se constitutes the structuring of a clinical problem within a therapeutic perspective. Second, the principal aspects of the psychiatric clinical picture are considered; these allow definition of the specific objectives of every intervention along with the general nature of the problem. The indication for usable tools is provided in terms of pharmacologic classes and is arrived at on the basis of diagnosis and of the principal objective of every intervention.

In the present prototype, the system is assumed to operate in the particular case of a patient with a schizophrenic condition, in which the problem is to choose the most indicated neuroleptic drug. Therefore, the strategic aim that reaches the inferior level is to select a neuroleptic drug for an antipsychotic intervention (first-level subgoal).

The subsequent subgoal of this intervention (second-level subgoal) can be either to reduce negative symptomatology or to minimize the patient's activation, accordingly to the relation observed between negative and positive symptoms. For definition of such a subgoal, therefore, heuristic decisional elements intervene, which refer to the aforementioned interpretive model of schizophrenic conditions.

Finally, the third-level subgoal is defined on the basis of other clinical findings. In fact, this level defines the traits toward which to further direct the intervention, optimizing the clinical impact of collateral neuroleptic drug activities.

In the prototype presently realized, the heuristic rules that support the consideration at the base of the definition of such subgoals are not yet active, and the same objects are left to be defined by the user. The user can enter them into a file, from which they can be read directly by the system, or can communicate them interactively to the system during consultation.

Once the type of intervention, drug class, and objectives are defined, they must be translated into concrete therapeutic action. For this, it is necessary that such directives are transformed in tactic operations of choice. The realization of the whole requires that such informative criteria guide the evaluation of the different options of choice in relation to the context of intervention, as evaluated in all its specific components. Such components concern the patients' current condition (psychiatric status, neurologic and physical examination), history (both psychiatric and medical), and current therapies (psychopharmacologic and specifics of other specialities).

However, heuristic rules provided by experts, as a rationalization of their considerations, do not cover exhaustively the knowledge necessary for making such choices. Instead, these groups of rules constitute a cluster placed around a central skeleton represented by preknowledge, which is necessary to connect them logically in a congruent KB. Thus, a kind of logical connective has been defined in Beta (preknowledge) capable of ordering different groups of rules on the basis of the level of subgoals they refer to and of orienting them towards the ultimate aim, i.e., choice of the best drug.

The different groups of assessing rules are logically connected on the basis of the level to which their subgoals belong. Thus, the different implicit operations are ordered according to a logical sequence, that can provide a sense of the different goals of every intervention. Therefore, the meaning of an *inclusive* criterion is attributed to the first-level subgoal; that is, the drugs that are adequate for achieving it are included in the list of drugs to consider for the subsequent evaluations.

The meaning of an *exclusive* criterion is attributed to the second-level subgoal; this defines which clinical elements and which pharmacodynamic characteristics must be compared to exclude clinically inadequate drugs. To this same level converge other rule clusters that concern other aspects of the clinical context (status, history, current treatments) that may single out absolute contraindications to the use of a given drug.

To the third-level subgoal is attributed a meaning of assessment criterion; this subgoal defines the weight of the evaluation coefficient attributed to the considerations that permit a preferential ordering between the options still remaining in the list. The second-level subgoal also possesses an assessment criterion meaning of this type that is consistently elicited with that of the third level. In this way, the second- and third-level subgoals concur in defining preference order between the different therapeutic options, thus contributing to achievement of the final goal. The latter is subsequently reached by comparing the conclusions of this process with the eventual psychopharmacologic therapy, evaluated in its efficacy with regard to both to dosage and treatment duration.

The system allows a feedback control of the decision process: if evaluations prove inadequate to pursue the goal of the process of choice, the latter is automatically revised according to criteria modified in restrictiveness. The process may thus be recursive until an adequate result is achieved, and involves only those evaluations that concern psychiatric status. This last point stems from the fact that other evaluation groups usually involve factors related to the safety of therapy, and the system assumes as its own absolute metarule the principle of "primum non nocere" (first do no harm); in this regard, no "variations of restrictivity" are available.

The prototype presently realized is limited to the choice of the most adequate drug. However, the project entails the formalization of knowledge related to the definition of the therapeutic protocol of the chosen drug and, thereafter, writing of a prescription, in the same way as was the case with the Alpha Project (15–17). The prescription is the moment in which the tactical procedures of the various interventions are translated into a project of therapeutic actions, which realization is usually forwarded to the patient or to the paramedical personnel. The value of automatic prescription is both that of eliciting the meaning of tactical indications deduced from the system until the final act of the consultation (therapeutic prescription), as well as that of providing a detailed written prescription for the patient. This is, in fact, to contain not only an elicitation of therapeutic schemes for all days before reaching maintenance dosage, but also indications about the active principle (for an international prescription), side effects, and warnings to the patient about pharmacologic and/or dietary interactions.

The Heuristic Nucleus of Evaluation of the Clinical Context

Turning our attention to the structures that bear knowledge sustaining the clinical heuristic evaluations, KB is presently structured to contain the rules necessary to take into consideration six specific clinical contexts: (i) the psychiatric clinical picture; (ii) psychiatric history; (iii) medical clinical picture; (iv) medical history; (v) present medically centered pharmacotherapy; and (vi) present psychiatrically centered pharmacotherapy.

At present, only the rules related to the evaluation of neuroleptics on the basis of the clinical psychiatric picture have been introduced in the KB. This cluster of explicit knowledge constitutes the heuristic for neuroleptic drug choice criteria on the basis of elements of psychiatric status.

The heuristic assumption at the base of relations between pharmacodynamic characteristics and clinical traits derives both from the previously explained interpretive model of schizophrenic conditions, and from clinical experience. The first offers a rationale for the connection between antiserotonergic activity and the clinical effect on negative symptoms, or between the $5\text{-HT}_2/D_2$ activity ratio and the relationship between negative and positive symptoms. Clinical experience and basic pharmacologic studies provide evidence for a relationship between anticholinergic activity and anti-Parkinson effect, as well as between antihistaminic activity and sleep induction. Instead, the assumption that antinoradrenergic activity is related to inhibition of motor activity and asthenia is purely heuristic and founded on personal opinion. Such heuristic relations thus enable comparison of the clinical profile of the patient with the pharmacodynamic profile of the drug. This comparison takes place at two levels: at one level, drugs that are inadequate to the clinical context are excluded; at the other level, "surviving" drugs are ordered according to preference value (certainty factor).

In the comparison between the pharmacodynamic profile of a drug and the clinical picture presented by a patient, there is an implicit subjective evaluation of intensity related to two reference populations: that of prescribable drugs and that of patients affected by the same disease. This relative evaluation renders operational an affirmation of the following type:

IF a patient has an "elevated intensity" of negative symptoms

THEN
choose the drug that possesses "elevated" antiserotonergic "activity."

An "elevated intensity" (or "elevated activity") means, for example, an intensity ranking towards the upper extreme of the intensity (or activity) distribution curve in the population considered. A possible way to express this ranking is the standard score. In Beta, the T-transformation of standard scores has been used, thus obtaining always positive values. This was necessary because the plus or minus signs are used with a different symbolic meaning from the usual one in pharmacodynamics. In fact, they are used to indicate whether the drug exerts an agonistic or antagonistic activity on a receptor, respectively.

Clinical symptomatology can also be expressed in T-scores, using assessment scales for quantification. Alternatively, the user can directly supply to the system his or her own judgment of symptom intensity on a severity scale ranging from 0 to 100.

At present, the only requirement for the user is to indicate the intensity of clinical symptomatology, either objectively or subjectively defined, whereas information regarding the pharmacological side can be obtained autonomously by the system by calculating pharmacodynamic activity T-scores of the prescribable drugs present in the data base. This calculation is repeated at every consultation by reading in a data base the names and the properties of drugs. This ensures flexibility of the system. In fact, in this way the possibility of updating the list of drugs is guaranteed without implying any modification in KB. To reach the final score, the system first calculates the ratio between the affinity of the considered receptor and the affinity of the receptor correlated with the first-level subgoal; the value thus obtained is transformed into a natural logarithm to improve discrimination of the various drugs at the extremes of the curve. Thus, the transformation in T-scores (Ts) is brought about based on the following formula:

$$Ts = [(U_o - U_m)/SD)*10] + 50$$

where U_o is the original value, U_m is the mean value in the reference population, and SD is standard deviation.

The exclusion of inadequate drugs is then based on the comparison between pharmacodynamic and clinical T-scores. Prescribable drugs are similarly evaluated. The difference is that during exclusion, all drugs below a critical pharmacodynamic T-score level are excluded, whereas during "survivor" evaluation, drugs are preferred (increasing their advisability by a factor CF) when their pharmacodynamic T-score is within a given range. The ranking of the different thresholds based on T-scores of correlated clinical variables is modifiable on the basis of the final result of the evaluation. The eventual modification is at the basis of the revision of the evaluation process just mentioned.

SIMULATION OF A CLINICAL PROBLEM

Now let us consider a hypothetic case in which the clinical picture is characterized by the prevalence of negative symptomatology. We will follow the Beta decisional process on the descriptive level to see how the events, triggered by the active rules at the reasoning level, evolve the state of knowledge about known facts.

The system first receives the strategic indications for the intervention (Fig. 1a); at present these are retrieved from a data base where they were previously stored by the user. Then Beta reads from the pharmacologic archives all available psychopharmacologic substances (Fig. 1b) and introduces into the list of the prescribable drugs those whose pharmacodynamic activity is in agreement with the first-level subgoal. Targets of this inclusion are drugs with antidopaminergic activity, clinically associated with an antipsychotic effect (neuroleptic drugs).

At this point the system calculates pharmacodynamic T-scores and excludes from the list all drugs with an anti–5-HT$_2$/anti-D$_2$ activity ratio that is inadequate for the clinical picture. In particular, the second-level subgoal being a reduction in negative symptomatology, in this case only two drugs with elevated anti–5-HT$_2$/anti-D$_2$ activity ratio remain in the list (in this example, clorpromazine clozapine).

The system thereafter begins to evaluate these two drugs in relation to the different clinical symptoms, giving a higher weight to symptoms correlated with the second- and third-level subgoals (in this case, to negative and extrapyramidal symptoms). To adequately discriminate between the two drugs, in the example the system must reconsider its own evaluations three times,

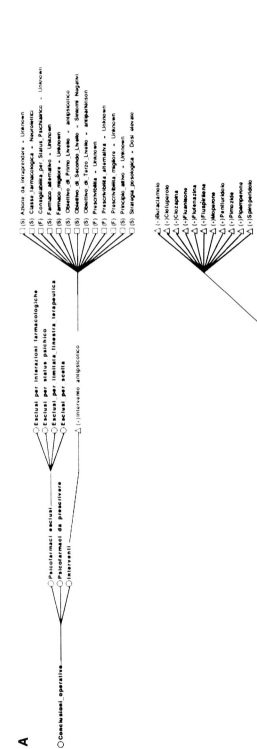

A

○ Conclusioni_operative

○ Psicofarmaci esclusi
○ Psicofarmaci da prescrivere
○ Interventi

Esclusi per interazioni farmacologiche
Esclusi per status psichico
Esclusi per limitata_finestra terapeutica
Esclusi per scelta

△ (-)interveno antipsicotico

(S) Azione da intraprendere – Unknown
(S) Classe farmacologica – Neurolettici
(F) Consigliabilita per Status_Psichiatrico – Unknown
(S) Farmaco_alternativo – Unknown
(S) Farmaco_migliore – Unknown
(S) Obiettivo_di_Primo_Livello – antipsicotico
(S) Obiettivo_di_Secondo_Livello – Sintomi Negativi
(S) Obiettivo_di_Terzo_Livello – antiparkinson
(F) Prescrivibilita – Unknown
(F) Prescrivibilita alternativa – Unknown
(F) Prescrivibilita migliore – Unknown
(F) Principio attivo – Unknown
(S) Strategia_posologica – Dosi elevate

△ (-)Butaclamolo
△ (-)Cloluperolo
△ (-)Clozapina
△ (+)Fluanisone
△ (+)Flufenazina
△ (+)Fluspirilene
△ (+)Moperone
△ (+)Penfluridolo
△ (+)Pimozide
△ (-)Pipamperone
△ (-)Spiroperidolo

B

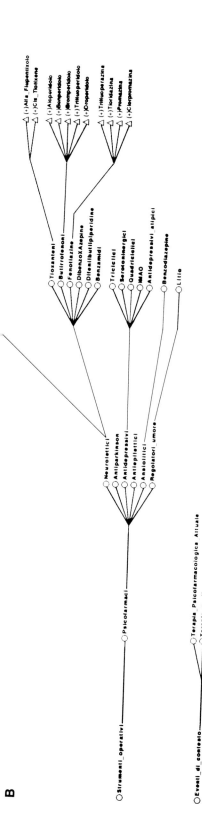

FIG. 1. All the entities of Beta KB are symbols. The main logic entities of Beta KB are objects which are represented in figures as triangles followed by a symbolic name (it is possible to use every kind of name, except a few reserved words). A class (represented in figures by a circle + symbolic name) is a set of objects that share one or more common proprieties (represented by a square + symbolic name + their present value). The logic linkages between objects, classes and attributes are represented as lines in the figures. In Beta KB, objects are not predefined but are dynamically created run time. In this figure we can see an early state of knowledge in the descriptive plane during a test session. (**A**) In the class of "conclusioni operative" ("operational conclusions") the object "intervento antipsicotico" is classified ("antipsychotic intervention"), which is described by the values of its proprieties which represent the strategic indication taken into account for the choice of the best drug. (**B**) In the class "Strumenti operativi" ("tools") objects are classified as the drugs available in the database. Drugs are subclassified by Beta following both clinical and chemical criteria. Objects representing drugs are named using Italian names as symbols.

169

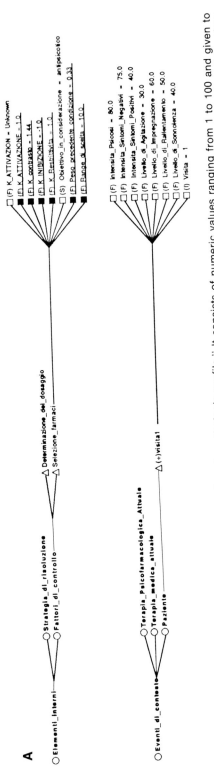

FIG. 2. The present clinical case is described as "psychopathologic profile." It consists of numeric values ranging from 1 to 100 and given to attributes representing psychopathologic dimensions. (**A**) In the present version of Beta KB, the clinical case is classified as a member of the class "paziente" ("patient"). (**B**) In the class of "conclusioni operative" ("operational conclusions") many drugs are excluded taking into account the present psychopathologic profile and they are subclassified as "esclusi per status psichico" ("excluded for psychic state"). Clozapine and chlorpromazine remain classified as "farmaci da prescrivere" ("prescriptable drugs"). They are also classified as available drugs for present intervention ("intervento antipsicotico" = "antipsychotic intervention"). The different rank in which they are ordered for final choice is reached taking into account the clinical picture and the present value of the "fattori di controllo" ("control factors") which determine the strength of discrimination criteria between drugs (see **A**).

170

B

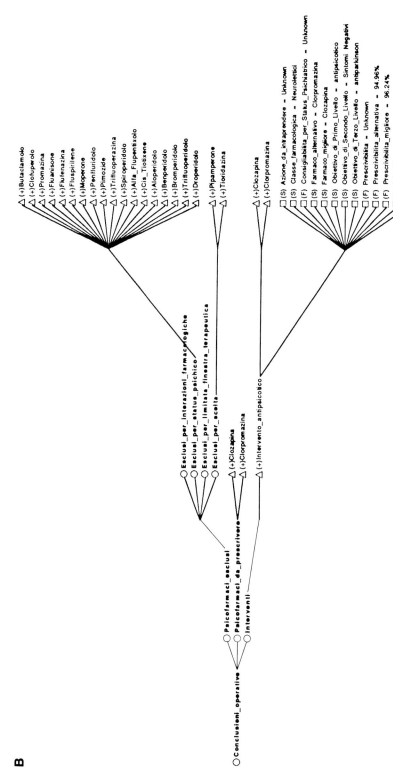

△ (+)Butaclamolo
△ (+)Clofuperolo
△ (+)Promazina
△ (+)Fluanisone
△ (+)Flufenazina
△ (+)Fluspirilene
△ (+)Moperone
△ (+)Pentluridolo
△ (+)Pimozide
△ (+)Trifluoperazina
△ (+)Spiroperidolo
△ (+)Alfa_Flupentixolo
△ (+)Cis_Tiotixene
△ (+)Aloperidolo
△ (+)Benperidolo
△ (+)Bromperidolo
△ (+)Trifluoperidolo
△ (+)Droperidolo

△ (+)Pipamperone
△ (+)Tioridazina

△ (+)Clozapina
△ (+)Clorpromazina

□ (S) Azione_da_intraprendere = Unknown
□ (S) Classe_farmacologica = Neurolettici
□ (F) Consigliabilita_per_Status_Psichiatrico = Unknown
□ (S) Farmaco_alternativo = Clorpromazina
□ (S) Farmaco_migliore = Clozapina
□ (S) Obiettivo_di_Primo_Livello = antipsicotico
□ (S) Obiettivo_di_Secondo_Livello = Sintomi Negativi
□ (S) Obiettivo_di_Terzo_Livello = antiparkinson
□ (F) Prescrivibilita = Unknown
□ (F) Prescrivibilita_alternativa = 94.96%
□ (F) Prescrivibilita_migliore = 96.24%
□ (S) Principio_attivo = Unknown
□ (S) Strategia_posologica = Dosi elevate

Esclusi_per_interazioni_farmacorlogiche
Esclusi_per_status_psichico
Esclusi_per_limitata_finestra_terapeutica
Esclusi_per_scelta

Psicofarmaci_esclusi
Psicofarmaci_da_prescrivere
Interventi

○ (+)Clozapina
○ (+)Clorpromazina

△ (+)Intervento_antipsicotico

○ **Conclusioni_operative**

FIG. 2. *Continued.*

171

increasing by 44% its resolution (Fig. 2a). Finally, it defines an order of preference between the two drugs (Fig. 2b) and, considering the absence of current neuroleptic treatment, chooses the best drug (in the example, clozapine).

This therapeutic choice appears to be in agreement with the observed clinical activity reported in the medical literature. To reach this solution, the system operates on an elevated number of properties defined for every drug.

CONCLUSIONS

The evolution of ES in general, and in medicine in particular, elicited some operational requirements, deriving from the specific applied perspective, which go beyond the aims of the first experimental prototypes developed in AI laboratories.

After a first phase of easy enthusiasm and a second of disappointment, we are having a new resurgence of projects to which ES can be applied and new horizons are now being opened. However, the need to define implicit reasoning reference models in ES construction is becoming increasingly evident; at the same time, it is necessary to define standard descriptors to discriminate among characteristics of the various systems. In this way, the specific characteristics that may render an ES more adequate to a particular application can be defined.

We can reasonably expect that the evolution of ES will better enable us to achieve three goals: (i) a better diffusion of clinical knowledge of "difficult formalization"; (ii) a greater flexibility of clinical reasoning by the single physician, overcoming conditioning due to prejudices and expectations; and (iii) a better utilization of knowledge as well as available information.

Finally, further possibilities offered by systems such as Beta should not be overlooked, as they propose a structure for preknowledge which is given as implicit in communication of heuristic clinical knowledge. In fact, they may constitute valuable supports for comparing such knowledge according to standardized procedures (16).

ACKNOWLEDGMENT

Beta Project is supported by a special grant from the Italian Foundation for Study of Schizophrenia (FIS). Eng. Fabrizio Ricci and Dr. Adriana Valente of ISRDS of the National Research Council (CNR) gave technical and scientific support to the NEXPERT version of Beta.

REFERENCES

1. Snyder SH. Amphetamine psychosis: a model of schizophrenia mediated by catecholamines. *Am J Psychiatry* 1973;120:61–7.

2. Lee T. Postmortem studies of dopamine receptors in schizophrenia. In: Sen AK, Lee T, eds. *Receptors and ligands in psychiatry*. Cambridge: Cambridge University Press, 1988: 11–28.
3. Farde L, Wiesel FA, Hall H, Halldin C, Stone-Elander S, Sedvall G. D2 receptors increase in PET study of schizophrenia. *Arch Gen Psychiatry* 1987;41:671–2.
4. Nair NPV, Lal S, Bloom DM. Cholecystokinin and schizophrenia. In: Van Ree JM, Matthysse S, eds. *Psychiatric disorders: neurotransmitters and neuropeptides*. Amsterdam: Elsevier, 1986:237–58. (Progress in Brain Research, Vol. 65.)
5. Verhoeven WMA, Van Ree JM, De Wied D. Neuroleptic-like peptides in schizophrenia. In: Sen AK, Lee T, eds. *Receptors and ligands in psychiatry*. Cambridge: Cambridge University Press, 1988:147–66.
6. Van Kammen DP, Gelerntner J. Biochemical instability in schizophrenia II: the serotonin in gamma-aminobutyric acid systems. In: Meltzer HY, ed. *Psychopharmachology: the third generation of progress*. New York: Raven Press, 1987.
7. Karczmar AG. Schizophrenia and the cholinergic system. In: Sen AK, Lee T, eds. *Receptors and ligands in psychiatry*. Cambridge: Cambridge University Press, 1988:29–63.
8. Van Kammen DP, Slawsky RC. State dependency and dysregulation of norepinephrine activity in schizophrenia. In: Sen AK, Lee T, eds. *Receptors and ligands in psychiatry*. Cambridge: Cambridge University Press, 1988:93–126.
9. Bleich A, Brown SL, Kahn R, Van Praag HM. The role of serotonin in schizophrenia. *Schizophr Bull* 1988;14:297–315.
10. Lozonczy MF, Song IS, Mohs RC, et al. Correlates of ventricular size in schizophrenia II: Biological measures. *Am J Psychiatry* 1986;143:1113–8.
11. Pancheri P. Neuroleptics and 5HT receptors: a working hypothesis for antipsychotic effect (submitted).
12. Pancheri P. Side-effects in course of neuroleptic treatment: a clinical overview. In: *Psychopharmacology: an up to date*. Rome, September 1988.
13. Bronzino JD, Morelli RA, Goethe JW. OVERSEER: a prototype expert system for monitoring drug treatment in the psychiatric clinic. *IEEE Trans Biomed Eng* 1989;36:533–40.
14. Neuron Data. *NEXPERT Object: User Manual*. Palo Alto, CA: 1990.
15. Marconi PL, Pancheri P, Valigi R. ALFA, sistema esperto sulla psicofarmacoterapia degli attacchi di panico su personal computer. *Abstracts "Attualita e Prospettive dell'Informatica in Medicina."* Florence, October, 26–29, 1988.
16. Pancheri P, Marconi PL. Applicazione dei sistemi esperti nella diagnosi e nella terapia psichiatrica. *Med Inform* 1989;6:22–6.
17. Ghirlanda L, Marconi PL, Valigi R, Pancheri P. ALFA: A.I. in medicina. Un sistema esperto per il trattamento farmacologico del disturbo da attacchi di panico. *Inform Oggi* 1988;43:12–8.

Psychiatry and Advanced Technologies,
edited by L. Ravizza, F. Bogetto, and
E. Zanalda. Raven Press, Ltd.,
New York © 1993.

17

Diagnostic Rationalization and Development by Means of Informatic Procedures with the Composite International Diagnostic Interview

G. Tacchini, M. T. Coppola, A. Musazzi,
and A. C. Altamura

Institute of Psychiatry, University of Milan 20122, Milan, Italy

Psychiatry has witnessed with growing interest the development of international systems for nosographical classification and standardized tools for diagnosis. Although early systems were rarely taken into consideration, ICD-9 (1) and DSM-III (2) not only have been widely quoted and utilized but also have been the object of much debate; it is easy to imagine that psychiatrists who were probably tired of nonfalsifiable and nonverifiable theories and of the relative failure of psychiatric research in the last 20 years found some satisfaction and stimulus in agreeing on the name to be attributed to the signs and symptoms they observed. An editorial in the *Lancet* (3) commented that the situation of modern psychiatry is paradoxical because clinical practice is in many aspects uncertain, whereas the scientific and methodological problems to which it gives rise are of great interest. The situation is one in which psychiatric diseases cannot be explained but can at least be described, thanks to international classifications. Nosography has dual aims: communication and prediction. Without the latter, diagnosis risks being nothing more than a trivial labeling of disorders, whereas the close link between prognosis and the validity of a diagnosis is obvious. However, for a diagnosis to be valid it must be reliable, even though reliability is not sufficient to ensure validity. The first of the two constraints to diagnosis, i.e., communicability, is a necessary premise for the second, predictability. From this point of view, the problem of transcultural psychiatric diagnosis takes on special importance: a diagnosis must be translatable into the different national cultures and, if a disease is present throughout the world, its transcultural stability is by itself an indirect criterion for validation, meaning that the disease is probably a "true" disease and not solely determined by cultural background. This does not mean that culturally determined diseases are not real. In fact, nosography must be a service and not an imposition; it must not replace national classifications which are often useful in local contexts (4).

Cultural influences on diagnosis are extremely relevant, as shown, for example, by the different approaches to the "mind–body" dichotomy (5). Comparison with psychiatry in the developing countries has cast some doubts on diagnostic certainties and on the expected prognosis (4). The technological innovations in survey tools seem to open extraordinary opportunities for development in psychiatry (6): These are some of the main factors that have inspired work on the Composite International Diagnostic Interview (CIDI), with the aim of accounting as much as possible for the impact of individual, social, and psychological variables. These variables are organized differently in different cultures, and not only determine psychopathologic manifestations of diseases but also the actual recognition of diseases.

A SHORT HISTORY OF THE INTERNATIONAL DIAGNOSTIC INTERVIEW

The CIDI was initiated in 1979 by a joint project of the WHO and AD-AMHA, the United States agency for mental disorders and drug and alcohol abuse (7). The aim of the project was to unify the diagnosis of mental disorders, alcoholism, and drug abuse.

The first phase, in 1980 and 1981, was dedicated to a study of the situation and identification of major problems. The second phase, in 1981 and 1982, prepared an International Conference which was to focus on the major problems. The third phase was initiated in 1982 and is now ended. This phase involved setting up an International Task Force which has developed diagnostic tools to be used together with the main nosographical classifications, ICD-9 and DSM-III. Two new tools, Schedules for Clinical Assessment in Neuropsychiatry (SCAN) (8) and CIDI, were conceived, to be used simultaneously with DSM-III and ICD-9.

Whereas SCAN has a more traditional clinical use, CIDI is a transcultural epidemiological tool. Its salient features are: (i) a high level of structuring, which is necessary to reduce variations in observer, content, and criteria. This makes it possible to compare very different areas of application and also allows use by nonmedical staff, which is an obvious necessity in epidemiologic studies, especially in developing countries where doctors are scarce; (ii) one of the consequences of the previous feature is the way questions are formulated: they are all completely filled out and "blind-ended," i.e., with answers that are part of a predetermined framework; they are simply stated and avoid all idiomatic forms so as to adapt to the different cultures; and (iii) the third feature is speed, because an interview in epidemiology cannot last for hours. In addition external information and key informants are not required. The interview is based only on what the proband personally affirms.

The Diagnostic Interview Schedule (DIS) has similar characteristics to those described above: both cover 40 of the 122 diagnoses contained in DSM-III, as can be seen in Table 1. The other diagnoses of DSM-III cannot be translated into blind-end questions. The characteristics of DIS are well known. It is sufficient to recall that it has been applied to 20,000 subjects in the ECA (Epidemiologic Catchment Area) program (9), has been translated into many languages and used in many countries with good results, and finally, the 40 diagnoses included in the DIS cover the bulk of psychiatric disorders.

CIDI also considers the European tradition and therefore includes part of the ninth edition of the Present State Examination (PSE-9), as well as the questions from DIS. Merging these two tools led to the development of CIDI,

TABLE 1. *DSM-III diagnoses covered by CIDI-C*

Eating disorders	Other specific affective disorders
Anorexia nervosa	Dysthymic disorders
Bulimia	Atypical affective disorders
Organic mental disorders	Atypical bipolar disorder
Dementia (unspecified)	Anxiety disorders
Substance use disorders[a]	Phobic disorders
Alcohol abuse	Agoraphobia with panic attacks
Alcohol dependence	Agoraphobia without panic attacks
Barbiturate, sedative abuse	Social phobia
Barbiturate, sedative dependence	Simple phobia
Opiate abuse	Anxiety states
Opiate dependence	Panic disorder
Cocaine abuse	Generalized anxiety disorder
Amphetamine abuse	Obsessive–compulsive disorder
Amphetamine dependence	Somatization disorders
Hallucinogen abuse	Somatization disorder
Cannabis abuse	Psychosexual dysfunction
Cannabis dependence	Pathologic gambling
Tobacco dependence	
Schizophrenic disorders	
Schizophrenia	
Psychotic disorders NEC	
Schizophreniform	
Affective disorders	
Major affective disorders	
Manic depressive episode	
Manic episode	
Bipolar disorder	
Major depression, single episode	
Major depression, recurrent	

CIDI, Composite International Diagnostic Interview; NEC, Not elsewhere classified.
[a] According to criteria of ICD-10 and DSM-III-R.

TABLE 2. *Comparison between CIDI-C and PSE-9: list indicates PSE-9 items included in CIDI-C*

Physical health	Anergia and retardation[a]
Physical illness	Early waking[a]
Psychosomatic symptoms	Loss of libido[a]
Worrying[a]	Irritability[a]
Tension pains	Expansive mood
Tiredness[a]	Subjective ideomotor pressure
Muscular tension[a]	Grandiose ideas
Restlessness[a]	Obsessional checking[a]
Hypochondriasis[a]	Obsessional cleanliness
Nervous tension[a]	Thought insertion
Free-floating anxiety[a]	Thought broadcast
Anxious foreboding[a]	Thought block
Panic attacks[a]	Delusion of thoughts read
Situational anxiety[a]	Verbal hallucinations
Anxiety on meeting people[a]	Dissociative hallucinations
Specific phobias[a]	Olfactory hallucinations
Avoidance of anxiety[a]	Other hallucinations
Inefficient thinking[a]	Delusions of control
Poor concentration[a]	Delusions of reference
Neglect due to brooding[a]	Delusions of misinterpretation[a]
Depressed mood	Delusions of persecution
Hopelessness	Delusions of grandiose ability[a]
Suicidal	Delusions of grandiose identity[a]
Morning depression[a]	Delusional explanations[a]
Social withdrawal[a]	Slowness and underactivity[a]
Self-depreciation[a]	Behaves as if hallucinated
Lack of self-confidence[a]	Blunted affect
Simple ideas of reference[a]	Slowness of speech[a]
Guilty ideas of reference[a]	Neologisms
Pathologic guilt[a]	Incoherence of speech
Loss of weight	Adequacy of interview
Delayed sleep[a]	

CIDI, Composite International Diagnostic Interview; PSE, Present State Examination.
[a] Questions were added to cover these; other items were adequately covered by questions from the Diagnostic Interview Schedule.

which required 5 years of efforts by Prof. Wing from London and Prof. Robins from St. Louis. Table 2 shows the items of PSE that are included in CIDI. The others cannot be translated into the "blind-end" format and concern delusion and perception; 28 PSE items were already present in the DIS, and only an evaluation of severity and of the last occurrence of the symptom, which are required by PSE, were added. The other 35 items of the PSE were reformulated in the DIS format. This effort was far from simple, because it was also necessary to match the time criteria of PSE (1 month) with the scalar criteria of DIS. This, however, was made easier by the fact that the diagnostic program CATEGO of the PSE is dichotomic.

The questions were modified also many times to take into account Asian cultures and the animistic cultures of South America. Figure 1 shows these results and a question of CIDI which integrates PSE and DIS: the PRB codes

```
                                           EVER IN
SLOW/RESTLESS                              LIFETIME
┌─────────────────────────────────────────────────────────────┐
│ 80. Has there ever been a period of                          │
│     two weeks or more when you talked                        │
│     or moved [Did you talk or move]                          │
│     more slowly than is normal for you?                      │
│                                                               │
│                                  ┌──────────────────────────┐ │
│                                  │ PRB:   1    3 4 5 *       │ │
│                                  └──────────────────────────┘ │
│         MD: _____   OTHER: _____                         │
│                                                               │
│                                    REC:  1 2 3 4 5 6          │
│         SEV: In the last month                               │
│              were you so slowed    AGE REC:    __/__          │
│              down that things                                │
│              around you seemed to  SEV:  1      2            │
│              go too fast?                                    │
│                                                               │
│ IF Q. 80 SEV = 1 OR 2: SKIP TO 81.                           │
│                                                               │
│ 80.A. In the last month, have you                            │
│       been bothered by a lack of                             │
│       energy or feeling slowed     ┌──────────────────────┐  │
│       down?                        │ PRB:  1          5    │  │
│                                    └──────────────────────┘  │
│                                                               │
│       SEV: In the last month, have                           │
│            you been moving much less                         │
│            than is normal for you?                           │
│                                    SEV:  1      2            │
└─────────────────────────────────────────────────────────────┘
```

FIG. 1. An example of the CIDI-C question format.

refer to the cause of disease, and only the "5" is a psychiatric symptom. The REC codes refer to the last manifestation of the disorder; if this occurred within the last month, the severity of the disorder is also asked (SEV code). Because DSM-III requires a duration of 2 weeks or longer for this symptom, which is not required by PSE, question 80 A was added to solve the problem.

Figure 2 shows part of the Probe Flow Chart that the interviewer uses to ascertain the different codes without ever suggesting the answer to the proband.

Preliminary tests (10) were carried out in the different countries listed in Table 3, and these also suggested modifications to the nosographical criteria (11). These were included in DSM-III-R (12), in ICD-10 (13) and in the draft criteria of DSM-IV. In particular, the sections on alcoholism and drug abuse were described in more detail and were also enlarged (14). For this reason, CIDI adopted an independent modular structure.

The degree of correlation with PSE and DIS has also been examined in preliminary tests, along with the degree of reliability of each single diagnosis

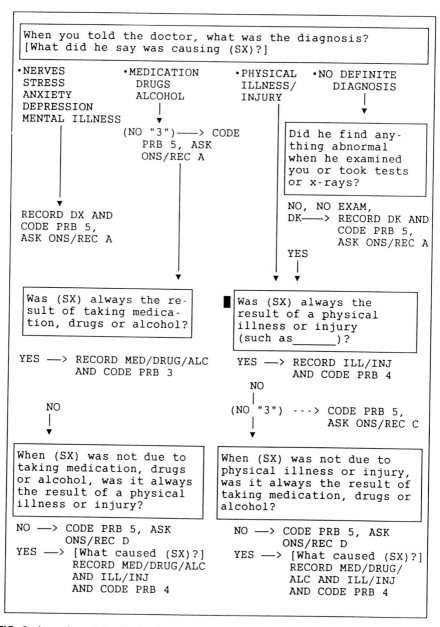

FIG. 2. A portion of the Probe Flow Chart (PFC) of CIDI-C: the PFC is used to assess whether symptoms reported by probands are of psychiatric relevance.

TABLE 3. *List of the centers participating in the CIDI-C Field Trial: Wave I*

Country	Name of center	Editor
Netherlands	Amsterdam	Dr. R.M.W. Smeets
Greece	Athens	Prof. G.C. Lyketsos
U.S.A.	Baltimore	Prof. J. Halikas
India	Bangalore	Dr. M. Isaac
China	Beijing	Dr. Xu You Xin
Great Britain	Cardiff	Dr. A. Farmer
Sweden	Hudding	Prof. C. Allgulander
G.D.R.	Jena	Prof. G.E. Kuhne
Luxembourg	Luxembourg	Prof. C. Pull
F.R.G.	Mainz	Dr. W. Maier
Italy	Milan	Dr. G. Tacchini
U.S.A.	Minneapolis	Dr. B. Grant
F.R.G.	Munich	Prof. H.U. Wittchen
Portugal	Porto	Dr. A. Droux
Norway	Oslo	Dr. I. Sandanger
Puerto Rico	San Juan	Dr. G. Canino
Brazil	São Paulo	Dr. C. Torres de Miranda
U.S.A.	St. Louis	Dr. L. Cottler
Australia	Sydney	Dr. G. Andrews

CIDI, Composite International Diagnostic Interview.

and items. At present, the R version of CIDI covers the nosographical systems listed in Fig. 3 and the Feighner Criteria, and can be correlated, with good results, with the other diagnostic tools shown in the figure.

INTERNATIONAL VALIDATION STUDY

Each country participating in the study prepared its own preliminary version of CIDI, and the national translations were then submitted to a reiterated back-version procedure until a good match was achieved with the English original, including graphics and page layout. In 1987, the members of the Task Force met and were trained together, after which they initiated the final field trial in their respective countries. This allowed a certain degree of freedom in the protocol, but in most cases they had to include clinical and nonclinical interviewers according to a balanced pattern and to follow the model illustrated in Fig. 4. The first part is a classical interviewer–observer protocol with all of the necessary precautions to prevent bias between interviewer and observer.

The second part of the protocol is more innovative: it includes readministration of doubtful or incorrect parts by the observer and a subsequent debate between interviewer and observer to identify the cause of the discordance. This meets a specific characteristic of CIDI: because each answer of the proband is "blind-ended" and the interview is completely structured, it is possible that all discordances are procedural errors and that the entire relia-

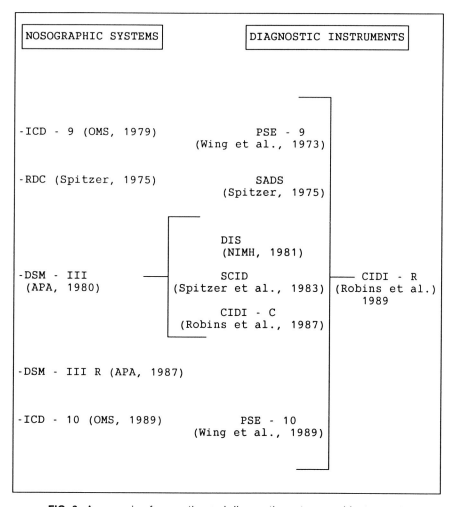

FIG. 3. A synopsis of currently used diagnostic systems and instruments.

bility study can be assimilated into a study of procedural validity and frequency of procedural errors. This is exactly what happens with the Discrepancy Resolution Module.

PRELIMINARY RESULTS

The data from 18 of 20 participating centers have been processed, for a total of 575 interviews. Table 4 shows a synthesis of the distribution of interviewers in the different centers, together with data concerning the type

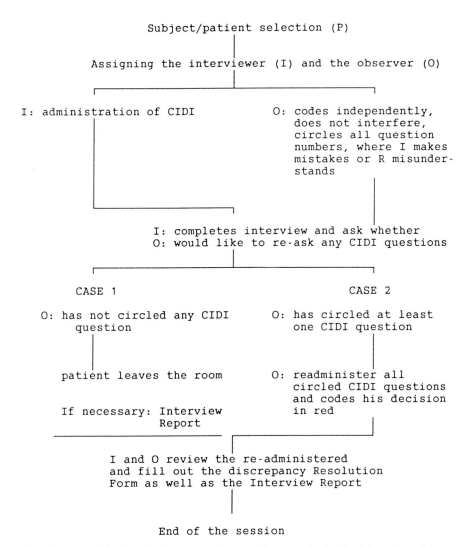

FIG. 4. Scheme of the interviewing procedure used for assessing CIDI-C inter-rater reliability during the Field Trial—Wave I.

of interviewer–observer pair, i.e., both clinical, both nonclinical, or one clinical and one nonclinical. Overall, interviews carried out by a clinical interviewer with a clinical observer comprised 13%; those with a clinical interviewer and a nonclinical observer, or vice versa, comprised 79%; and interviews with both nonclinical observers represented 8%. The procedure also called for evaluation of acceptance of the interview by patients and by interviewers and observers. This evaluation was provided by participants to

TABLE 4. *Types of interviewer pairs at each of the Centers participating in the CIDI-C field trial: Wave I*

Center	Both clinician		Clinician–nonclinician		Both nonclinician	
	n	%	n	%	n	%
Darlinghurst (Australia)	—	—	16	50.0	16	50.0
Cardiff (Great Britain)	—	—	32	100.0	—	—
Bangalore (India)	—	—	32	100.0	—	—
Jena (GDR)	9	36.0	16	64.0	—	—
Athens (Greece)	4	10.8	33	89.2	—	—
Luxembourg (Luxembourg)	32	100.0	—	—	—	—
San Juan (Puerto Rico)	—	—	40	100.0	—	—
Beijing (China)	—	—	32	100.0	—	—
Minneapolis (U.S.A.)	—	—	35	94.6	2	5.4
St. Louis (U.S.A.)	—	—	25	100.0	—	—
São Paulo (Brazil)	—	—	29	100.0	—	—
Amsterdam (Holland)	2	5.0	37	92.5	1	2.5
Paris (France)	7	28.0	18	72.0	—	—
Mainz (F.R.G.)	3	9.4	18	56.3	11	34.4
Milan (Italy)	6	18.8	20	62.5	6	18.8
Porto (Portugal)	9	28.1	23	71.9	—	—
Munich (F.R.G.)	—	—	16	55.2	13	44.8
Oslo (Norway)	—	—	32	100.0	—	—
Total	72	13.0	454	79.0	49	8

the study after completion of all of the interviews. The length of CIDI was judged to be excessive in most cases, and acceptable only in a minority (Table 5). This is because the entire CIDI was asked, which contained the two long sections on alcoholism and drug abuse, which by themselves constitute more than one-half of the CIDI.

Duration of the single interviews was 1 to 2 h in 33.8% of cases and from 2 to 3 h in 33% of cases out of 478 interviews. It must also be borne in mind that these data are influenced by the fact that most centers used probands who did not belong to the general population but were clinical, and were therefore affected by a significant number of psychiatric symptoms and disorders. They were also slower and more difficult to interview because of the high incidence of positive answers. All of this contributed to making the interviews longer. Interviewers, however, assessed the patient's acceptability of CIDI to be good or moderate in the vast majority of cases (92.8%). Moreover, CIDI was judged to range from very appropriate to appropriate both for nonclinical and clinical patients which, however, are not those for whom CIDI was conceived in 82% of cases, as is shown in Table 6.

TABLE 5. *Applicability of the CIDI-C as judged by the interviewers of the field trial: Wave I*

The length of the CIDI was (*n*)	
Much too long	7
Too long	40
Acceptable	9
Duration of the CIDI	
Less than 1 h	44
1–2 h	162
2–3 h	158
3–4 h	71
More than 4 h	43
Number of interviews	478

CIDI, Composite International Diagnostic Interview.

An evaluation of length, acceptability, and suitability, of each single section of CIDI from a cultural point of view was then requested. These results are shown in Table 7. On a scale of 1 to 3, length was judged to be good for almost all the sections of CIDI except for those concerning alcohol, where the average score was 1.8, i.e., between excessively long and too long. Acceptability for all sections was between 2 and 3, i.e., between moderate and good, except for the alcohol section which scored 1.1 (insufficient) and the section on drugs, where the average score was 1.5, between insufficient and moderate. This result was influenced not only by the length of these two sections but also by the fact that some questions were formulated in a very direct fashion, which in certain cultures or to some patients may seem to be offensive or indiscreet. The suitability of individual sections scored between 2 and 3 in all cases, i.e., between appropriate and very appropriate, except for the section concerning somatization, in which problems of conceptualization and nosographic classification in ICD-9 and DSM-III persisted. The average score in these cases was 1.5, between inappropriate and appropriate. For the section concerning alcoholism the average score was 1.4, and for drug abuse the average score was 1.9. A special case is the average score of

TABLE 6. *Acceptability and appropriateness of the CIDI-C as reported by the interviewers of the field trial: Wave I*

Poor			4
Moderate			25
Good			27
Clinical settings		Epidemiological settings	
Very appropriate	5	Very appropriate	14
Appropriate	31½	Appropriate	32
Not appropriate	16½	Not appropriate	7
No response	3	Not applicable	1
		No response	2

CIDI, Composite International Diagnostic Interview.

TABLE 7. *Synopsis of the main performance features of each section of CIDI-C after the field trial: Wave I*

Diagnostic section	Length[a]	Acceptance[a]	Appropriateness[b]	Cultural[b]	Recency and onset[a]
Tobacco	2.9	2.9	3.0	2.1	
Somatization	1.4	2.3	1.5	1.7	
Panic, GAD	2.4	2.7	2.1	2.1	
Phobias	2.1	2.8	2.2	2.7	
Depression	1.8	2.1	1.8	2.3	
Mania	2.1	2.3	2.2	2.8	
Schizophrenia	2.5	2.0	2.1	2.1	
Anorexia	2.6	2.8	3.0	1.9	
Bulimia	2.6	2.7	3.0	1.9	
Alcohol	1.2	1.1	1.4	1.4	1.8
Obsessive–compulsive	2.3	2.1	2.1	2.5	
Drugs	1.8	1.5	1.9	1.9	1.8
Gambling	2.8	2.7	1.6	1.8	
Organic brain	2.3	2.1	2.3	2.8	

CIDI, Composite International Diagnostic Interview: GAD, generalized anxiety disorder.
[a] Rating code. Length and recency/onset: 1, much too long; 2, too long; 3, acceptable. Acceptance: 1, poor; 2, moderate; 3, good.
[b] General and cultural appropriateness: 1, not appropriate; 2, appropriate; 3, very appropriate.

1.6 reported for the section concerning gambling. Cultural suitability was considered to be good for almost all CIDI sections, scoring around 2, except for somatization (average score 1.7), alcoholism (average score 1.4), drug abuse (average score 1.9), and gambling (average score 1.8). The latter result is due to the difficulty in defining pathological gambling, which varies enormously within different cultural contexts. Some cultures, such as the Anglo-Saxon, accept widespread betting in money, on horses, and on lotteries as traditional and this is not considered gambling, whereas in other countries, especially the developing countries, this is very infrequent.

The sections on alcoholism and drug abuse deserve special attention. The section on drugs requires a very documented and careful survey, and therefore becomes very long. That on alcohol gives rise to a special problem owing to different cultural definitions and cultural acceptance of alcoholism. In Anglo-Saxon cultures, in which beer and distilled alcohol are generally consumed, alcoholism is linked more directly to consumption of alcohol without any distinction concerning modalities. On the other hand, wine-producing cultures unanimously tolerate alcohol consumption when it takes place in certain situations, e.g., during meals and in amounts between two and three glasses of wine per meal. These amounts, however, are sufficient to meet the international criteria for alcohol abuse.

Subsequent analyses no longer concerned acceptability and suitability of the single CIDI sections but instead focused on the specific objective of this

TABLE 8. *Discordant codings of each section of CIDI-C during the field trial: Wave I*

CIDI section	From question no. to question no.	Mean number of discrepant codings/interview	No. of C-questions of that section
Tobacco	C15 → C15E	0.2	13
Somatization	C16 → C602	2.5	43
Panic	C61 → C671V	0.8	44
Phobia	C68A → C71	0.7	27
Depression	C72 → C98	2.2	74
Mania	C100 → C116	0.9	38
Schizophrenia	C1180 → C143C	2.8	56
	C260 → C265		
Anorexia nervosa	C144 → C148	0.5	9
Bulimia	B1 → B15A	0.2	23
Alcohol abuse/			
dependence	C1491 → C1705	1.4	61
Obsessive–compulsive	C172 → C179	0.9	20
Drug abuse/dependence	C181 → CD353	0.9	417
Psychosexual			
dysfunction	C210 → C212	0.4	5
Pathological gambling	C235 → C238	0.1	7
Organic brain syndrome	C239 → CPP	2.1	34
Overall number of discrepant PRB codings/interview		15.4	

CIDI, Composite International Diagnostic Interview.

study, i.e., reliability of the interview itself. A first evaluation of general reliability is shown in Table 8, in which the average number of discordances between interviewer and observer is reported section by section, together with the number of questions included in the different CIDI sections. The average number of discrepancies per interview is 15.4 over 871 questions, equal to a rough index of 1.76 errors/100 questions. Of course, this number must be correlated not only to the number of questions in that section but also to the number of positive answers given by the patients in each section, because the probability of discordances in the case of positive and negative answers is different, especially as CIDI requires that the cause of the reported disorders be identified. In particular, CIDI asks if the disorder is relevant to the patient's life, if it is due to alcohol or drug consumption, to physical diseases or accidents, and whether the disorder is to be considered a true psychiatric symptom. As a result, together with the number of questions in each section of CIDI reported in Table 8, it is also necessary to take into account the number of positive answers per section. This situation is illustrated in Table 9, which reports the lifetime diagnoses of all centers participating in the study. The diagnoses listed in this table are not necessarily mutually exclusive: for example, one of the most frequent diagnoses is tobacco abuse, which is undoubtedly compatible with other diagnoses. The

TABLE 9. *Lifetime diagnoses obtained during the CIDI-C field trial: Wave I*

CIDI sites	Overall
Tobacco	139
Somatization	4
Panic	74
Phobia	216
Generalized anxiety disorder	56
Depression	166
Bipolar I	26
Bipolar II	21
Schizophrenia	39
Anorexia	2
Bulimia	19
Obsessive–compulsive	59
Pathological gambling	8
Organic brain syndrome	46

CIDI, Composite International Diagnostic Interview.

source of discordances between interviewer and observer was discussed at the end of each interview on the basis of a section of the interview called Discrepancy Resolution Module, which identifies the causes according to predefined codes. Table 10 shows that the most frequent cause of discordance is represented by Code 1 (interview mistake by the interviewer) and the second most frequent is Code 5 (patient change of opinion). These results

TABLE 10. *Sources of disagreement of each section of CIDI-C resulting from the field trial: Wave I*

CIDI section	Sources of disagreement[a]										No. of questions	No. of total discrepancies
	1	2	3	4	5	6	7	8	9	Other		
Demographies	1	1			1						1–14E	3
Tobacco	9				6						15	15
Somatization	71	22	7	47	80		1				16–60.2	228
Panic–GAD	17	2		12	6						61–67	37
Phobia	41	17	4	5	26				1		68–71	94
Depression	54	4	9	6	53						72–99	126
Mania	15	1	5	1	15	4					100–118	41
Schizophrenia	24	3	1		24	3				3	119–143	58
Anorexia	2	5	2	1	7						144–148	17
Bulimia	1				2						131–15	3
Alcohol	26	3		1	10	1		2			149–170.2	43
Obsessive–compulsive	9	4			9						171–179	22
Drug	3			1	3						180–191.3	7
Sexual dysfunction	15				3	1					210–212	19
Pathological gambling											235–238	
Organic brain MMSE	1				2					1	239–259	4
Total	289	62	28	74	247	9	1	2		5		

[a] 0, no resolution; 1, interviewer: mistake in the Probe Flow Chart; 2, observer: mistake in the Probe Flow Chart; 3, "R" misunderstood question; 4, problem with question (ambiguous/cultural); 5, "R" changed his mind; 6, difference in the presentation of question; 7, Coding mistake; 8, Other (specify).
CIDI, Composite International Diagnostic Interview; GAD, generalized anxiety disorder; MMSE, Mini-Mental State Examination.

must be correlated with the high incidence of psychiatric patients included in the study, i.e., psychotic patients who easily change their minds, and this is the main difficulty with probands of this type. Of course, this takes place much less frequently when the probands are part of the general population, in which the frequency of psychotic disorders is low.

Table 11 shows how further statistical analysis can be performed on a single section of CIDI, in this case the psycho–organic syndrome section. This table shows the number of positive subjects for this diagnosis observed in each of the centers participating out of the total 575 interviews. These diagnoses were obtained through computerized diagnostic algorithms of the program that formulates diagnoses according to DSM-III criteria. In this case, the psycho–organic syndrome was present in a mild form in 34 of interviewees (5.9%) whereas it was more serious in only 11 interviewees (1.9%). Table 12 shows how the percentages of concordance of each of the different CIDI sections were processed, and shows κ values for all of the sections, the participating centers, and the interviews, regardless of whether

TABLE 11. *An example from the CIDI-C field trial: Wave I regarding the DSM-III diagnosis of Organic Brain Syndrome: number of subjects that in each centre fulfilled the diagnosis at its different levels of certainty*

	DSM-III diagnoses (1) Organic brain syndrome (orgbrain)											
Code center	No diagnosis		Definitely mild		Definitely severe		Possibly severe/ definitely mild		Maybe absent/ possibly mild		Could be severe, mild, or absent	
	%	n	%	n	%	n	%	n	%	n	%	n
01 (n = 32)	100	32	—	—	—	—	—	—	—	—	—	—
03 (n = 32)	75	24	9.4	3	—	—	3.1	1	3.1	1	9.4	3
04 (n = 32)	56.3	18	6.3	2	9.4	3	12.5	4	—	—	15.6	5
05 (n = 25)	92.0	23	—	—	—	—	—	—	8.0	2	—	—
06 (n = 37)	86.5	32	8.1	3	—	—	—	—	2.7	1	2.7	1
07 (n = 32)	90.6	29	3.1	1	—	—	—	—	—	—	6.3	2
08 (n = 40)	95.0	38	5.0	2	—	—	—	—	—	—	—	—
09 (n = 32)	96.9	31	3.1	1	—	—	—	—	—	—	—	—
10 (n = 37)	97.3	36	—	—	—	—	—	—	2.7	1	—	—
11 (n = 25)	96.0	24	—	—	—	—	—	—	—	—	4.0	1
12 (n = 29)	69.0	20	24.1	7	3.4	1	—	—	—	—	3.4	1
13 (n = 40)	57.5	23	5.0	2	5.0	2	—	—	—	—	32.5	13
14 (n = 25)	92.0	23	—	—	—	—	—	—	—	—	8.0	2
15 (n = 32)	90.6	29	6.3	2	—	—	—	—	—	—	3.1	1
16 (n = 32)	84.4	27	6.3	2	6.3	2	—	—	—	—	3.1	1
17 (n = 32)	50.0	16	28.1	9	9.4	3	6.34	2	—	—	6.3	2
18 (n = 29)	96.8	28	—	—	—	—	—	—	—	—	3.4	1
21 (n = 32)	87.5	28	—	—	—	—	—	—	—	—	12.5	4
All centers (n = 575)	83.7	481	5.9	34	1.9	11	1.2	7	2.4	14	4.9	28

CIDI, Composite International Diagnostic Interview.

TABLE 12. *Another example from the CIDI-C field trial: Wave I regarding 11 DSM-III diagnoses drawn from the data of all the participating sites: overall diagnostic agreement and κ calculations*

Diagnoses	κ values	Percentage agreement	Interviewer/observer	
ORGBRAIN (n = 575)	0.82	95.0	461	9
			20	85
DSMMANIA (n = 550)	0.94	99.3	515	2
			2	31
DSMDEP (n = 560)	0.96	98.2	320	5
			5	230
DSDYSTHY (n = 562)	0.96	98.9	459	5
			1	97
DSMBIPOL (n = 550)	0.94	99.3	515	2
			2	31
DSMDEPSE (n = 557)	0.99	99.8	513	1
			—	43
DSMDEPRT (n = 557)	0.92	97.1	411	8
			8	130
DSMBIPII (n = 557)	0.94	99.5	531	2
			1	23
DSMSCHIZ (n = 550)	0.92	98.9	505	4
			2	39
DSMSZFRM (n = 541)	0.89	99.6	540	—
			2	8
DSMOBCOM (n = 541)	0.94	98.5	463	4
			4	70

CIDI, Composite International Diagnostic Interview.

the interviewer was clinical or not. It can be observed that κ values were especially high (always above 0.80), and this points out the sound reliability granted by structured interviews as compared with semistructured interviews, such as PSE-9, in which κ values range between 0.60 and 0.70 for most sections (15). The most highly reliable diagnosis is that of depression (κ = 0.99) and the least reliable is psycho–organic syndrome, since this is based on observations of behavior and skills that are usually better evaluated by clinical interviewers compared with nonclinicians, whereas CIDI has also the opposite objective, i.e., to formulate diagnosis with trained but nonmedical staff. A similar analysis was carried out section by section in all of the centers, breaking down the cases according to whether the interviewer–observer couple was mixed (clinical and nonclinical), both clinical, or both nonclinical. The results for all of the centers overlap, and in this case, too, κ values were greater than 0.80, ranging from a minimum of 0.83 for the diagnosis of psycho–organic syndrome to a maximum of 1 for the diagnosis of depression, when interviewer and observer were clinical and nonclinical. When both interviewers are clinical a minimum value of 0.66 for the diagnosis of bipolarity and mania is obtained, but the κ values for all are greater than 0.80 and reach a maximum of 1 in the diagnosis of schizophrenia.

CONCLUSIONS

The results of this multinational WHO study point to a number of issues that constitute a necessary basis for future development of diagnostic techniques and tools, as well as of nosographic categorization and validity understanding. The very good κ values of CIDI, never less than 0.80, are a sound argument that reliability can be achieved in psychiatry and therefore can allow nonambiguous communication. The traditional clinical diagnosis, which relies on a free dialogue with the patient, can be based on a common glossary, such as DSM-III or ICD-9, but by no means ensures good replicability, and quite often contributes to serious misunderstandings (13). This situation becomes unsustainable when research, either genetic, biochemical, pharmacologic, neurophysiologic, or clinical, is involved, because it prevents, to a remarkable extent, the real possibility of replicating, verifying, and falsifying a single hypothesis. These difficulties can be overcome with the use of reliable diagnostic instruments such as CIDI, the use of which will probably become in future years a must in psychiatric research. Related to the previous reasons is the fact that good reliability among all the 19 nations involved in the study certainly stems from the high quality and accuracy of the training received by all the field trial coordinators; although this fact once again proves the replicability of CIDI, on the other hand it constitutes a real basis for transcultural nosography that can now be based on factual rather than speculative clinical comparisons. This possibility can be regarded, therefore, as the first step toward nonspeculative validity analysis and comprehension, a challenging field in which CIDI, which also offers a direct comparison between ICD-10 and DSM-III-R with a single interview, will probably become more and more useful.

REFERENCES

1. World Health Organization. *International classification of diseases*, 9th ed. Geneva: WHO, 1979.
2. American Psychiatric Association. *Diagnostic and statistical manual of mental disorders*, 3rd ed. Washington, DC: American Psychiatric Association, 1980.
3. Editorial. *Lancet* 1987;2:10.
4. Sartorius N. International perspectives of psychiatric classification. *Br J Psychiatry* 1988; 152(suppl)1:9–14.
5. Jablensky A. Methodological issues in psychiatric classification. *Br J Psychiatry* 1988; 152(suppl 1):15–20.
6. Cooper B. Psychiatry in the era of "health for all". *Soc Psychiatr Psychiatr Epidemiol* 1988;23:2–5.
7. Robins LN, Wing J, Altamura AC, et al. The compisite international diagnostic interview: an epidemiology instrument suitable for use in conjunction with different diagnostic systems and in different cultures. *Arch Gen Psychiatry* 1988;45:1069–77.
8. Wing GK. *Schedules for clinical assessment in neuropsychiatry*. SCAN System, PSE-10, Part 1. Geneva: WHO, 1989.
9. Regier DA, Myers JK, Kramer R, et al. The NIMH epidemiologic catchment area (ECA)

program: historical context, major objectives and study population characteristics. *Arch Gen Psychiatry* 1984;41:934–41.

10. Semler G, Wittchen HU, Joschke K, et al. Test-retest reliability of a standardized psychiatric interview. *Eur Arch Psychiatr Neurol Sci* 1987;236:214–22.

11. Wittchen HU, Robins LN, Altamura AC, et al. Diagnostic and inter-rater reliability of the Composite International Diagnostic Interview (CIDI). In: Stefanis CN, et al., eds. *Psychiatry: a world perspective*, vol 1. Amsterdam: Elsevier, 1990:125–32.

12. American Psychiatric Association. *Diagnostic and statistical manual of mental disorders*, 3rd ed., revised. Washington, DC: American Psychiatric Association, 1987.

13. World Health Organization. *International classification of disease*, 10th ed. Draft of Chapter V. Geneva: WHO, 1988 (restricted distribution).

14. Cottler LB, Robins LN, Altamura AC, et al. The CIDI-core substance abuse and dependance questions: cross-cultural and nosological issues. *Br J Psychiatry* 1991;159:653–8.

15. Cooper JE, Copeland JRM, Brown GW. Further studies on interviewer training and inter-rater reliability of the Present State Examination (PSE). *Psychol Med* 1977;7:517–23.

Psychiatry and Advanced Technologies,
edited by L. Ravizza, F. Bogetto, and
E. Zanalda. Raven Press, Ltd.,
New York © 1993.

18

Contribution of Medical Informatics to Assessment and Rehabilitation of Cognitive Functions

S. Giaquinto

St. John Baptist Hospital SMOM, 00148 Rome, Italy

We believe that because the operations of the neuronal network are timed in milliseconds, tests are required that can explore the processing of simple tasks with the smallest number of variables and express the result as an objective physiologic measure rather than in some arbitrary form such as a rating scale. For this reason we are in favor of a cognitive microanalysis (1) with laboratory tests specifically designed for the study of one or more functions, to test particular information processing operations and specialized cerebral structures. A recent conference on Alzheimer's disease concluded that "illiterate subjects, or persons from different cultures, might perform poorly on a cognitive test, not because of illness and disability but because the difficulty and inappropriateness of the test procedures. Tests of first-order capabilities such as visual perception, reaction time, or motor ability might be closer to measuring substrate levels of [central nervous system (CNS)] integrity and disability without the complication of trying to measure abstract–conceptual–cognitive behavior" (2).

Performance speed is a flexible component of cognitive processing and represents an important dimension in understanding the reasons for age-dependent differences. The time or rate of processing is assumed to be the critical factor, at least for those cognitive activities that are minimally influenced by experience, as opposed to those that depend on cumulative knowledge and are presumed to either improve or remain stable with age (3). The "universal decrement principle" argues that slowing in the central nervous system accounts for virtually all age-dependent changes in behavioral activities (4), although this principle is challenged by many negative findings when accuracy or professional abilities are considered.

Psychologic observations have a neurochemical counterpart. Evidence that it is possible to increase the metabolism of catecholamines comes from a study carried out by Karlsson et al. (5) on the effect of external stimulation in moderately deteriorated patients. Groups of four or five subjects underwent two weekly sessions of motor and cognitive exercise, each lasting an hour, and also manipulations of emotional behavior. The cerebrospinal fluid showed an increase in the level of homovanillic acid, which is one of the terminal metabolites of catecholamine breakdown. This result was attributed to both dendritic and synaptic growth. Experimental data also emphasize the role of dopamine turnover in attention (6,7). Likewise, cerebral circulation is probably activated by training; in humans, Kobayashi et al. (8) showed that environmental stimulation increases cerebral blood flow to levels significantly greater than those found in the elderly residents in institutions that provide low levels of social stimulation.

NEUROPSYCHOLOGICAL TRAINING

It is important to assess cognitive performance under controlled situations. Probably, it is even more important to assess individual abilities to cope with tasks of increasing difficulty and to assess a cognitive gain with exercise. Previous unpublished observations for our group have shown that young controls (mean age 29 years) linearly improve after five sessions in a reaction time task.

Choice reaction times improved, and the regression line was expressed by the equation:

$$y = 375.78 \text{ ms} - 16.64 \times t (p < 0.01)$$

An improvement was also seen at tachistoscopic tasks. The best threshold value for 10 random digits in a double array was obtained at 468-ms time exposure by one of the subjects at the fifth session. The regression line was:

$$y = 1122 - 68.8 \times t (p < 0.05)$$

EFFECTS OF NEUROPSYCHOLOGIC TRAINING IN THE ELDERLY

In recent years, two important facts have been recognized by researchers in the field of experimental aging: shattering of the stock character of the doddering elder who has lost memory, and the positive effects of mental exercise of paced tasks on cognitive ability in the elderly.

Training has proved very effective in the elderly, even though it is normally presumed that the capacity for development is reduced and the ability of the system to cope with information is slowed. Neuropsychologic training can give more self-reliance to the elderly, just as reality therapy can effect small improvements in the daily life of the demented patients that lighten their burden.

With the dichoptic presentation of target and mask stimuli Hertzog et al. (9) found that the interval necessary to escape masking was reduced by about 33 ms after 5 days of practice, even though the difference between the elderly group and young controls persisted. Salthouse and Somberg (3) report that in a group of subjects with an average age of 66 years, training with tachisto-scopic stimuli brought about improvements not only in signal detection but in memory scanning and in visual discrimination over 50 hours of practice sessions. The capacity to increase the speed of central processing was con-firmed by Baron and colleagues (10,11), who applied operant conditioning reinforced by monetary reward. These investigations provide interesting re-sults because they reveal that motivation is as important as practice in bring-ing about improvement.

The improvement due to practice, common to both the young and the elderly, applies to many other situations of repeated learning over time, as, for example, the verbal learning curves for Rey's test. Baron and Menich (11) found that the improvement due to practice can be greater than the differences due to age.

PERSONAL RESULTS

By applying computerized trials, our research group tried to lower reaction times in old subjects. Fourteen normal elderly, right-handed subjects were studied. Their mean age was 67.9 years (SD 4.45) and the formal education was 5 years. The group of normal aged was organized on the basis of the following criteria: age over 65 years; no known illness of neuropsychiatric interest; no therapies affecting the nervous system, including hypnotics; a still active life with social relationships, even if in retirement phase. More-over, 22 elderly right-handed outpatients with chronic cerebrovascular dis-ease (CCVD) also underwent cognitive training. They had a mean age of 69.5 years (SD 6.9) and 6 years of formal education. Both inclusion and exclusion criteria followed the lines proposed by the ad hoc committee in Paris as essential in identifying CCVD patients. Twenty more CCVD patients were selected on the basis of matched age and education. They were similarly tested three times at intervals of 6 weeks and did not receive any training. Altogether, the CCVD group exhibited a mild deterioration, as determined with SCAG and MMS scales, which did not severely interfere with daily life. Two weekly sessions were allotted for each subject in the first two groups. Each session was of 40-min duration and was held in a sound-attenuated room. The first session started after the subjects had become fully familiar-ized with the entire experimental set and with the environment. Altogether, eight sessions were held. The subject was given a simple reaction time task:

A red flash lasting for 18 ms on the full screen of a 17-in. monitor was the stimulus. Vision was binocular. Fifteen stimuli were delivered at random intervals to the subjects, who had to press a knob in a conveniently located position. Discrimination in the case of the choice reaction time was based on two colors in a random succession: 15 red and 15 blue flashes were delivered by a microcomputer, the former having the value of imperative stimulus. The subject had 2 s to respond. The longest time interval between two successive stimuli was 7 s. Mean reaction time, standard deviation, errors and omissions, percent, and relative coefficient of variation (12) were calculated. Because of possible errors due to either lack of response or wrong choice, the mean value was regularly weighted by applying the following function:

$$f(Pe) = 13Pe^3 - 5.6Pe^2 + 1.5Pe + 1$$

Pe is the elementary probability of error, estimated by $1 - (nc/n)$, where n is the number of stimuli and nc the number of correct responses. It follows that the mean value is multiplied by 2 in the case of Pe = 0.5, and by 10 in the case of Pe = 1.

The third task consisted of the identification of 10 random selected digits appearing in two rows on the screen. The angle subtended by each digit was 1° 20′ in the vertical and 58′ on the horizontal direction. The lighting was 0.2 lux, full-moon type, very clear but not dazzling. The first exposure time was 1.8 s, successively increased by 10%. The subject had to identify the complete set, speaking aloud. The threshold was reached when three successive digit sets at the same exposure could be identified. Within a single session the sequence of tasks was repeated twice more. In other words, over 40 min the subject was given simple reaction time, choice reaction time, and tachistoscopy three times. Only the values corresponding to the first administration in each session were used for statistical analysis of the data. In this report we deal with reaction times and tachistoscopy. Single-factor analysis of variance for repeated measurements was performed. The Newman and Keuls method was then applied to test the difference between all possible pairs of mean values obtained in each training session. Finally, tests for trends were performed to subdivide training variations into linear, quadratic, and cubic components (13).

RESULTS

Simple reaction time had a mean value of 209 ms (SD 34) in normal elderly and 299 ms (SD 66) in the patients. Neither group showed a significant improvement of this parameter with training [analysis of variance (ANOVA) df 7.91; F 1.98, NS and df 7.147; F 1.15, NS].

Weighted simple reaction time had a mean value of 221 ms (SD 31) in normal elderly and 288 ms (SD 85) in the patients. Again, neither group

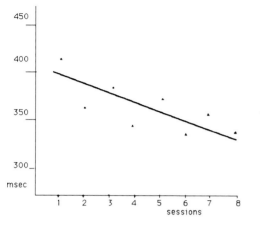

FIG. 1. Normal elderly. Choice reaction times under training.

showed significant improvement of this parameter with training (ANOVA df 7.91; F, 0.89, NS and df 7.147; F, 0.89, NS).

Choice reaction time had a mean value of 396 ms (SD 61) in normal elderly and 488 ms (SD 112) in the patients. Normal elderly benefit from training (ANOVA df 7.91; F, 3.17, $p < 0.01$). The test for linear trend was significant (df 1.91; F 20.02, $p < 0.001$) (Fig. 1). The other group also had a gain in performance (ANOVA df 7.147; F 4.5, p < 0.001). The test for linear trend was significant (df 1.147; F, 16.6, $p < 0.001$). The tests for quadratic and cubic trend were also significant (5.7, p < 0.05 and 4.4, $p < 0.05$) (Fig. 2).

Weighted choice reaction time, i.e., raw values multiplied by f (Pe), had a

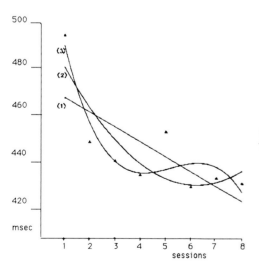

FIG. 2. CCVD patients. Choice reaction times under training.

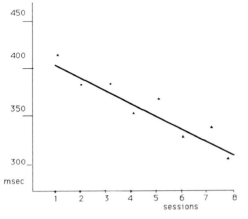

FIG. 3. Normal elderly. Weighted choice reaction times under training.

mean value of 453 ms (SD 68) in normal elderly. In this case, too, the analysis of variance showed high significance (ANOVA df 7.91; F 53.12, $p < 0.001$). The test for linear trend indicated high significance (df 1.91; F 53.12, $p < 0.001$) (Fig. 3). In the patients, the weighted choice reaction time had the mean value of 513 ms (SD 92). After training, improvement of this parameter was found (ANOVA df 7.147; F 4.5, $p < 0.001$). The test for linear trend was significant (df 1.147; F 20.4, $p < 0.001$). The test for quadratic trend provided negative results (3.4; NS). By contrast, a cubic trend was obtained (4.7; $p < 0.05$) (Fig. 4).

Tachistoscopic performances had a mean value of 2,963 ms (DS 795) in normal elderly. Training greatly improved the performance (ANOVA df 7.91; F 9.01, $p < 0.001$). The result obtained in the linear trend test was also

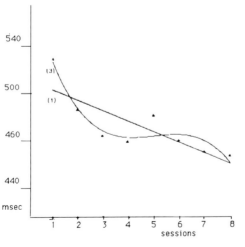

FIG. 4. CCVD patients. Weighted choice reaction times under training.

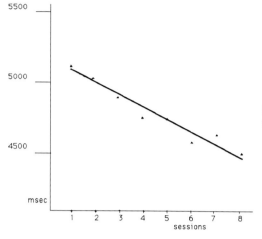

FIG. 5. CCVD patients. Tachisto-scopic training.

significant (df 1.91; F 56.89, $p < 0.01$). The patients showed a higher basal value of 5,072 ms (SD 1,377) but they significantly gained from training procedures (ANOVA df 7.147; F 10.5, $p < 0.001$). The linear model was applicable to this positive change (df 7.147; F 68.9, p < 0.05) (Fig. 5). The test for both quadratic and cubic trend provided negative results (2.4, NS and 0.1, NS).

In normal elderly the variation coefficient significantly decreased with training (ANOVA df 7.91; F 7.32, $p < 0.01$). However, the linear model was not sufficient to describe this trend and a significant quadratic component was also present (linear trend F 36.86, $p < 0.001$; quadratic trend F 8.81, $p < 0.01$). The Newman and Keuls test indicated that the percent variation coefficient decreased after the third session. In the cerebrovascular patients, values of the percent variation coefficient had random oscillations. However, percent variation coefficient had a baseline value of 6.11 but was 4.6 at the end of training (*t* test: $p < 0.05$).

In the untrained group, reaction time values did not improve (ANOVA df 2.38; F 2.95, NS) (Fig. 6). On the other hand, at tachistoscopy a slightly better performance was obtained at the retest (ANOVA df 2.38; F 4.8, $p < 0.05$) (Fig. 7).

POSSIBILITIES OF REVERSING A COGNITIVE DECLINE

Mean basal values calculated from normal elderly and cerebrovascular patients are significantly different, since the latter group shows the worse performance. Therefore, it can be stated that the negative effects of age on speeded tasks are certainly less than the effects induced by pathologic variables. However, the above results indicate that both normal elderly patients and patients with transient neurological disturbances can benefit from

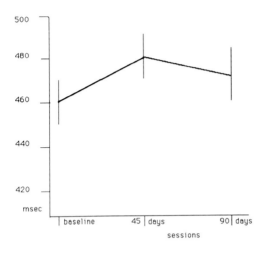

FIG. 6. Untrained CCVD patients. Choice reaction times.

training, albeit the latter group to a much lesser extent. Statistics indicate that improvement of performance in elderly subjects follows a linear course. Training therefore has the effect of accelerating central processing. We believe that this effect is not solely due to a better knowledge of the experimental setting. Three possible reasons exist: (i) measurements started when subjects were familiar with the experimental procedure; (ii) improvement of performance was still seen in the last sessions; (iii) control subjects failed to show a better performance with time, except for an initial gain at tachistoscopy.

Our experimental results support the so-called "disuse" theory to the extent that they reveal the possibility of reversing, at least in part, the decline

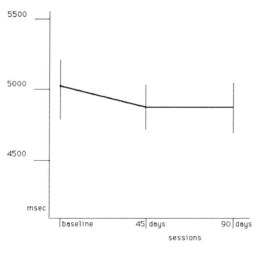

FIG. 7. Untrained CCVD patients. Tachistoscopy.

associated with aging. In normal elderly training could reveal reverse capacity and potential for improving psychologic functions and the management of new situations, which are called for by a paced daily life. The cerebrovascular patients had a less spectacular improvement of cognitive abilities.

The tasks that we have employed tap the mental abilities belonging to the so-called "fluid intelligence" in the Cattel–Horn theory (14). According to this theory, fluid intelligence declines with age and reflects primarily the biologic integrity of brain structures, whereas the so-called crystallized intelligence is the endproduct of cultural learning and professional skill, and this is considered to be age-independent.

First of all, an action locus at which the training procedure impinges seems to be the method of sensory storage at encoding level. Cerella et al. (15) have shown that there is an age-dependent slowing in the rate at which information is extracted from these buffers. Elderly subjects are slower by a factor of 1.31 compared with younger controls. The age effect is more intense when multielement displays are involved. Nevertheless, this simple extraction of information is relatively spared by age in comparison with the processes involved in transformation and storage of information, which are slowed by a factor of 1.7 to 1.8. Our results also show that simple reaction time, which does not involve discrimination, has no benefit from cognitive training. Therefore, a central activation of processing independent of peripheral input and motor speed is also involved. Better achievements can be explained by a better attention and an improvement of processing capabilities.

Anatomic regeneration is an unlikely process in the improvement of cognitive performance in a short-term rehabilitative plan, because it is supposed to take longer than the time covered by our training sessions.

COMPUTER-ASSISTED COGNITIVE RETRAINING

Finally, this research has a bearing on the problem of the so-called "computer-assisted cognitive retraining" (CACR). The computer provides increased opportunities for tight control over the rehabilitation strategy by automatically selecting the most appropriate material, monitoring performance, and providing feedback. The recent application of computer-assisted training in rehabilitative programs has its advocates. Story and Sbordone (16) hold that microcomputers are an effective and flexible tool for treating cognitive–communicative impairments. They offer the valuable advantage of amplifying the therapeutical resources of rehabilitation plans. The computer, by not being human, does not create a stressful environment in the therapeutic situation.

There are many possible CACR rehabilitative approaches, but we believe that few validation experiments have been carried out thus far. Lynch (17,18) has reviewed representative articles on this topic and argues that quantity is unparalleled by quality. Controversial issues are raised by Wood and Fussey (19), who found no evidence for improvement in cognitive tasks as a result of computer-assisted cognitive retraining. However, these negative results can be offset by the observed improvements in behavioral aspects of attention and by the serious impairment of brain functions in survivors of severe head trauma.

However, good results were observed when stroke patients suffering from unilateral neglect were treated with computerized sessions aimed at the improvement of lateral attention (20–22).

The effective use of the new colored graphics and the immediate feedback can be very motivating for patients. Microcomputers are now cheap and available everywhere. At Burden Neurological Institute in Bristol a network system has been developed which links each of the remote computers (in the patients' homes) to a central one at the Institute. This network uses the public telephone lines for the remote sites and dedicated lines for the local stations (23).

NEW COMPUTERIZED SYSTEMS (THE THINKᴀʙʟᴇ MACHINE)

In addition to aging, several pathologic conditions can affect the brain and necessitate rehabilitation. Head injury, vascular diseases, intoxication, and dementia are customarily represented in a rehabilitation center. A conference on Alzheimer's disease concluded that tests of first-order capabilities, such as visual perception, reaction time, or motor ability, might be closer to measuring substrate levels of CNS integrity and disability without the complication of trying to measure abstract–conceptual–cognitive behavior. Methods exploring first-order capabilities are also suitable for cognitive remediation, aiming at improvement of ability to take in and perceive sensory information, and to interact with the environment, retain information, solve problems, and make decisions.

Indeed, CACR is a new therapeutic tool, that can safely be applied in patients. Experimental work is in progress at our laboratories. Over the last 18 months we have customarily used a computerized system built by IBM and now officially announced in the United States. It provides clinical professionals with a new and amusing way of cognitive remediation. The system, which is called THINKable, uses instructions, colorful pictures, audio cues, and funny cartoons, and collects both right and wrong answers through a touch-screen. It also provides experimental settings, automatic data collection, and analysis. Subjects have to concentrate on tasks, not on the procedure.

The first model of cognitive processing outlines the hierarchy of some processes contributing to total cognition. Elements, treatment components, session plans, and workbooks are the steps enabling a therapeutic program.

The second model says that computer intervention can improve attention, discrimination, memory, and sequencing after an individual neuropsychologic assessment. These components are differently organized within the sessions to meet specific patients' cognitive capabilities.

THINKable is a unique software program that creates a structured environment in which a patient can practice skills in four focus areas, such as visual attention, visual discrimination, visual memory, and visual sequencing. Within each area there are four levels of difficulty. To date, seven patients have been treated by us; three with severe head trauma, two with subarachnoid hemorrhage, one with a stroke in the left hemisphere, and one with Alzheimer's disease. The treatment aimed at improvement of cognitive deficit.

Although work is still in progress, at present, the main results are (i) patients are very pleased to interact with a system in which no threatening examination is seen (one patient, who refused any kind of interpersonal approach after severe head injury accepted computerized remediation); (ii) every patient improved in performance, attaining higher levels; (iii) even the Alzheimer's patient improved in attention and discrimination; (iv) activities of daily living seemed to improve; and (v) neuropsychologic training gave more self-reliance to the patients.

We have observed improved self-confidence in the trainees. All of them exhibited better alertness and sense of mastery in their daily activities, with more prompt responses to environmental stimuli. Since the objectivity of anecdotal observations may be biased by a variety of variables, these aspects are worthy of further behavioral measurements. System requirement is a minimum of 4 Mb free memory and a 30-Mb hard disk. One full-size expansion slot and one color touch-sensitive screen are required. The machine is now officially announced.

ACKNOWLEDGMENT

The excellent cooperation of Jim Beluhe, Bruce Mahaffey, Piero Cecchini, Mauro Fini, Massimo Fiori, and Giuseppe Nolfe is greatly appreciated.

REFERENCES

1. Eisdorfer C, Cohen D. The assessment of organic impairment in the aged. In: Burdock EI, Sudilovski A, Gershon S, eds. *The behavior of psychiatric patients.* New York: Marcel Dekker, 1982;329–51.
2. Khachaturian ZS. Diagnosis of Alzheimer's disease. *Arch Neurol* 1985;42:1097–1105.
3. Salthouse TA, Somberg BL. Isolating the age deficit in speeded performance. *J Gerontol* 1982;37:59–63.
4. Botwinick J. *Aging and behavior.* New York: Springer, 1984.
5. Karlsson I, Brane G, Melin E, Nuth AL, Rybo E. Mental activation–brain plasticity. *Clin Neuropharmacol* 1984;7(suppl 1):336–7.

6. Marshall JF. Behavioral consequences of neuronal plasticity following injury to nigrostratial dopaminergic neurons. In: Scheff SV, ed. *Aging and recovery of function in the central nervous system*. New York: Plenum Press, 1984:101–28.

7. Stricker EW, Zigmond MJ. Recovery of function following brain damage: homeostasis at dopaminergic synapses. In: Goldstein G, ed. *Advances in clinical neropsychology*. New York: Plenum Press, 1984:161–82.

8. Kobayashi S, Yamaguchi S, Katsube T, Kitani T, Okada K, Kitamura J. Influence of social environment factors on cerebral circulation and mental function in the normal aged. In: Fieschi C, Lenzi GL, Loeb C, eds. *Monograph in neural sciences*, vol 11. Basel: Karger, 1984:163–8.

9. Hertzog CK, Michael VW, Walsh DA. The effect of practice on age differences in central perceptual processing. *J Gerontol* 1976;31:428–33.

10. Baron A, Menich SR, Perone M. Reaction times of younger and older men and temporal contingencies of reinforcement. *J Exp Anal Behav* 1983;40:275–87.

11. Baron A, Menich SR. Age-related effects of temporal contingencies on response speed and memory: an operant analysis. *J Gerontol* 1985;40:60–70.

12. Sachs L. *Applied statistics. A handbook of techniques*. New York: Springer-Verlag, 1982.

13. Winer BJ. *Statistical principles in experimental design*. New York: McGraw–Hill, 1971.

14. Horn JL. Psychometric studies of aging and intelligence. In: Gershon S, Raskin A, eds. *Aging*, vol 2. New York: Raven Press, 1975:19–43.

15. Cerella J, Poon LW, Fozard JL. Age and iconic read-out. *J Gerontol* 1982;37:197–202.

16. Story TB, Sbordone RJ. The use of microcomputers in the treatment of cognitive-communicative impairments. *J Head Trauma Rehab* 1988;3:45–56.

17. Lynch W. An update on research in computer-assisted cognitive retraining. *J Head Trauma Rehab* 1987;2:93–5.

18. Lynch W. Computers in neuropsychological assessment. *J Head Trauma Rehab* 1988;3:92–4.

19. Wood RLI, Fussey I. Computer-based cognitive retraining: a controlled study. *Int Disabil Studies* 1987;9:149–53.

20. Caltagirone C, Nocentini U, Troisi E. La riabilitazione del neglect con l'impiego di computers. In: Giaquinto S, ed. *La riabilitazione cognitiva assistita da computers*. Rome: Marrapese, 1989:85–105.

21. Cucinotta D, Godoli G, Angelini A. Il training computerizzato nell'anziano. In: Giaquinto S, ed. *La riabilitazione cognitiva assistita da computers*. Rome: Marrapese, 1989:73–84.

22. Giaquinto S, Nolfe G. Sul recupero del rallentamento cognitivo. In: Giaquinto S, ed. *La riabilitazione cognitiva assistita da computers*. Rome: Marrapese, 1989:55–71.

23. Curry SH. Un programma di riabilitazione cognitiva con microcomputer per i superstiti di gravi traumi cranici. In: Giaquinto S, ed. *La riabilitazione cognitiva assistita da computers*. Rome: Marrapese, 1989:227–38.

Psychiatry and Advanced Technologies,
edited by L. Ravizza, F. Bogetto, and
E. Zanalda. Raven Press, Ltd.,
New York © 1993.

19

The AMDP-Based Psychiatric Information System: A Proposal for a Computerized Clinical Record

Luciano Conti and Gabriele Massimetti

Institute of Clinical Psychiatry, University of Pisa, 56100 Pisa, Italy

The clinical record is the crux of clinical practice: It permits the combination of information from different sources and provides the basis for diagnostic, therapeutic, and prognostic decisions. The more the case history, clinical, psychologic, and laboratory information is plentiful, precise, detailed, and readily available, the more reliable are the diagnosis, prognosis, and therapeutic decisions.

Despite constant technological progress, it is difficult to exploit the potential of a computer in the creation and practical use of a clinical record because of the difficulties that arise in processing of the data involved and the necessary interaction between computer and clinician.

A preliminary data-processing problem is the organization of the records themselves, which must include, for each patient, a section of constant data (anamnestic and demographic) and a section of variable data that is updated with each patient visit. This means that records must be built up on the basis of "relational" structures within which subfiles of information, similar in sense, source, and purpose are cross-indexed according to key fields (e.g., code number of the patient, type of laboratory examination) so that it is not only possible to retain the logical unity of data derived from each patient but also to allow the separate management of subfiles in order to obtain high speed in data processing, to avoid duplication of data, and to safeguard patient privacy (1).

The computerization of clinical records would also ideally provide a computer-guided diagnostic interview as well as an automatic diagnosis and therapeutic protocol, possibly involving in the procedure the artificial intelligence systems presently being developed.

Another aspect of the problem of computerizing the clinical record lies in the clinician's reaction to and use of the record itself. First, to be useful the clinical record must assimilated into daily clinical practice without altering the charge/benefits ratio of this activity. It must not render the work tedious or complicated through the need for special keys and/or commands, and it must permit rapid retrieval of stored patient information in easily readable form.

From the patient's point of view, the use of the computer should not interfere with the relationship between the patient and the clinician and should not obstruct the psychiatric interview, which is the keystone of the therapeutic process.

Bearing in mind these difficulties and limitations, an attempt has been made at the Institute of Clinical Psychiatry of the University of Pisa to construct the basis for a computerized clinical record by creating the AMDP (Arbeitsgemeinschaft für Methodik und Dokumentation in der Psychiatrie) Psychiatric System (PISA system).

HISTORICAL BACKGROUND

At the Institute of Clinical Psychiatry of the University of Pisa (ICP), techniques have been developed since 1965, using the facilities of the Centro Nazionale Universitario di Calcolo Elettronico (CNUCE) of Pisa, for acquiring, organizing, storing, retrieving, processing, and analyzing of clinical psychiatric and clinical trial data in an increasingly flexible, rapid, and sophisticated way.

One of the most important applications developed has been the Data Bank for Psychopharmacology (BDP), which permits storage of clinical data collected in a standard format, selection of any group of patients and of any portion of the data, and statistical analysis of the selected data. To furnish the BDP of a comprehensive and explicit documentation scheme for data from clinical trials of psychotherapeutic drugs, it was decided in 1977 to install at the ICP the Biometric Laboratory Information Processing System (BLIPS), which had been developed by the Psychopharmacology Research Branch of the National Institutes of Mental Health (NIMH) and the Biometric Laboratory of the George Washington University between 1965 and 1977 (2). The two systems were integrated into a powerful new system, the BLIPS/BDP (3).

When the creation of a computerized clinical record for the monitoring of naturalistic treatment was planned in 1978, a careful study was undertaken of the Kachmont Monitoring System, a patient information system created at the Douglas Hospital of Montreal, that utilizes basic BLIPS forms and processing. At that time there were mostly available only computer terminals connected on a time-sharing basis with mainframes; for this reason, the main requirements of an efficient and usable computerized clinical record were not satisfied and this project was temporarily dropped.

Afterwards minicomputers became available, which seemed to satisfy almost all of the requirements of a computerized clinical record, and at the computer center of the ICP the development of a system for the computerization of the outpatient clinic on a DIGITAL PDP 11/23 PLUS began. This system, Syntactic–Semantic Data Entry (DESS), which adopted a new philosophy, permitted the entering of data with effective syntactic and semantic control and thus guaranteed the reliability of the stored data. Although the input, storage, and retrieval portions of the DESS were ready to function, the system was not completed at the output stage, because minicomputers were suddenly rendered obsolete, at least for the purpose of a computerized clinical record, by the arrival of personal computers (PCs).

The philosophy of the DESS, however, was applied to the new system HENRY/ETC (4) which was, practically speaking, the transfer of the BLIPS/ BDP from the mainframe to the PC. HENRY/ETC fully exploited the more user-friendly features of the Macintosh, which made available to everybody a complex but easy-to-use system for data entry, editing, storage, and retrieval without losing the possibility of utilizing the mainframe for complete data documentation or for more complex statistical analysis.

On the basis of all this experience, we decided, in 1990, to lay the foundations for a computerized clinical record, the PISA system.

THE PISA SYSTEM

The philosophy underlying this project was that of making available a flexible, easy-to-use system, not requiring any specific knowledge of data processing, employable during a psychiatric examination without causing any interference with the patient–clinician relationship or any significant increase in the workload of the clinician, while furnishing him with both a guide for a complete examination of the patient and rapid retrieval of any information already stored for the patient being examined. The intention was therefore that the PISA system, in its basic version, should be usable in either the psychiatric ward or private practice, but also, given its modular construction, that it be easily expandable with specific rating instruments for specific research purposes.

As a basis for the PISA system we chose an internationally standardized information tool, the AMDP system which was created by German-speaking psychiatrists in 1965. The basic German version was published in 1979 (5), the Spanish version was published in 1980 (6), and the French version in 1981 (7). The AMDP system has since been translated into many other languages (e.g., English, Portuguese, Japanese, Dutch) under the supervision of the

AMDP international secretariat. The Italian translation was published in 1990 (8).

The AMDP system was chosen because (a) it derives from the classic German psychopathology and therefore should not create any intercultural problems, either teminologically or conceptually, and should provide a common basis for understanding and agreement; (b) it avoids any preconceived theories by simply presenting the psychopathologic disturbances as they occur; (c) it defines the psychopathologic picture without any attempt at diagnosis and therefore can be used independently of any specific diagnostic–classification system; and (d) it assesses psychopathologic and somatic symptoms according to a five-point scale and is thus able not only to identify a psychopathologic feature but also to provide information on the symptom's severity.

All five AMDP forms—the three anamnestic forms (AMDP-1, -2, and -3), the psychopathologic scale (AMDP-4), and the somatic scale (AMDP-5)—were utilized in the original format (based on the French version). The order of presentation of the anamnestic items was changed to rationalize the interview, but the original format for stored data was followed exactly to avoid difficulties in analyzing the data.

For software support, we chose the commercial Data Base Management System (DBMS) FoxBASE+/Mac, produced by Fox Software, Inc. This DBMS was chosen for several reasons: it is the Macintosh database with the highest processing speed in all the most important functions (e.g., input and sorting of data, re-indexing, searching); the FoxBASE+/Mac has itself a highly user-friendly interface, which facilitates the personalization of the system and fully utilizes the user-friendly interface of the Macintosh without reducing the operational speed, as is common with most of the other DBMS. Fox achieves its high speeds through a complex memory- and processor-optimization scheme, as well as an understanding of the strengths of the original Macintosh ROM; all the commands can be executed not only from the keyboard but also from a simple pull-down menu and from different buttons appearing on the screen; multiwindow management is also possible; the "help" function can be consulted at any time during the personalization phase, to facilitate programming, or during the operative phase; the operational potential of the Fox DBMS can easily be expanded by loading and executing external programs; and the Fox system derives directly from an equivalent system operating on MS-DOS (IBM compatible) with which it has complete compatibility and, therefore, with the multiuser version, concurrent access to and updating of data files is possible on a network that supports both Macintosh and IBM computers.

The PISA system has been planned primarily for use during psychiatric examination, and for this reason keyboard use has been reduced as much as possible in favor of use of the mouse, which permits the input of data with a simple "click."

The amount of information required for the completion of an interview does not, as a rule, exceed that normally collected during a careful psychiatric examination, the only exception occurring during the first examination, when the case history information has to be obtained. The data can be acquired and entered at the same time, so that the psychiatrist's work load is limited and the stored data can then be utilized for study and research purposes without any further expense or loss of time.

The system ensures a high degree of quality control in the collection of data, in that the extensive use of pop-up menus and buttons, each associated with a clearly indicated specific value of the variables, prevents out-of-range errors; when the keyboard is used the appropriate syntactic controls are brought into action. The unintentional missing of data is prevented by the system's sequential data-entry procedure, which activates a new question only after the answer to the previous question has been received.

The system has a semantic control that checks input data against a logical correlation with previous information. For example, with the PISA system, if a patient answers that he has no siblings, the following question, regarding their order of birth, is automatically filled in as "only child," or if a patient has never married, a question regarding age at marriage is automatically answered as "not applicable."

Errors and/or omissions in the information already in the file can easily be corrected without interfering excessively with all the other data filed, and the same syntactic and semantic controls that apply during the input phase are maintained during the correction phase. To safeguard the privacy of the patient, a personal password is required to gain access to the data bank.

Finally, the PISA system has a context-sensitive "help" facility, which allows the user to check the exact meaning of any item and to read a clear and exhaustive definition of any psychopathologic term. This facility is derived from the AMDP manual, the result of the work of an international committee of experienced psychiatrists. When the "help" facility is called up, a window appears on the screen with explanations regarding the item active at that moment, and by pressing a button it is possible to call up the general index and to select the specific topic to be explained.

On first screening the PISA system (Fig. 1), only by giving the correct password is it possible to access the system. To avoid as much as possible any typewriting errors, the system requires the entry of only the first letters of the first and family name of the patient; a window then appears on the screen with a list of any patients with those initials currently stored in the data bank, together with the principal identification information (e.g., date and place of birth, address, fiscal code) (Fig. 2).

If the patient's record is not yet stored in the data bank (Fig. 3), the command "new" will initiate a new personal record by assigning a code inside the PISA system and by asking for all the identification information needed to complete the identification (ID) sector. The system initiates the anamnestic

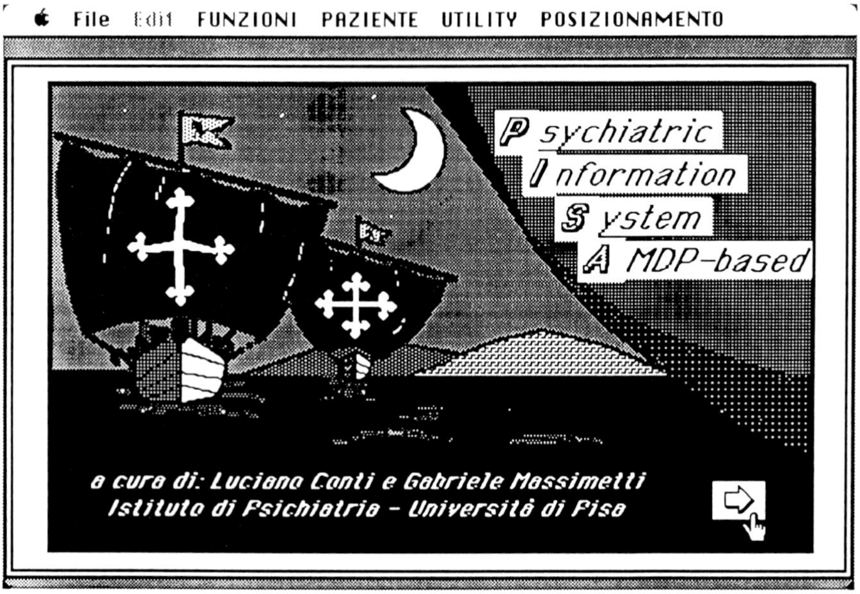

FIG. 1. First sceening of the PISA system. On clicking on the arrow, a password is required to access the system.

interview with the general anamnesis (AMDP-1), followed by the psychiatric history (AMDP-3) and the history of life events (AMDP-2). Once this section has been completed, the psychopathologic (AMDP-4) and somatic (AMDP-5) sectors are presented.

When the patient is identified as being already recorded in the data bank, the command "open" calls up the existing record, which is automatically updated (e.g., date, progressive number of the interview) and the psychopathologic (AMDP-4) and somatic (AMDP-5) scales are immediately presented. Before returning the patient's record to the files, the system asks whether any significant life events have occurred during the interval between the previous and the current interview and, if so, the AMDP-2 is presented.

For any record to be stored in the data bank, it must first be completed; if for any reason the interview is interrupted before its completion, the acquired information is stored in temporary memory.

For the moment, a satisfactory means of recording therapeutic information in a way that is practically useful for statistical analysis has not yet been found, given the difficulties encountered in documenting precisely the drugs (e.g., in terms of type, amount, frequency) actually taken by the patient during naturalistic treatment. Therefore, we decided to incorporate into the PISA system sufficient space only for the recording of the current prescribed treatment. If the psychiatrist requires more precise information regarding the

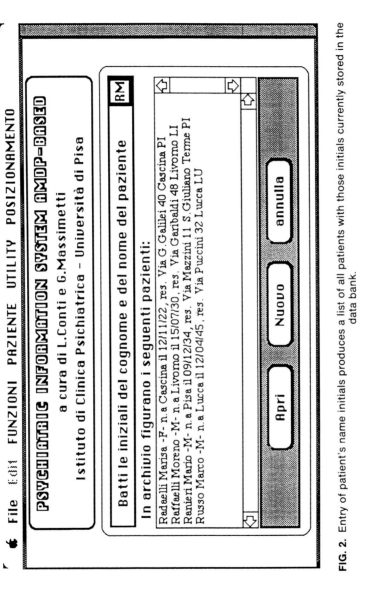

FIG. 2. Entry of patient's name initials produces a list of all patients with those initials currently stored in the data bank.

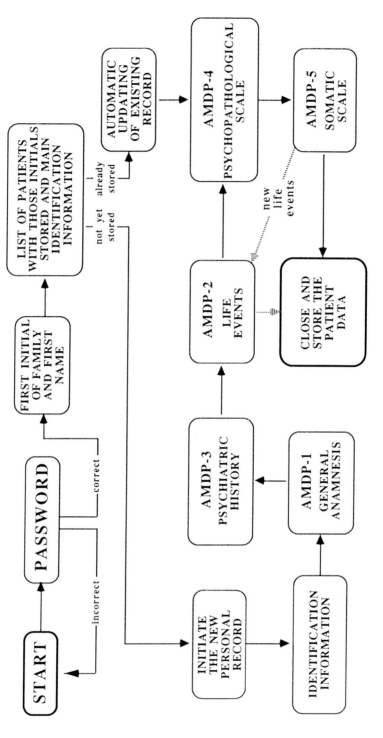

FIG. 3. Scheme of the general functioning of the PISA system.

therapeutic regimen, it is possible to add to the system instruments (such as the DOTES of the BLIPS system) specifically created for the provision of detailed drug documentation.

A principal aspect of the PISA system is the narrative report; for this purpose a procedure for decodification of codified data, the INDaCo (Interprete Narrativo di Dati Codificati), has been designed that although created for the PISA system, is capable of managing any type of data based on a FOX DBF (Data Base File).

INDaCo is easy to learn and utilizes a programming language that permits the construction of simple programs for the automatic interpretation of codified data. These programs, as well as the codified data, are stored as FOX DBF (each record of the DBF represents an instruction of the program) and can be edited and/or modified by means of the standard FOX procedures.

The grammatical DBF is composed of four fields: (a) the "label" field, which distinguishes between different instructions and which provides the logic for specific connections and the ordering of instructions; (b) the "conditions" field, which verifies the existence of the conditions required for the execution of the instructions; (c) the "command" field, consisting of one or more commands to be executed if the "conditions" field is satisfied; and (d) the "sentence" field, which consists of the sentences to be written in the narrative report when all the conditions are satisfied.

The general outline of the INDaCo is clearly explained in Fig. 4: The interpreter checks one instruction at a time against the patient data currently retrieved from the AMDP data bank. The sentences associated with the satisfied instructions are linked together in a buffer which, when the end of file (EOF) is reached, can be sent to the screen and/or to the printer and/or saved as a text file to be processed further by standard word processing.

In addition to the narrative report (complete with diagnosis and prescribed treatment), various optional outputs are available: a list of the "critical" items (i.e., the psychopathologic and somatic items rated as "severe" or "extremely severe"); a bar graph representing the psychopathologic profile of the patient, derived from a factor analysis of the AMDP-4 and -5 scales; a bar graph comparing the actual psychopathologic profile with any previous assessment; and a comparison, in tabular form, among the factor scores of up to 10 different assessments.

A selection program, which permits the retrieval of stored data on the basis of external criteria and the organization of the selected data for use with the most common statistical packages, is also available.

Apart from its use in psychiatric practice, the PISA system could serve as a useful teaching tool, both for its structural characteristics and for the presence of the on-line "help" facility. The structural characteristics of the system would guide the student to a systematic and complete collection of psychiatric information and the on-line "help" facility would make available to the student appropriate additional explanations of psychopathologic terms,

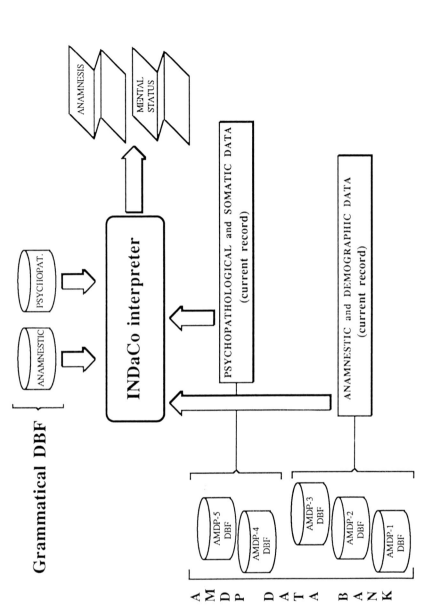

FIG. 4. General functioning scheme of INDaCo system.

derived from the AMDP manual, explanations which are based on the work of an international committee of experienced psychiatrists.

At present, 70% of the PISA system is ready to run: most of the subroutines have been tested successfully and some of them have already been assembled. A few more months are still required before a completed version of the system can be tested in actual psychiatric practice. We predict that by the end of 1991 the PISA system will be ready for extensive use.

REFERENCES

1. Marconi PL, Massimetti G, Mengali F, Conti L. Psichiatria e informatica. In: Cassano GB et al., eds. *Trattato italiano di Psichiatria*. Milan:Masson, 1993.
2. Guy W. *ECDEU Assessment manual for psychopharmacology*. DHEW Publication No. (ADM) -338, 1976.
3. Cassano GB, Conti L, Massimetti G, Mauri M, Dell'osso L. CCPDD—Un centro per la documentazione dei data in psicofarmacologia clinica. *Riv Psichiatria* 1985;20:1–17.
4. Conti L, Massimetti G, Mengali F, Cassano GB. Un sistema per la gestione automatica di dati psicofarmacologici su personal computer. *Med Inf* 1989;6:11–8.
5. *Arbeitsgemeinschaft für methodik und dokumentation in der psychiatrie*. Das AMDP-System, Berlin: Springer, 1979.
6. Lopez-Ibor Aliño JJ. *El sistema AMDP*. Madrid, Grupo Para El Progreso de la Psiquiatria, 1980.
7. Bobon DP. *Le système AMDP*, 2nd edition. Mardaga, Bruxelles, 1981.
8. Conti L, Dell'osso L, Cassano GB. Il Sistema AMDP. Mazzucchelli S.R.L., Milano, 1990.

Psychiatry and Advanced Technologies,
edited by L. Ravizza, F. Bogetto, and
E. Zanalda. Raven Press, Ltd.,
New York © 1993.

20

Computers and Psychiatric Nosology with Special Reference to the Code-DD

Thomas A. Ban

Department of Psychiatry, Vanderbilt University, Nashville, Tennessee 37232

Nosology is one of the two main disciplines that provide a solid foundation for modern psychiatry. *Psychopathology*, the other main discipline, is concerned with the identification, description, and classification of signs and symptoms of psychiatric disorders, whereas *nosology* deals with the integration of signs and symptoms into diseases and the classification of mental disorders.

Development of psychiatric nosology is intimately linked to the development of a methodology with the capability to separate distinctive categories within mental illness, and the current revival of interest in psychiatric nosology is the result of the recognition that a valid psychiatric nosology is an essential prerequisite for the interpretation of findings in research in which advanced technologies are employed.

Despite its utmost importance, it is not known which of the many classifications can provide a nosology, with a high predictive validity, of psychiatric disorders. To break the impasse created by this situation, a methodology was developed to render nosologic concepts accessible for validation, by allowing the comparison of conceptually different systems of diagnostic classifications. The methodology is referred to as Composite Diagnostic Evaluation, or CODE System.

THE CODE SYSTEM

The CODE System consists of a set of diagnostic instruments, one instrument for each nosologic entity, which, by specially devised algorithms, can assign patients to diagnosis in several diagnostic systems (within the particular nosologic category) simultaneously. To achieve its objective, each CODE within the system, dealing with a different nosologic entity, consists of a set of symptoms, referred to as "codes," which allow diagnoses in all the component diagnostic systems of the nosologic category; a semistructured interview suitable for elicitation of the symptoms and the establishment of whether "absent" or "present"; and a set of diagnostic decision trees that allow the organization of symptoms into distinctive psychiatric illnesses in all the component diagnostic systems.

The prototype of all CODEs is CODE-DD, the Composite Diagnostic Evaluation for Depressive Disorders (1). It consists of a Rating Scale for Depressive Diagnoses (RSDD) with its subscale, the Rating Scale for the Assessment of Severity in Depressive Disorders (RSASDD). The RSDD is based on 90 characteristic variables of depressive illness, presented in the order of the "dynamic totality" of psychiatric disease (2). Of the 90 variables of the RSDD, only 40 are employed in the RSASDD. They are grouped together under 10 headings, each representing a different affected area of mental functioning in depressive illness.

To obtain the information necessary for completing the RSDD, a Semi-Structured Interview for Depressive Disorders (SSIDD) was devised. It consists of 90 sets of questions, each set corresponding to one specific RSDD variable. For 63 of the 90 RSDD variables, the decisions, whether "present" or "absent," are based exclusively on the answers of the patient, whereas for another 12 RSDD variables they are based exclusively on the observations and/or judgment of the interviewer while administering the SSIDD. Of the remaining 15 variables, the decisions are based on both; the verbal responses of the patient can be overruled by the observations (judgments) of the interviewer.

CODE-DD can provide diagnoses within 25 diagnostic systems. This is achieved by a transformation of the component classifications in a manner to fit variables of the RSDD and the adoption of a decision tree model. Because the SSIDD contains the necessary information for all diagnostic decisions, by employing a simple algorithm 25 diagnoses can be obtained simultaneously. Of the 25 diagnostic systems included in CODE-DD, five are derived from the conceptual development of European classifications (although in the formulation of one of the five classifications, i.e., ICD-10, consensus of experts has played a prominent role); ten are empirical classifications, the results of factor or cluster analyses of psychiatric rating scales; five are research-oriented classifications (although in the formulation of one of the five classifications, i.e., DSM-III-R, consensus of experts has played a prominent role); four are classifications that have been in use in one or another country; and one is a composite diagnostic classification of depressive disorders (CDC of CODE-DD), based on the different other classifications.

USES: CLINICAL, EDUCATIONAL, AND RESEARCH

Administration of CODE-DD is based on a 30- to 40-min computer-prompted interview, which can be carried out at any location provided a laptop computer and the necessary diskette are available. The program presently in use is written in the Fortran programming language for the MS-DOS operating system and requires an IBM or IBM-compatible computer.

Administration of the semistructured interview begins with introductory questions (not used in the diagnostic decisions) restricted to information on demography and psychiatric history. It continues with 90 sets of questions starting with questions to the patient and ending with questions to the interviewer. The same program is employed for clinical, educational, and research purposes. However, when employed for clinical purposes exclusively the printout is restricted to information on the patient's demography, including psychiatric history, severity, and diagnostic profile, whereas when it is employed for educational purposes the printout also includes information on the patient's symptom profile and on the diagnostic decision-making process.

CODE-DD is a suitable instrument for multicenter clinical research. An early pilot study of inter-rater reliability, carried out with the participating investigators of a multinational clinical trial, revealed a median item agreement of 87.8%, with a higher than 80% agreement for 74 of the 90 items. Interpretation of kappa coefficient, however, was difficult, because of the widely varying distribution of patients in the different systems. For example, the highest kappa coefficients were encountered with the Vienna Research Criteria (0.795) and Winokur's Criteria (0.607), with an inter-rater agreement of 87.8% and 79.6%, respectively, whereas the lowest kappa coefficients were encountered with Robins and Guze's Criteria (0.000) and Klein's Criteria (0.000), with an inter-rater agreement of 95.5% in both. In more recent inter-rater reliability studies, it is not uncommon to attain a 100% inter-rater agreement.

Other investigations have revealed that the severity score of the RSASDD, derived by the administration of CODE-DD, highly correlated with the total score of frequently employed rating scales. Thus, for example, the correlation coefficient between the total scores of the RSASDD and the Hamilton Depression Scale was 0.7848, and between the RSASDD and the Beck Scale 0.6894. In other studies, again it was found that approximately one-third of the patients who fulfilled DSM-III-R criteria for a depressive illness did not fulfill the Vienna Research criteria, and approximately one-fifth of the same patients did not fulfill Kraepelin's criteria. From a practical and heuristic point of view, however, probably most important are the psychopharmacologic findings that responsiveness to treatment differs in the different subforms of depression and that there is a linear relationship between responsiveness to treatment with an inactive placebo and with antidepressant drugs.

CONCLUSION

It is increasingly recognized that a valid psychiatric nosology is an essential prerequisite for the interpretation of contributions from the neurosciences with possible relevance to mental illness. Such a nosology might also play a significant role in bridging the increasingly widening gap between neuropharmacologic research and its psychopharmacologic applications (1,2).

In the CODE system, a composite diagnostic evaluation of mental disorders is presented and a methodology put forward for the identification of clinically relevant forms and subforms of psychiatric illness. If any of the clinical forms and/or subforms represent biologically meaningful populations, the CODE system has fulfilled its role by providing the necessary endpoints for research in the neurobiology and molecular genetics of mental illness.

Finally, it should be noted that the CODE system is based on the contention that psychiatric illness, like any other medical illness, is the result of a specific disease process. As such, mental disease, like any other disease "is of antiquity and nothing about it changes. It is we who change, as we learn to recognize what was formerly imperceptable" (3).

REFERENCES

1. Ban TA. *Composite diagnostic evaluation of depressive disorders: CODE-DD*. Brentwood: JM Productions, 1989.
2. Ban TA. Prelegomenon to the clinical prerequisite: psychopharmacology and the classification of mental disorders. *Prog Neuropsychopharmacol Biol Psychiatry* 1987;11:527–80.
3. Charcot JM. *Lectures on the diseases of the nervous system: delivered at La Salpetriere by JM Charcot*. Translated by George Sigerson. London: New Sydenham Society, 1877.

Psychiatry and Advanced Technologies,
edited by L. Ravizza, F. Bogetto, and
E. Zanalda. Raven Press, Ltd.,
New York © 1993.

21

D$_2$ Receptor Heterogeneity: Molecular and Cellular Evidence

Cristina Missale, Sandra Sigala, and PierFranco Spano

Institute of Pharmacology and Experimental Therapeutics, School of Medicine, University of Brescia, 25124 Brescia, Italy

The classification of dopamine (DA) receptors is an extremely controversial subject. In 1978, Spano et al. (1) suggested the existence of two different populations of DA receptors, named D$_1$ and D$_2$, on the basis of biochemical and pharmacologic criteria. In this classification scheme, which was summarized by Kebabian and Calne in 1979 (2), D$_1$ was the receptor associated with stimulation of adenylate cyclase (AC), whereas D$_2$ defined receptors that were independent of the cyclic AMP (cAMP) generating system (Fig. 1). More recently, it has been shown that D$_2$ receptors may inhibit AC activity (3–5) and may activate potassium channels (6–8). The interpretation of these results, however, remains questionable, since it has not been conclusively defined whether a single receptor entity activates different intracellular signals or whether multiple D$_2$ receptor subtypes are involved. Indeed, pharmacologic studies have thus far provided only preliminary evidence for D$_2$ receptor subtypes (9), and the molecular biology approach has revealed that at least two forms of D$_2$ receptor may exist (10,11). These molecules, which appear to be generated by alternative splicing of primary transcripts of a single gene, differ from each other in the insertion of a stretch of 29 amino acids in the third cytoplasmic loop (11,12). Whether or not the "short" and the "long" molecular forms represent functionally distinct receptor subtypes remains to be elucidated.

TRANSDUCTION MECHANISMS AT D$_2$ DOPAMINE RECEPTORS

Dopamine D$_2$ receptors are involved in the regulation of major physiologic functions, particularly in the brain and pituitary gland. That D$_2$ receptor stimulation results in the inhibition of AC activity was first demonstrated by De Camilli et al. (3) in broken-cell prolactinoma preparations and subse-

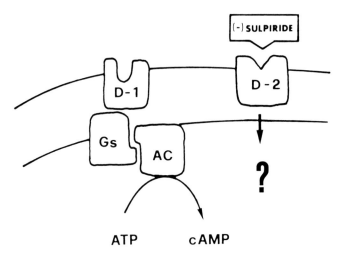

FIG. 1. Signal transduction at DA receptors as proposed by Spano et al. in 1978. DA receptors have been proposed to exist as two classes: D_1 (D-1), which are associated to stimulation of adenylate cyclase and D_2 (D-2), which are uncoupled to the cAMP generating system.

quently in rat anterior pituitary membranes (4,5,13,14). In intact lactotrophs, the increase of both cAMP formation and PRL secretion induced by VIP was found to be prevented by DA and selective D_2 agonists, these effects being stereospecifically blocked by sulpiride and other D_2 receptor antagonists (15). After these discoveries, the development of a selective antagonist for D_1 receptors, i.e., SCH 23390, made it possible to definitively demonstrate an AC coupled to D_2 receptors through an inhibitory Gi protein in most of the CNS regions innervated by dopaminergic fibers (4,16,17) (Fig. 2).

The DA-inhibited AC has therefore been widely used as a unique model to study the pharmacology of D_2 receptors. Recent observations, however, have pointed out that D_2-mediated effects may not be entirely explained by AC inhibition. Such a paradigm has thus being changed by new evidence suggesting multiplicity of signal transduction at D_2 receptors.

The first evidence that DA may inhibit spontaneous Ca^{2+} action poten-

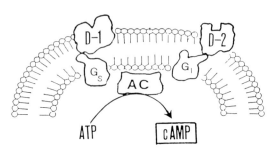

FIG. 2. The dual regulation of adenylate cyclase system by DA receptors.

tials in lactotrophs was reported by Taraskevich and Douglas in 1978 (18). More recently, it was shown by voltage-clamp experiments with neurons from *Lymnaea stagnalis* that DA inhibited a calcium-inward current in a sulpiride-reversible and cAMP-independent manner (19,20). DA was also found to prevent both basal and neurotensin-stimulated Ca^{2+} influx into rat pituitary cells, this effect being mediated by D_2 receptors which appeared to be independent of the cAMP generating system (15,21).

Intracellular recordings from bovine lactotrophs, on the other hand, have shown a hyperpolarizing response to DA associated with increased membrane conductance; this effect had a reversal potential close to -73 mV, suggesting an increase in K^+ permeability (6). Similar conclusions were drawn by studying the electrical properties of both isolated human prolactinoma cells (22) and lactotrophs from female rat pituitary (23). In line with these observations, by evaluating the 86Rb fluxes as a neurochemical index of K^+-channel activity (24,25), it has been recently shown that DA, by interacting with D_2 receptors, increases the K^+ permeability in a purified lactotroph preparation (7). In particular, two distinct K^+ channels appeared to be opened by DA. One of these was Ca^{2+} dependent, the effect of DA being blunted in the presence of cadmium; in addition, the stimulatory effect of DA on this component was prevented by forskolin, which increases intracellular cAMP levels (7), suggesting that in pituitary lactotrophs the activity of Ca^{2+}-dependent K^+ channels is under the control of cAMP and is therefore stimulated by DA as a consequence of AC inhibition. The second DA-stimulated 86Rb efflux component has been shown to be voltage activated, Ca^{2+} insensitive, and cAMP independent (7), suggesting a direct coupling between the channel and D_2 receptors. Single K^+-channel openings associated with D_2 receptor activation have also been recently described in acutely dissociated striatal neurons (8) and in neurons of rat substantia nigra pars compacta (26). Clearly, an effect of DA on K^+ conductance and membrane potential could explain the inhibition of Ca^{2+} influx previously described.

On the other hand, a number of observations have suggested that D_2 receptors could be associated with inhibition of phosphatidylinositolbisphoshate (PIP2) hydrolysis, leading to a decrease in the formation of inositoltrisphosphate (IP3) and diacylglycerol (DG). The available data, however, are rather controversial and no convincing proof has been generated for a direct link between D_2 receptors and this system. In particular, DA inhibition of PIP2 hydrolysis has been regarded as an indirect event in the signal transduction at D_2 receptors (for review see 27). Taken together, the data discussed here strongly suggest that D_2 receptors are associated with at least two different transduction mechanisms: inhibition of AC leading to opening of Ca^{2+}-activated K^+ channels, and activation of voltage-activated, cAMP-independent K^+ channels. These two mechanisms, which result in cell hyperpolarization, may account for the majority of cellular events in the signal cascade initiated by D_2-receptor activation.

PHARMACOLOGY OF D$_2$ RECEPTORS

Heterogeneity within DA receptors has been investigated by evaluating differences in the affinities of agonists and antagonists in binding studies or on AC activity or the different efficacies in various behavioral tests.

The first suggestion of D$_2$ receptor heterogeneity came from studies about the pharmacology and the function of DA autoreceptors. Autoreceptors and postsynaptic D$_2$ receptors have similar pharmacologic characteristics when the relative affinities and selectivities of antagonists are considered. However, concerning their sensitivity to agonists, differences in the pharmacology of the two receptor populations are possible. Behavioral (29,30), electrophysiologic (28), and biochemical observations indeed have suggested that DA agonists are more potent at D$_2$ autoreceptors than at D$_2$ postsynaptic sites. In general, the ED$_{50}$ values for DA agonist-induced sedation (presynaptic response) are, in fact, 10 times lower than those for agonist-induced stereotyped behavior (postsynaptic response) (29,30). Similarly, the ED$_{50}$ value for apomorphine-mediated inhibition of nigrostriatal cell firing is about 10 times lower than for apomorphine-elicited postsynaptic responses (28). In addition, some agents have been described, such as 3-PPP (31) and EMD 23448 (32), that have some selectivity for DA autoreceptors. Taken together, these observations addressed the issue of whether or not pre- and postsynaptic D$_2$ receptors are different molecular entities.

Recently, the higher potency of conventional agonists and the relative selectivity of compounds such as 3-PPP and EMD 23448 for autoreceptors have been related to the greater receptor reserve at presynaptic striatal sites or to the fact that pre- but not postsynaptic D$_2$ receptors might operate in vivo in the high-affinity state, rather than to receptor heterogeneity. In 1983, BHT 920 was developed as a compound stimulating preferentially presynaptic D$_2$ receptors (33). Recent studies in denervated animals and in rats, in which the degree of D$_1$ receptor stimulation was experimentally manipulated, suggested, however, that the concomitant D$_1$ receptor stimulation can easily uncover the postsynaptic activity of BHT 920, giving support to the idea of similarity between pre- and postsynaptic D$_2$ sites (34,35). Interestingly, a retrospective analysis of the literature on BHT 920 pointed out that this compound does not affect either basal or DA-stimulated striatal AC activity (36). This observation may be the first suggestion that BHT 920 does not interact with D$_2$ receptors associated with inhibition of AC. We have recently studied the pharmacology of BHT 920 in purified lactotrophs, in which D$_2$ receptors associated either with AC inhibition or with the modulation of voltage-dependent K$^+$ channels have been described (7). The results of this study suggested that BHT 920 does discriminate between the two populations of D$_2$ receptors. The compound was indeed as potent as quinpirole in inhibiting neurotensin-induced prolactin release and in opening voltage-dependent K$^+$ channels; in contrast, it did not inhibit both basal and VIP-stimulated AC activity in lactotroph homogenates, nor did it affect VIP-induced prolactin release and the activity of the Ca^{2+}-activated, cAMP-dependent K^+ channels in intact cells (9). The first pharmacologic evidence has thus been generated suggesting heterogeneity within D_2 receptors.

CONCLUSIONS

The data obtained by measuring the transduction capability of D_2 receptors in different systems and with different approaches have suggested that two main mechanisms may account for the majority of cellular events in the signal cascade initiated by the receptor activation: inhibition of cAMP formation leading to opening of Ca^{2+}-activated, cAMP-dependent K^+ channels and to opening of voltage-activated, cAMP-independent K^+ channels. The finding that a known D_2 agonist, BHT 920, may discriminate between the two D_2 receptor systems is the first pharmacologic evidence giving essential support to the idea of D_2 receptor heterogeneity (Fig. 3). This assumption has been recently confirmed by data generated by the application of molecular biology to receptor research, showing that two isoforms of D_2 receptors are generated in human and rat pituitary and in rat brain by alternatively spliced mRNAs (37).

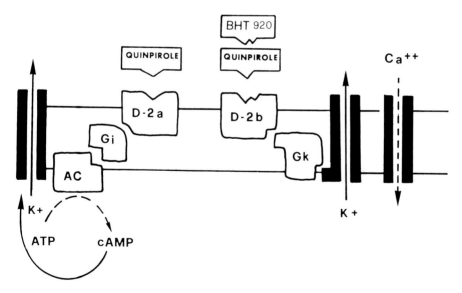

FIG. 3. Signal transduction at D_2 receptors. According to the sensitivity to BHT 920 D_2 receptors have both divided into D_{2a} (D-2a) and D_{2b} (D-2b) subtypes. Activation of D_{2a} receptors results in inhibition of AC; this effect, in turn, increases the permeability of Ca^{2+}-activated potassium (K^+) channels. Activation of the D_{2b} receptor subtype increases potassium permeability through voltage-dependent K^+ channels to hyperpolarize the cell membrane and decrease Ca^{2+} influx.

Whether or not the "short" and the "long" molecular forms represent the D_2 receptors associated with AC or coupled to potassium channels is still a matter of investigation.

REFERENCES

1. Spano PF, Govoni S, Trabucchi M. Studies on pharmacological properties of dopamine receptors in various areas of the central nervous system. *Adv Biochem Psychopharmacol* 1978;19:155–63.
2. Kebabian JW, Calne DB. Multiple receptors for dopamine. *Nature* 1979;277:93–6.
3. De Camilli P, Macconi D, Spada A. Dopamine inhibits adenylate cyclase in human prolactin-secreting pituitary adenomas. *Nature* 1979;278:252–4.
4. Onali P, Schwartz JP, Costa E. Dopaminergic modulation of adenylate cyclase stimulation by vasoactive intestinal peptide (VIP) in anterior pituitary. *Proc Natl Acad Sci USA* 1981; 78:6531–4.
5. Enjalbert A and Bockaert J. Pharmacological characterization of the D-2 dopamine receptor negatively coupled to adenylate cyclase in rat anterior pituitary. *Mol Pharmacol* 1983;23: 576–84.
6. Ingram CD, Bicknell RJ, Mason WT. Intracellular recordings from bovine anterior pituitary cells: modulation of spontaneous activity by regulators of prolactin secretion. *Endocrinology* 1986;119:1508–18.
7. Castelletti L, Memo M, Missale C et al. Potassium channels involved in the transduction mechanism of dopamine D-2 receptors in rat lactotrophs. *J Physiol* 1989;410:251–65.
8. Freedman JE, Weight FF. Single K channels activated by D-2 dopamine receptors in acutely dissociated neurons from rat corpus striatum. *Proc Natl Acad Sci USA* 1988;85:3618–22.
9. Pizzi M, Valerio A, Benarese M, et al. Selective stimulation of a subtype of dopamine D-2 receptors by the azepine derivative BHT 920 in rat pituitary. *Mol Neuropharmacol* 1990;1:37–42.
10. Bunzow JR, Van Tol HHM, Grandy DK, et al. Cloning and expression of a rat D-2 dopamine receptor cDNA. *Nature* 1988;336:783–7.
11. Dal Toso R, Sommer B, Ewert M et al. The dopamine D-2 receptor: two molecular forms generated by alternative splicing. *EMBO J* 1989;8:4025–34.
12. Monsma FJ, McVittie CD, Gerfen CR, et al. Multiple D-2 dopamine receptors produced by alternative RNA splicing. *Nature* 1989;342:926–9.
13. Cote TE, Grewe CW, Kebabian JW. Stimulation of a D-2 dopamine receptor in the intermediate lobe of rat pituitary gland decreases the responsiveness of beta adrenoceptors: biochemical mechanism. *Endocrinology* 1981;108:420–6.
14. Swennen L, Denef C. Physiological concentrations of dopamine decrease adenosine 3′,5′-monophosphate levels in cultured rat anterior pituitary cells and enriched populations of lactotrophs: evidence for a causal relationship to inhibition of prolactin release. *Endocrinology* 1982;111:398–404.
15. Memo M, Castelletti L, Missale C, et al. Dopaminergic inhibition of prolactin release and calcium influx induced by neurotensin in anterior pituitary is independent of cyclic AMP system. *J Neurochem* 1986;47:1689–95.
16. Stoof JC, Kebabian JW. Opposing roles for D-1 and D-2 dopamine receptors in efflux of cyclic AMP from rat neostriatum. *Nature* 1981;294:366–8.
17. Memo M, Missale C, Carruba MO, et al. Pharmacology and biochemistry of dopamine receptors in the central nervous system and peripheral tissue. *J Neural Transm* 1986;22: 19–32.
18. Taraskevich PS, Douglas WW. Catecholamine of supposed inhibitory hypophysiotropic function suppress action potentials in prolactin cells. *Nature* 1978;276:832–4..
19. Stoof JC, Werkman TR, Lodder JC, et al. Growth hormone producing cells in Lymnaea stagnalis as a model for mammalian dopamine receptors? *Trends Pharmacol Sci* 1986;1: 7–9.
20. De Vlieger TA, Lodder JC, Werkman TR, et al. Dopamine receptor stimulation has multiple

effects on ionic currents in neuroendocrine cells of the pond snail Lymnaea stagnalis. *Neurosci Lett Suppl* 1985;22:418.

21. Memo M, Carboni E, Trabucchi M, et al. Dopamine inhibition of neurotensin-induced increase in Ca influx into rat pituitary cells. *Brain Res* 1985;347:253–7.

22. Israel JM, Jaquet P, Vincent JD. The electrical properties of isolated human prolactin-secreting adenoma cells and their modification by dopamine *Endocrinology* 1985;117:1448–55.

23. Israel JM, Kirk C, Vincent JD. Electrophysiological responses to dopamine of rat hypophysial cells in lactotroph-enriched primary cultures. *J Physiol* 1987;390:1–22.

24. Bartschat DK, Blaustein MP. Potassium channels in isolated presynaptic nerve terminals from rat brain. *J Physiol* 1985;361:419–40.

25. Bartschat DK, Blaustein MP. Calcium-activated potassium channels in isolated presynaptic nerve terminals from rat brain. *J Physiol* 1985;361:441–57.

26. Lacey HG, Mercuri NB, North RA. Dopamine acts on D-2 receptors to increase potassium conductance in neurones of the rat substantia nigra zona compacta. *J Physiol* 1987;392:397–416.

27. Vallar L, Meldolesi J. Mechanisms of signal transduction at the dopamine D-2 receptor. *Trends Pharmacol Sci* 1989;10:74–7.

28. Skirboll LR, Grace AA, Bunney BS. Dopamine auto- and postsynaptic receptors: electrophysiological evidence for differential sensitivity to dopamine agonists. *Science* 1979;206:80–2.

29. Iversen SD. *Handbook of psychopharmacology.* 1977.

30. Strombom U. Antagonism by haloperidol of locomotor depression induced by small doses of apomorphine. *J Neural Transm* 1977;40:191–4.

31. Hjorth S, Carlsson A, Clark D, et al. 3-PPP, a new centrally acting dopamine receptor agonist with selectivity for autoreceptors. *Life Sci* 1981;28:1225–38.

32. Seyfried CA, Fuxe K, Wolf HP, et al. Neurochemical and functional studies with EMD 23448, a novel dopamine agonist. *Acta Physiol Scand* 1982;116:465–8.

33. Anden NE, Golembiowska-Nikitin K, Thornstrom U. Selective stimulation of dopamine and noradrenaline autoreceptors by BHT 920 and BHT 933, respectively. *Naunyn Schmiedebergs Arch Pharmacol* 1982;321:100–4.

34. Hjorth S, Carlsson A. Postsynaptic dopamine (DA) receptor stimulatory properties of the putative DA autoreceptor-selective agonist BHT 920 uncovered by co-treatment with the D-1 agonist SKF 38393. *Psychopharmacol* 1987;93:534–7.

35. Pifl C, Hornykiewicz O. Postsynaptic dopamine agonist properties of BHT 920 as revealed by concomitant D-1 receptor stimulation. *Eur J Pharmacol* 1988;146:189–91.

36. Jennewein HM, Bruckwick EA, Hanbauer I, et al. Evidence for a specific effect of BHT 920, an azepine derivative, on tyrosine hydroxylase in the dopaminergic system of the rat. *Eur J Pharmacol* 1986;123:363–9.

37. Giros B, Sokoloff P, Martres MP, et al. Alternative splicing directs the expression of two D-2 dopamine receptor isoforms. *Nature* 1989;342:923–6.

Psychiatry and Advanced Technologies, edited by L. Ravizza, F. Bogetto, and E. Zanalda. Raven Press, Ltd., New York © 1993.

22

GABA$_A$-Receptor Complex: A Target Site for General Anesthetics and Ethanol

A. Concas, E. Sanna, M. Serra, G. Santoro, and G. Biggio

Department of Experimental Biology, Division of Pharmacology, University of Cagliari, 09123 Cagliari, Italy

The GABA$_A$ receptors are the molecular sites of the most abundant inhibitory neurotransmitter present in the central nervous system (1). Electrophysiologic studies have established that the interaction of GABA with these sites induces the opening of a chloride channel that is functionally associated with these receptors (2). Furthermore, the GABA$_A$ receptor is known to be a site of action for several pharmacologically important classes of drugs. A wide variety of centrally acting depressant, convulsant, anticonvulsant, anxiolytic, and anxiogenic drugs exert their pharmacologic effects by modulating GABAergic synapses through a specific interaction with high-affinity recognition sites localized at the level of the GABA$_A$/benzodiazepine/Cl$^-$ ionophore receptor complex (3–5). Thus, pharmacologic and biochemical studies have allowed identification of different types of binding sites on this receptor: (i) a recognition site for GABA agonists (muscimol) and antagonists (bicuculline); (ii) a recognition site for both anxiolytic and anxiogenic drugs; (iii) a recognition site for convulsant drugs such as picrotoxin or *t*-butylbicyclophosphorothionate (TBPS); and (iv) a recognition site for the anticonvulsant barbiturates.

More recently, a large number of experimental data have also demonstrated that the GABA$_A$ receptor complex is involved in the pharmacology of some general anesthetics (6–12) and ethanol (13–16). In fact, these compounds have been shown to alter many of the biochemical, electrophysiologic, and behavioral parameters currently used to study the function of the GABA$_A$ receptor complex.

The present chapter will review some studies recently carried out in our laboratory to characterize biochemically the action of propofol (2.6-diisopropylphenol), a novel short-acting general anesthetic, pentobarbital, alphaxalone, and ethanol on the function of the GABA$_A$ complex.

MATERIALS AND METHODS

Animals

Male Sprague–Dawley CD rats (Charles River, Como, Italy) weighing 180–200 g were used. They were housed six per cage for at least 1 week before preparation for experiments at 24°C with lights on from 0800 to 2000 h, and were allowed water and standard laboratory food ad libitum.

In Vitro Studies

Stock solutions of alphaxalone (10 nM) and propofol (56 nM) were dissolved in dimethyl sulfoxide and serial dilutions were made with the incubation buffer. Pentobarbital was dissolved in buffer. All drugs were added to the reaction mixture at the beginning of the incubation. The control groups were incubated with an equivalent amount of solvent.

In Vivo Studies

Ethanol in a 20% (w/v) aqueous solution was injected intragastrically 45–60 min before sacrifice to animals deprived of food and water for 12–15 h before the experiment. Isoniazid was dissolved in distilled water and administered subcutaneously 60 min before sacrifice. Ro 15-4513, Ro 15-1788, diazepam, and FG 7142 were suspended in saline with a drop of Tween 80/5 ml and administered intraperitoneally 70, 70, 30, and 30 min before sacrifice, respectively. β-CCE was suspended in saline with a drop of Tween 80/5 ml and administered intravenously 15 min before sacrifice.

Biochemical Assays

The rats were killed and the brains were rapidly removed and the cerebral cortex was dissected out and used to measure [^{3}H]GABA binding, [^{35}S]TBPS binding, and ^{36}Cl$^-$ uptake (17).

For [^{3}H]propofol binding the tissue was homogenized in 20 vol of ice-cold 0.32 M sucrose in a glass homogenizer fitted with a Teflon pestle. The P$_2$ pellet was resuspended in 10 vol 50 mM Tris-HCl buffer, pH 7.4, and incubation was carried out in the presence of [^{3}H]-propofol (specific activity 23.3 Ci/mmol), using 200–250 μg proteins in a total incubation volume of 500 μl. After 7 h at 37°C the incubations were terminated by rapid filtration through glass fiber filter strips (Whatman GF/B), which were rinsed twice with 4 ml of ice-cold Tris-HCl buffer. Nonspecific binding was defined as the binding in the presence of 30 μM propofol. Saturation studies were based on 12 different concentrations of ligand (50–3,200 nM). The specific activity of [^{3}H]propofol was kept constant at 50 nM and then diluted with unlabeled propofol dissolved in dimethyl sulfoxide.

ANESTHETICS AND GABA$_A$-RECEPTOR FUNCTION

The enhancement of the inhibitory synaptic transmission mediated by the neurotransmitter γ-aminobutyric acid (GABA) is believed to be a general feature of many anesthetic drugs. Accordingly, electrophysiologic and biochemical data have clearly shown that chemically different nonvolatile and inhalation anesthetics produce a marked and persistent enhancement in the function of the GABA$_A$-receptor complex (6–12). Thus, a good correlation has been found between the pharmacologic potency of these compounds and their capability to alter different biochemical parameters ([^{3}H]muscimol binding, [^{35}S]TBPS binding, ^{36}Cl$^-$ uptake) currently used to evaluate in vitro the action of positive and negative modulators of the GABA$_A$-receptor complex.

Recently, propofol, a sterically hindered phenol derivative, has been introduced into clinical practice as an intravenous anesthetic agent characterized by its short recovery time either after a single bolus injection or after infusion (18). The pharmacology of propofol has been broadly reviewed with regard to its pharmacokinetics and pharmacodynamic properties, but little is known about its neurochemical mechanism of action. Electrophysiologic data have indicated a possible interaction of propofol with the GABA$_A$-receptor complex (19). In fact, it has been shown that propofol potentiates the GABA-evoked neuronal inhibition in central neurons.

On the basis of this evidence the present study was undertaken to investigate the possible interaction of propofol with the GABA$_A$-receptor complex. For this purpose, the effect of propofol on [^{3}H]GABA binding, [^{35}S]TBPS uptake, and on muscimol-stimulated ^{36}Cl$^-$ uptake was studied in a membrane preparation of rat cerebral cortex and was compared with the effects of alphaxalone and pentobarbital, two nonvolatile general anesthetics known to enhance GABAergic transmission via the activation of allosteric recognition sites located at the level of the Cl$^-$ channel coupled to GABA$_A$ receptors (10,20,21). As shown in Fig. 1, propofol, like alphaxalone and pentobarbital, enhanced in a concentration-dependent manner the specific binding of [^{3}H]GABA to washed, frozen, and thawed membrane preparations from the rat cerebral cortex. The maximal effect was observed in the presence of 300 μM propofol (59 ± 10% above the control value), 100 μM alphaxalone (70 ± 12%), and 1 mM pentobarbital (78 ± 6.5%). To clarify whether the propofol-induced increase of [^{3}H]GABA binding was related to enhanced activity of the GABA$_A$-receptor–gated chloride channel, we studied the effect of propo-

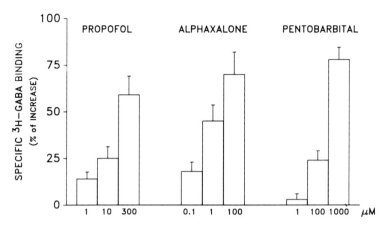

FIG. 1. Increase of [^{3}H]GABA binding induced by alphaxalone, propofol, and pentobarbital in frozen-thawed membrane preparations from rat cerebral cortex. [^{3}H]GABA was measured in frozen-thawed membrane preparations from rat cerebral cortex with 10 nM [^{3}H]GABA. Data are the means ± SEM from three to seven separate experiments, each run in quadruplicate.

fol on [^{35}S]TBPS binding and on muscimol-stimulated ^{36}Cl$^-$ uptake in the rat cerebral cortex.

As shown in Fig. 2, the in vitro addition of propofol, alphaxalone, and pentobarbital to unwashed membrane preparations from rat cerebral cortex inhibited [^{35}S]TBPS binding in a concentration-dependent manner. However, although these drugs showed the same efficacy (maximal inhibition 100%), they differed markedly in potency, being in rank order of potency alphaxalone (IC$_{50}$ 0.3 μM) > propofol (IC$_{50}$ 4 μM) > pentobarbital (IC$_{50}$ 40 μM).

Consistent with these results, propofol enhances muscimol-stimulated ^{36}Cl$^-$ uptake in membrane vesicles from rat cerebral cortex in a concentration-dependent manner (Fig. 3): an effect similar to that induced by alphaxalone and pentobarbital.

Taken together, these data suggest that propofol, like other general anesthetics and several hypnotics, enhances the function of the GABA$_A$ receptor complex. However, the molecular mechanism involved in the action of this anesthetic at the level of the GABAergic synapses remains to be clarified.

The potent and selective enhancement elicited by propofol of GABAergic transmission suggests that the effect of this compound might be mediated through a direct interaction with a specific molecular component of the GABA$_A$-receptor complex.

The failure of propofol to affect [^{3}H]flunitrazepam binding, together with the failure of Ro 15-1788 and PK 11195, a central and a peripheral benzodiazepine receptor ligand (22,23), to antagonize its effect on [^{35}S]TBPS binding

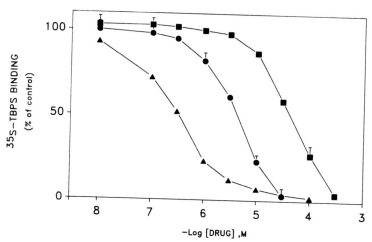

FIG. 2. Decrease of [^{35}S]TBPS binding by propofol (●), alphaxalone (▲), and pentobarbital (■). [^{35}S]TBPS binding was measured in fresh, unwashed membrane preparations from rat cerebral cortex with 2 nM [^{35}S]TBPS. Data are expressed as the percentage decrease in binding from control values and are the means ± SEM from four separate experiments, each run in triplicate. Specific binding of [^{35}S]TBPS in the control group was 51 ± 4.6 fmol/mg protein (mean ± SEM, $n = 16$). (From ref. 17 with permission.)

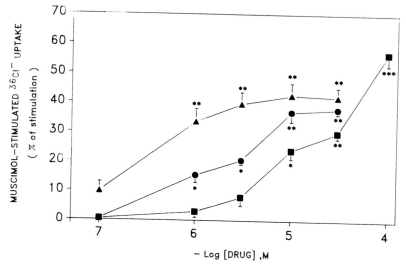

FIG. 3. Enhancement of muscimol-stimulated ^{36}Cl$^-$ uptake into membrane vesicles from rat cerebral cortex by propofol (●), alphaxalone (▲), and pentobarbital (■). Membrane vesicles were preincubated for 10 min at 30°C in the presence of increasing concentrations of drugs or solvent. Data are expressed as the percentage increase in uptake above the muscimol (5 μM)-stimulated ^{36}Cl$^-$ uptake. Data are the means ± SEM from four to seven experiments, each run in quadruplicate. *$p<0.05$; **$p<0.01$; ***$p<0.001$ compared with the control value. (From ref. 17 with permission.)

TABLE 1. *Propofol decreases the density and the affinity of [*^{35}*S]TBPS binding sites in rat cerebral cortex*[a]

	B_{max} (fmol/mg protein)	K_D (nM)
Solvent	1,823 ± 122	83 ± 7
Propofol 5 μM	1,380 ± 119*	117 ± 11*

[a] [^{35}S]TBPS binding was measured using eight concentrations (2.5–500 nM) of [^{35}S]TBPS. Data are the mean ± SEM from four separate experiments, each run in triplicate.
* $p < 0.05$ vs. solvent.

excludes a direct interaction at the level of benzodiazepine recognition sites (17). On the other hand, the finding that propofol completely inhibits [^{35}S]TBPS binding suggests a competitive interaction of this compound on picrotoxin/TBPS recognition sites. However, saturation studies of [^{35}S]TBPS binding indicated that propofol inhibited this parameter in an allosteric manner. In fact, both the apparent K_D and B_{max} of [^{35}S]TBPS binding were altered by propofol (Table 1). Furthermore, the result that the effect of propofol at the level of the GABA$_A$-receptor complex was completely antagonized by the specific GABA$_A$-receptor antagonist bicuculline (17) suggests a possible direct interaction of propofol with the GABA$_A$ recognition site. However, the evidence that propofol enhances rather than reduces [^{3}H]GABA binding should rule out this hypothesis.

Finally, the similarities in the qualitative effect of propofol, pentobarbital, and alphaxalone on GABAergic synapses suggest that recognition sites for steroids and/or barbiturates might be also involved in the action of propofol on the GABA$_A$-receptor complex. To clarify this issue, we evaluated the effect of alphaxalone and pentobarbital in combination with propofol. As shown in Table 2, the concomitant in vitro addition of propofol with either alphaxalone or pentobarbital produced a simple additive enhancement of [^{3}H]GABA binding and muscimol-stimulated ^{36}Cl$^-$ uptake, as well as an additive inhibition of [^{35}S]TBPS binding, suggesting separate sites of action for these drugs.

Taken together, these results strongly suggest that the GABA$_A$-receptor complex may have a relevant role in mediating the anesthetic effect of propofol as well as that of other general anesthetics. Moreover, the finding that propofol fails to competitively interact with the recognition sites at the level of the GABA$_A$-receptor complex might also be evidence for a specific site of action of this drug.

[^{3}H]PROPOFOL BINDING SITE IN THE RAT BRAIN

More recently, to detect putative recognition sites for propofol we examined the binding of the radiolabeled propofol ([^{3}H]propofol) to rat cortical

TABLE 2. *Additive effect of alphaxalone and pentobarbital on the propofol-induced changes of [³H]GABA binding, [³⁵S]TBPS binding, and muscimol-stimulated ³⁶Cl⁻ uptake in rat cerebral cortex[a]*

[³H]GABA binding (% of solvent)	Solvent	+ Alphaxalone (1 μM)	+ Pentobarbital (100 μM)
Solvent	100 ± 5.9	148 ± 4.5*	120 ± 3.1*
Propofol 10 μM	128 ± 4.2*	175 ± 6.3**	147 ± 3.8**

³⁶Cl⁻ uptake (% of solvent)	Solvent	+ Alphaxalone (0.3 μM)	+ Pentobarbital (30 μM)
Solvent	100 ± 6.2	121 ± 4.6*	127 ± 3.9*
Propofol 1 μM	119 ± 3.9*	136 ± 4.2**	146 ± 4.4**

[³⁵S]TBPS binding (% of solvent)	Solvent	+ Alphaxalone (0.1 μM)	+ Pentobarbital (30 μM)
Solvent	100 ± 6.7	71 ± 3.9*	59 ± 4.4*
Propofol 0.3 μM	62 ± 5.8*	35 ± 2.0**	23 ± 4.8**

[a] Data are the means ± SEM from three to seven separate experiments, each run in triplicate.
* $p < 0.05$ vs. solvent; ** $p < 0.05$ vs. propofol.

membranes. [³H]Propofol binding to a crude synaptosomal preparation was highly specific (80–90% of specific binding), increased linearly with the protein concentration, and reached equilibrium within 7 h at 37°C. Saturation studies in the rat cerebral cortex showed that propofol binds to two populations of binding sites (Table 3). Regional distribution studies showed that propofol binding was higher in the cerebellum, cerebral cortex, and hippocampus and lower in the striatum and spinal cord, and is also present in peripheral tissue such as heart and liver (data not shown). Furthermore, [³H]propofol binding is completely inhibited by pretreatment of membranes with proteinase K, suggesting an interaction of propofol with proteins rather than with other components of membrane.

In conclusion, our biochemical data suggest that propofol is a new, suitable tool to investigate the role of GABAergic synapses in the mechanism of action of anesthetic drugs. Moreover, the finding that specific binding sites for propofol exist in the rat brain may constitute a new field of research to

TABLE 3. *[³H]-Propofol binding parameters in rat cerebral cortex[a]*

High affinity	Low affinity
B_{max} 7.8 ± 2 pmol/mg protein	B_{max} 55 ± 12 pmol/mg protein
K_D 112 ± 8 nM	K_D 6.4 ± 1.1 μM

[a] [³H]Propofol binding was measured using 12 concentrations (50–3,200 nM) of [³H]-propofol. Data are the means ± SEM from three separate experiments, each run in triplicate.

study the molecular mechanism involved in the pharmacologic action of general anesthetics.

ETHANOL AND [³⁵S]TBPS BINDING

A large number of behavioral, biochemical, electrophysiologic, and pharmacologic data suggest that GABAergic neurotransmission plays an important role in some of the central actions of ethanol (13–16). One of the major contributions to the understanding of the molecular mechanism involved in the neurochemistry of ethanol has been recently made by several authors who showed that the in vitro addition of ethanol enhances the permeability of the GABA-coupled chloride channel, as revealed by the increase of GABA-mediated influx of $^{36}Cl^-$ measured in brain membrane preparations or in cultured neurons (24–27), an effect similar to that of benzodiazepines and barbiturates and opposite to that of negative modulators of GABAergic transmission (28,29).

In the present report we illustrate some of the biochemical and pharmacologic data obtained by evaluating the effect of the in vivo administration of ethanol on the ex vivo binding of [³⁵S]TBPS measured in unwashed membrane preparations from rat cerebral cortex. Figure 4 shows that the intragastric injection of ethanol (0.5–4 g/kg) produced a dose-related inhibition of [³⁵S]TBPS binding to cortical membranes. This effect was detected 60 min

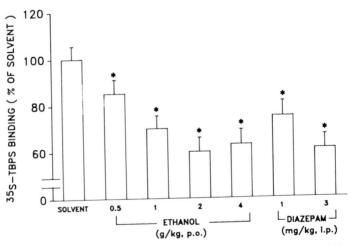

FIG. 4. Acute administration of ethanol and diazepam decreases in a dose-related manner [³⁵S]TBPS binding in the cerebral cortex. Rats were killed 60 and 30 min after the administration of ethanol and diazepam, respectively. Values are the means ± SEM of five separate experiments. *$p < 0.05$ vs. solvent-treated rats (ANOVA followed by Scheffe's test).

after the administration of ethanol and was maximal at the dose of 2 g/kg, which caused in the animals a marked sedation or a slight ataxia.

The ethanol-induced decrease of [^{35}S]TBPS binding was similar to that elicited by the acute administration of diazepam (Fig. 4), suggesting that ethanol, like anxiolytic benzodiazepines, enhances the function of the GABA-coupled Cl$^-$ channel. However, as shown in Fig. 5, Scatchard plot analysis of the saturation isotherms of [^{35}S]TBPS binding revealed that whereas diazepam decreased the density of [^{35}S]TBPS recognition sites, the effect of ethanol was due to a reduction of the apparent affinity of the binding sites for the radioligand, with no change in the receptor density. This result suggests that ethanol and diazepam do not share a common molecular mechanism in the activation of the GABA-coupled Cl$^-$ channel and that different sites of action may be involved. This conclusion is further supported by evidence that pretreatment of rats with flumazenil (8 mg/kg) failed to prevent the effect of ethanol but completely antagonized the diazepam-induced decrease of [^{35}S]TBPS binding (Table 4). Conversely, the previous administration of the imidazodiazepine derivative Ro 15-4513 (8 mg/kg), a benzodiazepine receptor partial inverse agonist known to prevent some of the behavioral, electrophysiologic, biochemical, and pharmacologic effects of ethanol (30–32), completely reversed the effect of both ethanol and diazepam on [^{35}S]TBPS binding, whereas administered alone it increased (+ 28%) this

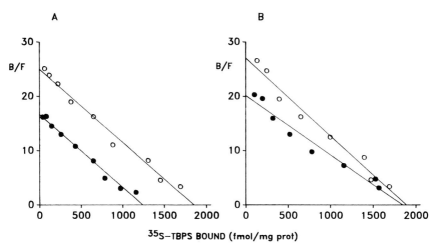

FIG. 5. Differential kinetic characteristics of [^{35}S]TBPS binding in cortical membranes of diazepam **(A)**- and ethanol **(B)**-treated rats. Rats were killed 60 and 30 min after the administration of ethanol (1 g/kg p.o.) and diazepam (3 mg/kg i.p.). Shown are the Scatchard plots corresponding to a typical experiment repeated five times with very similar results. B_{max} (fmol/mg prot) and K_D (nM) in the cerebral cortex of the two groups were: **(A)**, solvent-treated (○): $B_{max} = 1850.8$, $K_D = 74.1$; diazepam-treated (●): $B_{max} = 1240.2^*$, $K_D = 74.5$; **(B)** solvent-treated (○): $B_{max} = 1882.4$, $K_D = 69.5$; ethanol-treated (●): $B_{max} = 1838.8$, $K_D = 91.3$. (From ref. 36 with permission.)

TABLE 4. *Failure of Ro 15-1788 to prevent ethanol-induced decrease of [³⁵S]TBPS binding in rat cerebral cortex[a]*

	[³⁵S]TBPS binding (fmol/mg prot)	
	Solvent	Ro 15-1788 (8 mg/kg)
Control	39.6 ± 2.0	38.0 ± 2.3
Ethanol (1 g/kg)	25.7 ± 1.8*	26.9 ± 2.2*
Diazepam (1 mg/kg)	23.8 ± 2.1*	40.4 ± 2.6

[a] Rats were sacrificed 70, 60, and 30 min after the administration of Ro 15-1788, ethanol, and diazepam, respectively. Values are the means ± SEM of four separate experiments.
* $p < 0.05$ vs. control rats.

parameter (Fig. 6). Moreover, administration of the anxiogenic and proconvulsant β-carboline derivatives FG 7142 (12.5 mg/kg) and β-CCE (0.6 mg/kg), like Ro 15-4513, reversed the effect of ethanol, but administered alone markedly enhanced [³⁵S]TBPS binding in the same membrane preparation (Fig. 6).

To further clarify the action of ethanol on the function of the GABA-coupled Cl⁻, we studied the effect of this compound in rats in which the GABAergic transmission had been inhibited by previous treatment with isoniazid. In agreement with our previous data (33), isoniazid (350 mg/kg) induced in 60 min a marked increase (+62%) of [³⁵S]TBPS binding to rat

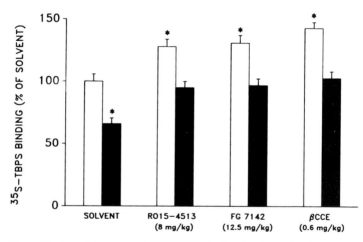

FIG. 6. Ethanol-induced decrease of [³⁵S]TBPS binding in rat cerebral cortex: reversal by Ro 15-4513 and anxiogenic β-carbolines; □, control; ■, ethanol. Rats were killed 70, 60, 30, and 15 min after the administration of Ro 15-4513, ethanol, FG 7142, and β-CCE, respectively. Each value represents the mean ± SEM of five separate experiments. *$p < 0.05$ vs. solvent-treated rats (ANOVA followed by Scheffe's test).

TABLE 5. *Diazepam potentiates the inhibitory action of ethanol on isoniazid-induced increase of [^{35}S]TBPS binding in rat cerebral cortex*[a]

		[^{35}S]-TBPS binding (fmol/mg prot)
Control		39.0 ± 2.3
Isoniazid	(350 mg/kg)	63.2 ± 3.1*
Isoniazid + ethanol	(0.5 g/kg)	50.7 ± 2.9**
Isoniazid + ethanol	(1 g/kg)	46.8 ± 2.9**
Isoniazid + ethanol	(2 g/kg)	44.8 ± 2.6**
Isoniazid + ethanol	(4 g/kg)	46.0 ± 3.0**
Isoniazid + diazepam	(0.25 mg/kg)	56.2 ± 3.3*
Isoniazid + diazepam + ET	(0.5 g/kg)	40.9 ± 2.8

[a] Rats were sacrificed 60, 45, and 30 min after administration of isoniazid, ethanol, and diazepam, respectively. Data are the mean ± SEM from four separate experiments.
* $p < 0.05$ vs. control rats; ** $p < 0.05$ vs. isoniazid-treated rats.

cortical membranes (Table 5). Ethanol (0.4–5 g/kg) administered 15 min after isoniazid significantly reduced in a dose-dependent manner the increase of [^{35}S]TBPS binding induced by isoniazid (Table 5). Moreover, ethanol (0.5 g/kg) markedly potentiated the effect of the injection of a low dose of diazepam (0.25 mg/kg), which per se was ineffective in reducing the increase of [^{35}S]TBPS binding produced by isoniazid. In fact, the concomitant administration of the two drugs completely reversed the effect of this GABAergic inhibitor (Table 5).

Finally, ethanol completely antagonized the tonic–clonic convulsions elicited by isoniazid (350 mg/kg subcutaneously). In fact, as shown in Table 6, the subsequent administration of ethanol (0.5–4 g/kg) markedly reduced the number of rats that exhibited seizures, significantly prolonged the latency period of the convulsive episodes, and attenuated the severity of the seizures.

TABLE 6. *Isoniazid-induced tonic–clonic seizures in rats: antagonism by ethanol*[a]

	Dose (g/kg)	Latency of convulsions (min)	% of rats presenting convulsions	Pattern of convulsions	
				Clonus	Tonus
Saline		56 ± 6	100	18/20	7/20
Ethanol	0.5	63 ± 7	85	16/20	6/20
Ethanol	1	76 ± 11*	60	12/20	4/20
Ethanol	2	90 ± 8*	30	6/20**	2/20
Ethanol	4	180 ± 23*	10	2/20**	0/20**

[a] Rats were injected subcutaneously with isoniazid (350 mg/kg) and 30 min later ethanol (0.5–4 g/kg) was administered intragastrically. Rats were then observed for the following 4 h during which latency and pattern of tonic–clonic seizures were recorded. Values in the columns of pattern of convulsions (clonus–tonus) are expressed as a number of rats affected per total number of animals in the given group. (From ref. 36 with permission.)
* $p < 0.05$ vs. saline-treated rats (ANOVA followed by Scheffe's test); ** $p < 0.05$ vs. saline-treated rats (Fisher's exact probability test).

CONCLUSIONS

The present results suggest that the in vivo administration of ethanol enhances the function of the $GABA_A$ receptor-coupled chloride ionophore in the rat brain. Accordingly, we found that the intragastric injection of ethanol induces a dose-related decrease of [^{35}S]TBPS binding measured ex vivo in cortical membrane preparations. This effect is similar to that elicited by diazepam and is reversed by the negative modulators of GABAergic transmission Ro 15-4513 and β-carbolines. These findings are in line with several previous reports showing that in vitro addition of high concentrations of ethanol increases $GABA_A$ receptor-mediated $^{36}Cl^-$ uptake (16,25,27) and decreases [^{35}S]TBPS binding in rat brain membranes (34,35).

Taken together, these data strongly suggest that some of the pharmacologic actions exerted by ethanol are mediated through a positive interaction at the level of the $GABA_A$-receptor complex. However, the exact nature of this interaction remains to be clarified. Considering the different kinetic profiles of [^{35}S]TBPS binding found in the action of ethanol (decrease in the apparent affinity of [^{35}S]TBPS binding sites for the ligand) and diazepam (decrease in the [^{35}S]TBPS binding site density), we can conclude that different molecular mechanisms are involved in the effects of these compounds at the level of the $GABA_A$ receptor coupled. This conclusion is further supported by the fact that pretreatment of rats with the specific benzodiazepine receptor antagonist Ro 15-1788 does not abolish the inhibitory effect of ethanol on [^{35}S]TBPS binding, whereas it completely antagonized that of diazepam.

These results suggest that the action of ethanol is not mediated by a direct activation of benzodiazepine receptors. This conclusion is also supported by data showing that the concomitant administration of ethanol and diazepam results in a dramatic potentiation of the inhibitory effects on [^{35}S]TBPS binding, indicating that the two drugs have a mutual synergistic action. Conversely, the data showing that the benzodiazepine receptor ligand Ro 15-4513 reverses the ethanol-induced decrease of [^{35}S]TBPS binding could be explained by a partial inverse agonist property of this compound at the benzodiazepine recognition site. In fact, the benzodiazepine receptor partial inverse agonists FG 7142 and β-CCE prevent, similarly to Ro 15-4513, ethanol-induced inhibition of [^{35}S]TBPS binding. These findings, together with previous in vitro (16,25,34) and in vivo (27) studies, support the idea that ethanol potentiates GABAergic transmission by enhancing the function of the $GABA_A$-receptor–coupled chloride ionophore.

This conclusion is supported further by the antagonistic effect of ethanol on the biochemical and pharmacologic actions of isoniazid, an inhibitory of GABAergic transmission. Accordingly, ethanol, like diazepam, prevents in a dose-related manner both the enhancement of [^{35}S]TBPS binding and the convulsive activity elicited by the administration of isoniazid, further suggesting that ethanol potentiates GABAergic transmission.

In conclusion, our data indicate that the in vivo administration of ethanol, with an effect similar to that of the anxiolytic and anticonvulsant diazepam, decreased [^{35}S]TBPS binding in the rat cerebral cortex and antagonized the convulsive pattern induced by isoniazid.

Finally, these data strongly suggest that ethanol exerts its actions through a rather specific interaction at the level of the GABA$_A$-receptor–coupled chloride ionophore, an event that might play a crucial role in the pharmacology of ethanol.

REFERENCES

1. Enna SJ. In: Enna SJ, ed. *The GABA receptors*. Clifton, NJ: Humana Press, 1983:1–23.
2. Bormann J, Hammill OP, Sackman B. Mechanisms of anion permeation through channels gated by glycine and gamma-amino-butyric acid in mouse cultured spinal neurons. *J Physiol* 1987;385:243–86.
3. Biggio G, Costa E. *Benzodiazepine recognition site ligands: biochemistry and pharmacology*. New York: Raven Press, 1983. (Advances in biochemical psychopharmacology, vol. 38).
4. Olsen RW, Venter JC, eds. *Benzodiazepine/GABA receptors and chloride channel: structure and functional properties*. New York: Alan R Liss, 1986.
5. Biggio G, Costa E, eds. *Chloride channels and their modulation by neurotransmitters and drugs*. New York: Raven Press, 1988. (Advances in biochemical psychopharmacology, Vol. 45).
6. Keane PE, Biziere K. The effects of general anaesthetics on GABAergic synaptic transmission. *Life Sci* 1987;41:1437–48.
7. Moody EJ, Suzdak PD, Paul SM, Skolnick P. Modulation of the benzodiazepine/γ-aminobutyric acid receptor chloride-channel complex by inhalation anaesthetics. *J Neurochem* 1988; 51:1386–93.
8. Robertson B. Actions of anaesthetic and avermectin on GABA$_A$ chloride channels in mammalian dorsal root ganglion neurones. *Br J Pharmacol* 1989;98:167–76.
9. Huidobro–Toro JP, Bleck V, Allan AM, Harris RA. Neurochemical actions of anesthetic drugs on the γ-aminobutyric acid receptor-chloride channel complex. *J Pharmacol Exp Ther* 1987;242:963–969.
10. Turner DM, Ransom RW, Yang JS-J, Olsen RW. Steroid anaesthetics and naturally occurring analogs modulate the γ-aminobutyric acid receptor complex at the site distinct from the barbiturates. *J Pharmacol Exp Ther* 1989;248:960–66.
11. Harrison NL, Vicini S, Barker JL. A steroid anesthetic prolongs inhibitory postsynaptic currents in cultured rat hippocampal neurons. *J Neurosci* 1987;7:604–9.
12. Allan AM, Harris RA. Anesthetic and convulsant barbiturates alter γ-aminobutyric acid-stimulated chloride flux across brain membranes. *J Pharmacol Exp Ther* 1986;238:763–8.
13. Liljequist S, Engel JA. Effects of GABAergic agonists and antagonists on various ethanol-induced behavioral changes. *Psychopharmacology* 1982;78:71–5.
14. Hunt WA. The effect of ethanol on GABAergic transmission. *Neurosci Biobehav Rev* 1983; 7:87–95.
15. Mereu G, Gessa GL. Low doses of ethanol inhibit the firing of neurons in the substantia nigra pars reticulata. A GABAergic effect? *Brain Res* 1985;360:325–30.
16. Allan AM, Harris RA. Gamma-aminobutyric acid and alcohol actions: neurochemical studies. *Life Sci* 1986;39:2005–15.
17. Concas A, Santoro G, Serra M, Sanna E, Biggio G. Neurochemical action of the general anaesthetic propofol on the chloride ion channel coupled with GABA$_A$ receptors. *Brain Res* 1991;542:225–32.
18. Langley MS, Heel RC. Propofol: a review of its pharmacodynamic and pharmacokinetic properties and use as an intravenous anaesthetic. *Drugs* 1987;35:342–72.

19. Collins GGS. Effects of the anaesthetic 2,6-diisopropylphenol on synaptic transmission in the rat olfactory cortex slice. *Br J Pharmacol* 1988;95:939–49.
20. Gee KW, Chang W, Brinton RE, McEwen B. GABA-dependent modulation of the Cl⁻ ionophore by steroids in rat brain. *Eur J Pharmacol* 1987;136:419–23.
21. Lambert JJ, Peters JA, Cottrell GA. Actions of synthetic and endogenous steroids on the GABA_A receptor. *Trends Pharmacol Sci* 1987;8:224–7.
22. Hunkeler W, Mohler M, Pieri L, et al. Selective antagonists of benzodiazepines. *Nature* 1981;290:514–6.
23. Le Fur G, Vander N, Perrier ML, et al. Differentiation between two ligands for peripheral benzodiazepine binding sites [³H]Ro 5-4864 and [³H]PK 11195, by thermodynamic studies. *Life Sci* 1983;33:449–57.
24. McQuilkin SJ, Harris RA. Factors affecting actions of ethanol on GABA-activated chloride channels. *Life Sci* 1990;46:527–41.
25. Suzdak PD, Schwartz RD, Skolnick P, Paul SM. Ethanol stimulates gamma-aminobutyric acid receptor mediated chloride transport in rat brain synaptoneurosomes. *Proc Natl Acad Sci USA* 1986;83:4071–5.
26. Ticku MK, Lowrimore P, Lehoullier P. Ethanol enhances GABA-induced ³⁶Cl⁻ influx in primary spinal cord in cultured neurons. *Brain Res Bull* 1986;17:123–6.
27. Allan AM, Harris RA. Acute and chronic ethanol treatments alter GABA receptor-operated chloride channels. *Pharmacol Biochem Behav* 1987;27:665–70.
28. Concas A, Serra M, Atsoggiu T, Biggio G. Foot-shock stress and anxiogenic β-carbolines increase ³⁵S-TBPS binding in the rat cerebral cortex, an effect opposite to anxiolytics and GABA mimetics. *J Neurochem* 1988;51:1868–76.
29. Malatynska E, Serra M, Ikeda M, Biggio G, Yamamura HL. Modulation of GABA-stimulated chloride influx by β-carbolines in rat brain membrane vesicles. *Brain Res* 1988;443: 395–97.
30. Suzdak PD, Glowa JR, Crawley JN, Schwartz RD, Skolnick P, Paul SM. A selective imidazobenzodiazepine antagonist of ethanol in the rat. *Science* 1986;234:1243–7.
31. Bonetti EP, Burkard WP, Gabl M, et al. Ro 15-4513: a partial inverse agonism at the BZR and interaction with ethanol. *Pharmacol Biochem Behav* 1989;31:733–49.
32. Kulkarni SK, Mehta AK, Ticku MK. Comparison of anticonvulsant effect of ethanol against NMDA-, kainic, acid- and picrotoxin-induced convulsions in rats. *Life Sci* 1990;46:481–7.
33. Serra M, Sanna E, Biggio G. Isoniazid, an inhibitor of GABAergic transmission, enhances ³⁵S-TBPS binding in rat cerebral cortex. *Eur J Pharmacol* 1989;103:91–7.
34. Liljequist S, Culp S, Tabakoff B. Effect of ethanol on the binding of ³⁵S-t-butylbicyclophosphorothionate to mouse brain membranes. *Life Sci* 1986;38:1931–9.
35. Liljequist S, Culp S, Tabakoff B. The effect of ethanol on ³⁵S-TBPS binding to mouse brain membranes in the presence of chloride. *Pharmacol Toxicol* 1989;65:362–7.
36. Sanna E, Concas A, Serra M, Santoro G, Biggio G. Ex vivo binding of t-[³⁵S]butylbicyclophosphorothionate: a binding tool to study the pharmacology of ethanol at the γ-aminobutyric acid-coupled chloride channels. *J Pharmacol Exp Ther* 1991;256:922–8.

Psychiatry and Advanced Technologies,
edited by L. Ravizza, F. Bogetto, and
E. Zanalda. Raven Press, Ltd.,
New York © 1993.

23

Refractory Depression: Biological and Pharmacologic Bases

Patrice Boyer

Department of Research, Paris V University, 75014 Paris, France

Basic strategies in the pharmacologic treatment of refractory depression can be summarized as (i) optimization of the current drug regimen; (ii) substitution of the antidepressant used; (iii) combination of two or more different drugs, each one acting through different biochemical modifications; and (iv) withdrawal of undesirable drugs.

Most of these strategies appear to be empirical and are based on everyday clinical practice. Nevertheless the third strategy corresponds to an attempt at rationalizing the use of drugs at the neurotransmitter level. This approach, even if considered as "reductionist," is one of the only options allowed by the present status of our knowledge. This chapter will only examine the extent to which the so-called "mechanisms of action" of antidepressants at the serotonergic and noradrenergic levels can be of some relevance for the understanding of refractory depression (1).

SEROTONERGIC (5-HT) FUNCTION AND REFRACTORY DEPRESSION

If we consider the effects of repeated administration (i.e., the long-term effect) of antidepressants on the indices of serotonergic function in laboratory animals, we can collect a large amount of data from studies using such techniques as receptor binding methods, measurement of brain second-messenger induction (cAMP induction), single-unit electrophysiologic studies, and behavioral responsiveness to antagonists. The different categories of antidepressants can be tested on this 5-HT general functioning model, as shown in Table 1.

There is no consistent change after a long-term antidepressant therapy in binding of the 5-HT_1 receptors (the different subtypes of 5-HT_1 receptors are included in this category) (2). In contrast, the 5-HT_2 receptor binding shows

TABLE 1. *Effects of repeated administration of antidepressant treatments on indices of serotonergic system function in laboratory animals*

Antidepressant category	Receptor binding			Neurophysiological responsiveness to agonists	
	5-HT$_1$	5-HT$_2$	IMI	Presynaptic	Postsynaptic
Specific 5-HT–uptake inhibitors	0	↑ 0	↑	↓	0
Specific NE-uptake inhibitors	↓ 0	↓ 0	↓ 0	0	↑
Nonspecific uptake inhibitors	0	↓	↓ 0	0	↑
MAO inhibitor	↓	↓	↑ 0	↓	0
ECT	0	↑	↓ 0	↓	↑ I

From ref. 1.
↑ = increase, ↓ = decrease, 0 = not affected.

a general decrease after the same long-term therapy, with the important exception that some 5-HT-uptake inhibitors produce an upregulation in this system (the same result is obtained with ECT use) (3). The imipramine binding receptor, which in many studies has been found to be reduced in the platelets of depressed patients, is also upregulated by chronic 5-HT–uptake inhibitor treatment. In the same way, the long-term antidepressant (ADT)-induced decreased physiologic responsiveness to serotonin in presynaptic neurons is specific to the 5-HT–uptake inhibitors and to the monoamine oxidase (MAO) inhibitors (4). The norepinephrine (NE)-uptake inhibitors and the nonspecific serotonin and NE uptake inhibitors produce, conversely, an increased responsiveness to 5-HT in postsynaptic neurons. The behavioral responsiveness to serotonin agonists demonstrates a decrease in activity after longterm treatment with most ADTs (5). In general, the major findings from laboratory animal studies of long-term ADT treatment indicate that the most uniform changes involve a reduced 5-HT$_2$ receptor number at the receptor binding level, a reduced presynaptic sensitivity, and increased postsynaptic sensitivity at the physiologic level.

SEROTONIN HYPOTHESIS OF ANTIDEPRESSANT DRUG ACTION AND OF REFRACTORY DEPRESSION

The previous observations have led to the formulation of the serotonin hypothesis of antidepressant drug action. The acute affect of treatments with MAO inhibitors or 5-HT–uptake inhibitor drugs is to increase synaptic serotonin. This may initially augment serotonin function but because of the stimulation of the presynaptic receptors that are inhibitory to serotonin release, the release in response to the nerve impulse may be less than normal. After longer-term treatment with MAO inhibitors or 5-HT–uptake inhibitors, the increased synaptic 5-HT results in downregulation of the presynaptic receptor; therefore each nerve impulse releases more serotonin (6). A failure in the presynaptic receptor desensitization can account for a first explanation of some depressive states refractory to 5-HT–uptake inhibitor treatment. The absence of presynaptic 5-HT receptor desensitization can itself be due either to lack of a sufficient amount of serotonin in the synaptic cleft or to the maintenance of a hypersensitive state of the receptor. In the first case, the proper therapy would be co-treatment with a 5-HT precursor or with lithium. Major supports for this hypothesis derive both from the parachlorophenylalanine (PCPA) studies and from the low tryptophan diet amino acid study, which provide strong evidence that a sufficient amount of 5-HT at the synaptic level is necessary, although not totally sufficient, for effective antidepressant treatment (7). In the second case, the best strategy would probably consist of administering an NE-uptake inhibitor, the long-term action of which results in an increased responsiveness to serotonin in postsynaptic neurons, as shown by Blier and de Montigny (8).

NORADRENERGIC FUNCTION AND REFRACTORY DEPRESSION

It can be seen in Table 2 that long-term ADT therapy with all compounds thus far tested markedly and reliably reduces β-receptor binding and β-adrenergic–stimulated cyclic AMP accumulation (9). The changes in the α_1 and α_2 adrenergic systems are somewhat more variable but also tend to follow a general pattern of increased physiologic responsiveness in the α_1-adrenergic system (10). This contrasts with the variable but generally decreased neurophysiologic receptor binding responsiveness and behavioral responsiveness to agonists of the α_2-system (11).

TABLE 2. *Effects of repeated administration of antidepressant treatments on indices of noradrenergic function in laboratory animals*

Antidepressant category	Receptor binding			Agonist stimulated cAMP accumulation	Neurophysiological responsiveness to agonists		
	β	α_1	α_2		β	α_1	α_2
Specific 5-HT–uptake inhibitors	↓0	↑0	0	↓ 0	0	—	↓
Specific NE-uptake inhibitors	↓↓	↑0	↓↑0	↓↓	↓0	↑	↓
Nonspecific uptake inhibitors	↓↓	↑0	↓↑0	↓	↓0	↑	↓0
MAO inhibitors	↓↓	↑0	↓	↓	↓	—	—
ECT	↓	↑	↓0	↓	0	—	—

From ref. 1.
— = Not tested.

Thus, the pattern of upregulating the α_1-system and downregulating the α_2-system suggests that, since the inhibitory presynaptic α_2-receptors are less sensitive and the postsynaptic α_2-receptor are more sensitive, an overall increase in postsynaptic α_1-noradrenergic function would occur after ADT.

Drugs with important noradrenergic uptake–blocking properties, such as desmethylimipramine and amitriptyline, produce some α_2-decreased responsiveness of the α_2-system in humans. Responses obtained with the α_2-agonist clonidine (pre- and postsynaptically) are corroborating the previous findings in laboratory animals. Nevertheless, a large number of studies have failed to confirm an antidepressant-induced reversal of the blunted growth-hormone response to clonidine.

In depressed patients, an increased response of cortisol to the α_2-antagonist yohimbine has been shown, together with increased blood pressure and a normal plasma 3-methoxy-4-hydroxy-phenylglycol (MHPG) response. These effects have not been studied after longterm ADT treatment (2). Finally there are very few results, if any, supporting the evidence that increasing the rate of production of norepinephrine precursors or directly stimulating the postsynaptic α-receptor is of help in the treatment of refractory depression. These facts are easily understandable if we consider that after repeated administration the α-receptor postsynaptic down-regulation induced by agonists results in an attenuation of the signal. Administration of MAO inhibitors can reverse these results. Conversely, the use of an α_2-adrenoceptor presynaptic antagonist results in the enhanced release of norepinephrine, and consequently stimulates signal transduction. When given chronically, there is a moderate degree of α_2-autoreceptor upregulation, but this is compensated by the availability of sufficient α_2-antagonist. Thus, there is a sustained enhancement of signal transmission.

Substitution for or combination with an α_2-antagonist seems to be fully justified in the case of therapeutic failure with the use of more classical norepinephrine or mixed NE/5-HT–uptake inhibitors.

CONCLUSION

We cannot assume that a better knowledge of the respective receptor binding affinities, pre- and postsynaptic neurophysiologic and behavioral-induced responsiveness of the different long-term antidepressant therapies will lead us consistently to the proper choice of better treatment in refractory cases. However, because the pre- and postsynaptic serotonin receptor regulatory mechanisms probably play a central role in refractory depression, we will conclude by stressing some of the effects induced by long-term treatment with 5-HT inhibitors. These include neurophysiologic and behavioral serotonin presynaptic receptor desensitization, 5-HT_2 upregulation, and imipramine binding site upregulation. Further hypotheses will certainly be tested with new compounds such as 5-HT$_{1A}$, 5-HT$_2$, and 5-HT$_3$ agonists and antagonists.

REFERENCES

1. Heninger GR, Charney DS, Delgado PL. Neurobiology of treatments of refractory depression. In: American Psychiatric Association, ed. *Review of psychiatry*, Vol 9, Cap 2. Washington, DC: American Psychiatric Association. 1990.
2. Heninger GR, Charney DS, Sernberg DE. Mechanisms of action of antidepressant treatments. In: Meltzer HI, ed. *Psychopharmacology: the third generation of progress*. New York: Raven Press, 1987.
3. Andree TH, Mikuni M, Tong CY. Differential effect of subchronic treatment with various agents on serotonin-2 receptors in rat cerebral cortex. *J Neurochem* 1986;46:191–7.
4. Blier P, de Montigny C. Serotoninergic but not noradrenergic neurons in rat central nervous system are affected by repeated administrations of MAO inhibitors. *Eur J Pharmacol* 1985; 113:85–9.
5. Goodwin GM, De Souza RJ, Green AR. Attenuation by electroconvulsive shock and antidepressant drugs of the 5-HT1A receptor mediated hypothermia and serotonin syndrome produced by 8-OH-DPAT in the rat. *Psychopharmacology* 1987;91:500–5.
6. Sanders–Bush E, Conn PJ. Neurochemistry of serotonin neuronal system: consequences of serotonin receptor activation. In: Meltzer H., ed. *Psychopharmacology: the third generation of progress*. New York: Raven Press, 1987.
7. Shopsin B, Freidman E, Gershon S. Parachlorophenylalanine reversal of tranylcypromine effects in depressed patients. *Arch Gen Psychiatry* 1976;33:811–19.
8. Blier P, de Montigny C. Short term lithium treatment enhances serotoninergic neurotransmission: electrophysiological evidence in the rat CNS. *Eur J Pharmacol* 1985;113:69–77.
9. Costa E, Ravizza L, Barbaccia ML. Evaluation of current theories on the mode of action of antidepressants. In: Bartholini G, Lloyd KG, Morselli PL eds. *Mode of action of antidepressant*. New York: Raven Press, 1986.
10. Hong KV, Rhim BJ, Lee WS. Enhancement of central and peripheral alpha 1 adrenoceptor sensitivity and reduction of alpha 2 adrenoceptor sensitivity following chronic imipramine treatment in rats. *Eur J Pharmacol* 1986;120:275–83.
11. Cohen RM, Aulakh CS, Campbell JC, et al. Functional subsensitivity of alpha 2 adrenoceptors accompanies reductions in yohimbine binding after clorgyline treatment. *Eur J Pharmacol* 1982;81:145–8.

Psychiatry and Advanced Technologies,
edited by L. Ravizza, F. Bogetto, and
E. Zanalda. Raven Press, Ltd.,
New York © 1993.

24

Peripheral-Type Benzodiazepine Receptors Are Decreased in Lymphocytes of Untreated Patients with Generalized Anxiety Disorder: Effects of Chronic Benzodiazepine Treatment and Withdrawal

Patrizia Ferrero, *Paola Rocca, *Concetta De Leo,
*Anna Maria Milani, Bruno Bergamasco, and *Luigi Ravizza

*Departments of Neurology and *Psychiatry, University of Turin,
10126 Turin, Italy*

Few experimental biologic models are available for understanding anxiety-related neurobiologic processes and for testing putative anxiolytic treatments in vivo on the patients. Most of what is known of the biochemistry of anxiety has come from studying the action of anxiety-reducing or anxiolytic drugs, particularly benzodiazepines (BDZs) (1–3). BDZs elicit their primary therapeutic action in the central nervous system through specific binding sites located in a subunit of the γ-aminobutyric acid ($GABA_A$) receptor (cBDZr) (4,5). In addition to these sites, another class of BDZ recognition sites was identified in peripheral tissues and has been referred to as "peripheral type" BDZ receptors (pBDZr) (for reviews see refs. 6 and 7). The primary subcellular localization of pBDZr appears to be the mitochondrial compartment. Consistent with these findings are recent reports demonstrating effects of pBDZr in steroid biosynthesis, possibly by mediating the delivery or availability of cholesterol to enzymes situated into the inner layer of the mitochondrial membranes (8,9).

The connections between pBDZr and GABA mediated activities are poorly understood. In vitro GABA does not alter the binding affinity or the density of pBDZr and neither do chloride ions (10), whereas systemic administration of drugs with high affinity for the various components of the $GABA_A$ receptor has been shown to alter the density of pBDZr in both peripheral tissues and brain (11,12). Ligands that can bind to the pBDZR with high affinity have been reported to induce convulsions and exhibit proconflict actions (13,14). Moreover, alterations in pBDZr have been assessed in several stress paradigms in animals and humans (7,15–17).

There are relatively few reports on the status of pBDZr in human pathology. An increase in their number was reported in brain during carcinogenesis, Huntington's chorea, and Parkinson's disease, which was associated with events of glial proliferation (18–20). By contrast, a reduced density of pBDZr was demonstrated in nonabstinent alcoholics and patients chronically treated with neuroleptics (21–23). Interestingly, a decrease of pBDZ binding sites labeled by the selective ligand [^{3}H]PK11195 has been described in platelets (24) and lymphocytes (25) from patients with generalized anxiety disorder (GAD) as compared with healthy controls.

This study was undertaken to further assess the characteristics of pBDZr in pathological anxiety. Densities and affinities of the selective pBDZr ligand [^{3}H]PK11195 were measured comparatively in preparations of lymphocyte membranes from patients with anxiety disorders (GAD and panic disorder), other neuropsychiatric diseases, and normal healthy controls. In some of the anxious patients we repeated our binding assay during BDZ treatment and 1 month after cessation of therapy.

MATERIALS AND METHODS

Subjects

Data from 73 patients and 35 healthy controls were available for analysis. The patients were in- or outpatients attending the Psychiatric Clinic and the Department of Neurology, University of Turin, from January 1989 to July 1990. The controls were healthy volunteers recruited from the hospital staff. Informed consent was obtained from all subjects or from the patient's family after the procedure was fully explained. Before inclusion in the study all individuals were examined by at least one research clinician and had a complete history and physical examination, including detailed neurologic and psychiatric evaluations. Electroencephalogram (EEG) analysis and computed tomography (CT) scan of the head were performed in all the demented, Parkinsonian, and epileptic patients but not in those with GAD, panic disorder, or alcoholism or in controls. The subjects were grouped according to the clinical diagnosis into three groups. Group 1 consisted of 23 outpatients with a Diagnostic and Psychiatric Manual of Mental Disorders criteria 3rd edition, revised (DSM-III-R) (1987) diagnosis of anxiety disorders. Subjects with a history of major mental illness, including major depression or a recent history of substance abuse, were excluded. Of the 23 anxious patients, 15 fulfilled the criteria for GAD and eight for panic disorder and had had at least one panic attack in the week before entering the study. For patients with GAD, a rating of 18 or above on the Hamilton Rating Scale of Anxiety (HRSA) and 38 or above on the Trait Form of the State–Trait Anxiety Inventory was required for enrollment in the study. The Hamilton Depression Scale and the Schedule for Affective Disorders and Schizophrenia-Lifetime version were available for panic disorder patients only. None of the patients had received psychoactive drugs before the investigation. For the 15 patients with GAD, blood samples were taken on the day before BDZ administration and while undergoing anxiolytic treatment for 3–6 months (clordemetildiazepam, 2–4 mg/day) as monotherapy. In 10 patients, binding parameters were reexamined at least 1 month after cessation of therapy. Both second and third determinations were carried out when the patients had recovered from anxiety to the extent of having HRSA values within the normal range (mean ± SEM: treated patients 9.1 ± 1.0, withdrawn patients 6.2 ± 0.9).

Group 2 included 50 neuropsychiatric patients. Their diagnoses were as follows: dementia of Alzheimer type (DAT) ($n = 10$), Parkinson's disease (PD) ($n = 10$), Down's syndrome (DS) ($n = 10$), epilepsy ($n = 10$), and alcoholism ($n = 10$). All diagnoses were made according to current established criteria and in the case of DAT met DSM-III-R (1987) criteria for primary degenerative dementia and those of NINCDS-ADRDA group as having "probable" Alzheimer's disease (AD) (26). Current alcoholics met DSM-III-R (1987) criteria for alcohol dependence, degree of severity moderate or severe. At the time of the study, none of the patients with AD and alcoholism was receiving psychoactive drugs for at least 3 months. All the patients with idiopathic PD, stage II–IV according to Hoehm and Yahr, were treated with L-dopa + dopadecarboxylase inhibitor. All the epileptic patients were under chronic treatment with phenobarbital. For all drugs, the average daily dosages were those used currently for therapeutic activity, and every treatment was discontinued at least 12 h before the blood sampling.

Group 3 consisted of 35 healthy controls. The subjects were free of somatic or psychiatric disorders, with no previous family history of psychiatric disturbances, and were receiving no psychoactive medication.

T-lymphocyte subpopulations in blood were also analyzed in each subject by direct immunofluorescence on an automated laser flow cytometry system (Ortho-Spectrum). Monoclonal antibodies of the OKT series were used (Ortho-Immune): OKT_3 defines mature T-cells, OKT_4 marks the helper/inducer subsets, and OKT_8 the cytotoxic/suppressor subset. In our laboratory the normal percentages (mean ± SD) for OKT_3, OKT_4, and OKT_8 were respectively 73 ± 7, 43 ± 7, and 33 ± 7%. Mean white cell counts, as well as the percentage of total T-lymphocytes and that of the various cell subsets, were similar in all the groups examined. The corresponding values (mean ± SD) obtained in GAD patients, other neuropsychiatric patients, and controls were, respectively: white cells (total 1×10^3) 5.0 ± 1.8, 5.2 ± 1.8, and

5.9 ± 1.6; OKT$_3$ 75.8 ± 4.2, 74.3 ± 5.0, and 73.1 ± 6.8; OKT$_4$ 48.2 ± 6.3, 45.7 ± 4.9, and 43.6 ± 6.1; OKT$_8$ 26.7 ± 5.4, 28.3 ± 4.7, and 30.7 ± 6.1.

Lymphocyte Preparations and [^{3}H]PK11195 Binding Assay

Blood samples (30–50 ml) by antecubital venipuncture were collected into heparinized (10 UI/ml blood) glass tubes between 0900 and 0100 h and then processed for lymphocyte purification no later than 2 h after drawing. Lymphocytes were isolated according to the method of Boyum (27). [^{3}H]PK11195 binding was performed according to our previously described method (28). Binding activity was assayed in 50 mM Tris-HCl, pH 7.4, in a final volume of 500 μl, containing 400 μl of lymphocyte membranes (50 μg of protein), 50 μl of [^{3}H]PK11195 (New England Nuclear; specific activity 82.3 Ci/mmol, final concentration 1–50 nM), and 50 μl of buffer in the absence (total binding) or presence (nonspecific binding) of 1 μM PK11195. After a 30-min incubation time at 4°C, the reaction was terminated by the addition of 3 ml of ice-cold buffer and filtration under vacuum over prewetted Whatmann GF/C filters.

RESULTS

Lymphocyte [^{3}H]PK11195 Binding in Generalized Anxiety Disorder

Representative saturation isotherms and relative Scatchard plots of [^{3}H]PK11195 binding to crude lymphocyte membranes from untreated anxious patients and controls are shown in Fig. 1. [^{3}H]PK11195 bound in a specific and saturable manner to a single population of pBDZr in both diagnostic groups. Nonspecific binding increased linearly and was identical in controls and patients (data not shown). GAD produced a significant decrease of the density of lymphocyte [^{3}H]PK11195 binding sites without changing the binding affinity. The maximal number of recognition sites of [^{3}H]PK11195 in lymphocyte crude membrane preparations from GAD patients was decreased by approximately 50%, whereas the average K_d value did not differ significantly from that of the age-matched controls (Table 1).

[^{3}H]PK11195 binding parameters to lymphocytes were then reexamined during anxiolytic treatment and in 10 patients 1 month after BDZ withdrawal. Both these determinations were carried out when anxiety was sufficiently improved, as judged by the clinical assessment and the Hamilton rating scores in the range of normal values. The scattergrams of individual B_{max} values to lymphocyte membranes from nontreated, treated, and drug-free remission anxious patients, as compared with their respective controls, are shown in Fig. 2. The decreased binding capacity was a characteristic feature

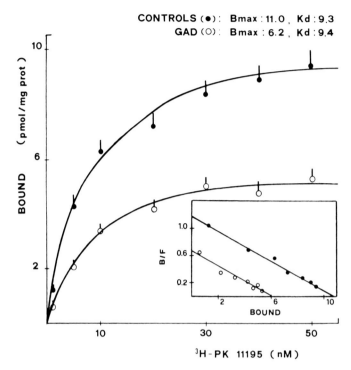

^{3}H-PK 11195 (nM)

FIG. 1. Representative saturation isotherms and Scatchard plots **(inset)** of [^{3}H]PK11195 specific binding to lymphocyte membranes from untreated anxious patients and age-matched controls. Data are mean values from five different experiments. Scatchard analysis shows that the affinity of the binding (slope) did not change, whereas the maximal number of binding sites (intersect at the x-axis) was remarkably reduced in lymphocyte membranes from generalized anxiety disorder (GAD) patients.

TABLE 1. *Specific binding of [^{3}H]-PK11195 to lymphocyte membranes of neuropsychiatric patients and controls[a]*

			[^{3}H]-PK11195 specific binding	
Group	No.	Age (yr)	B_{max} (pmol/mg prot)	K_d (nM)
Controls	35	43.5 ± 2.8	10.0 ± 0.5	9.8 ± 0.6
Generalized anxiety disorder	15	41.1 ± 4.3	5.7 ± 0.4*	10.3 ± 0.6
Panic disorder	8	31.8 ± 2.2	9.4 ± 0.5	10.6 ± 0.9
Alzheimer's disease	10	65.1 ± 2.2	9.8 ± 0.6	9.9 ± 0.6
Parkinson's disease	10	64.6 ± 2.8	10.7 ± 0.8	9.3 ± 0.5
Alcoholism	10	44.8 ± 4.3	9.1 ± 0.8	10.1 ± 1.0
Epilepsy	10	45.8 ± 7.8	9.0 ± 1.5	9.5 ± 0.4
Down's syndrome	10	30.0 ± 5.1	9.7 ± 0.6	9.9 ± 0.7

[a] Values are mean ± SEM.
* $p < 0.001$ if compared with controls and all the other disease groups.

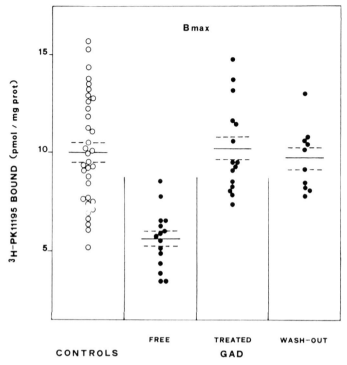

FIG 2. Scattergram of B_{max} values of [^{3}H]PK11195 binding to lymphocyte membranes for patients with generalized anxiety disorder (GAD) and controls. Untreated and treated patients: $n = 15$, mean age $\pm$ SEM, 41.1 $\pm$ 4.3; withdrawn patients: $n = 10$, mean age $\pm$ SEM, 38.3 $\pm$ 4.4. Controls: $n = 35$, mean $K_d \pm$ SEM 9.8 $\pm$ 0.6; untreated patients: $n = 15$, mean $K_d \pm$ SEM 10.3 $\pm$ 0.6; treated patients: $n = 15$, mean $K_d \pm$ SEM 10.5 $\pm$ 0.8; withdrawn patients: $n = 10$, mean $K_d \pm$ SEM 11.1 $\pm$ 1.9. Each point represents an individual subject. The difference in B_{max} value is statistically significant ($p < 0.001$).

in untreated GAD patients, as the numbers of pBDZr returned to the range of control values in anxious patients that were under anxiolytic therapy and remained at this normal level during the drug-free remission period. Neither chronic pharmacologic intervention nor treatment withdrawal altered apparent K_d values. A comparison of the individual Hamilton rating scores (mean HRSA score $\pm$ SEM 27.5 $\pm$ 1.1) and B_{max} values for [^{3}H]PK11195 binding obtained in the untreated GAD patients shows a trend to a significant inverse correlation between these two variables ($r = 0.50$, $p < 0.05$).

Analysis of Lymphocyte [^{3}H]PK11195 Binding in Other Neuropsychiatric Patients

Binding parameters (mean B_{max} and K_d) for all the disease subgroups and correspondent controls are compared in Table 1. The dissociation constant values were the same in all controls and disease groups. Moreover, no significant differences were found between the [³H]PK11195 B_{max} values of the patients with AD, PD, DS, epilepsy, and alcoholism as well as with panic disorder, and their respective controls. No sex effect was observed for [³H]PK11195 binding parameters in any of the studied populations (data not shown). There was no significant correlation between individual B_{max} values and age either in controls ($r = 0.27$) or in the patients with GAD ($r = 0.033$), or in any of the other neuropsychiatric disease groups examined.

DISCUSSION

BDZ are among the most widely prescribed drugs because of their therapeutic action in relieving anxiety. Their anxiolytic effects have been attributed to a modulation of GABA-operated chloride channels (1–3). In addition to binding to this class of neurotransmitter receptors, BDZ have also been reported to bind with high affinity to several other proteins, of which the so-called pBDZr have been studied the most extensively. pBDZr are characterized pharmacologically by their high affinity for the 4'-chlorodiazepam analog Ro 5-4864 and by their very low affinity for other BDZ compounds such as clonazepam and flumazenil, which are high-affinity ligands of the central type GABA-linked BDZ recognition sites. In addition to BDZ, pBDZr exhibit a high affinity for isoquinoline carboxamide compounds, such as PK11195, although the binding domain for both ligands might be not identical in all tissues and species (6,7). pBDZr have been successfully characterized in circulating lymphocytes using the BDZ ligands [³H]diazepam and [³H]Ro 5-4864 (28). The non BDZ compound PK11195 has also been found to label pBDZr on this cell type (25,29). [³H]PK11195 was used in the present study to monitor the characteristics of pBDZr in lymphocyte membranes obtained from a relatively large population of neuropsychiatric patients and normal controls. Our results demonstrate that, first, nontreated patients with GAD exhibit a significant 50% decrease in the number of lymphocyte pBDZr that differentiate them not only from healthy individuals but also from other neuropsychiatric patients and particularly from those with panic disorder. Second, the abnormality in pBDZr associated with GAD is restored to a normal value after 1–3 months of medication with BDZ, which also coincided with recovery from anxiety as reflected by Hamilton rating scores. Furthermore, the biochemical effect seems in some way specific for BDZ recognition sites, because experiments with [³H]NMS binding for cholinergic muscarinic receptors showed no alterations in lymphocyte obtained from GAD patients (30).

The reduction of [³H]PK11195 binding sites in lymphocytes associated with GAD does not appear to be caused by nonspecific variables or other methodological factors. [³H]PK11195 was found to bind specifically and in a saturable manner to a single population of binding sites in all preparations, and no change in the absolute amount of nonspecific binding could be measured between patients and controls. Other possible confounding variables were either controlled for or excluded as an explanation of our findings. We have reported elsewhere and here confirmed that the binding is not affected by age or gender (29). Fasting blood samples were used, collected at the same time of day, and the binding assay performed no longer than 1 week after the membranes were frozen. Furthermore, total white cell blood counts as well as percentages of total T-lymphocytes or T-lymphocyte subsets in the GAD patients were comparable to those of other neuropsychiatric patients and controls, suggesting that the binding abnormality is not dependent on changes in the number or relative proportion of peripheral circulating lymphocytes.

Our results hinge on the general problem of regulation of pBDZr by anxiolytic drugs and anxiety as well. Several investigators have suggested that the GABA/BDZ receptor complex participates in the neurochemical events which mediate anxiety or fear-related behavior (2,31,32). Recent reports implicate pBDZr in anxiety (14,24,25), environmental stress (11,33,34), and convulsive states (35,36). Acute stress, like short-lasting swimming stress (34), surgical stress (15), or examination stress (16) significantly enhances the number of pBDZr. Chronic stress like sessions of inescapable tail-shock reduce pBDZr (7).

The general agreement of our data with those obtained by Weizman et al. (24) and Ferrarese et al. (25), who respectively found a decreased number of pBDZr in platelets and lymphocytes of GAD individuals, suggests that this reduction is a well-reproducible phenomenon not restricted to a single cell type. The finding that it occurs in lymphocytes may have some relevance for previous indications that both anxiety-related agents and stress can modulate immune responses (37). However, the present study clarifies certain aspects of this abnormality. First, we extended [³H]PK11195 binding investigation to another category of anxiety disorders and to several other neuropsychiatric diseases, some of which are associated with abnormality of central GABAergic transmission. Second, we analyzed [³H]PK11195 binding when the anxious patients recovered from their anxiety, whether they were under anxiolytic treatment or withdrawn from therapy. Our results indicate that the alteration of pBDZr seems highly associated with GAD, as the receptor density was not decreased in lymphocytes from patients with panic disorder, AD, PD, DS, epilepsy, and alcoholism. The difference in pBDZr status between GAD and panic disorder patients could prove valuable as a diagnostic criterion to distinguish subtypes of pathologic anxiety. Interestingly, in a recent study we found that pBDZr may distinguish a subtype of obsessive–compulsive disorder (30). Current concepts suggest the separation of the syndrome of panic disorder from other forms of anxiety disorders (38,39), and an extensive literature points to a relationship of affective disorder with panic disorder (40,41).

Two important (but as yet unanswered) questions arise from our findings. The first is whether modifications of lymphocyte pBDZr can represent a state or a trait marker of GAD. The normalization of the binding density observed in this study in response to drug treatment was positively associated with symptom recovery. Moreover, the number of binding sites present in lymphocytes before treatment correlated significantly with anxiety severity ratings. These data suggest that lymphocyte [^{3}H]PK11195 binding might be considered a state-dependent marker and could become a diagnostic aid, particularly useful in cases of unclear classical symptoms. The further study of patients who do not show a clinical improvement under anxiolytic therapies might validate this suggestion.

The other question concerns the mechanism(s) responsible for the GAD-induced reduction in [^{3}H]PK11195 binding. Possible mechanisms include a change in an endogenous BDZ receptor ligand, perhaps released into blood during the chronic anxiety condition. At present, the best-identified substances that are candidates for endogenous ligands of central and peripheral BDZ receptors and share the pharmacologic characteristics as anxiogenic compounds are a 10-kDa protein termed diazepam binding inhibitor (DBI) and some of its peptide fragment products (42). We have demonstrated that pBDZr and DBI coexist in the major sets and subsets of blood lymphocytes as well as in monocytes (43). Measurements of DBI concentration and pBDZr density in distinct peripheral blood mononuclear cells from anxious patients are currently under investigation.

In conclusion, regardless of the mechanism, our data support the view that pathologic anxiety is associated with a pronounced alteration in pBDZr. [^{3}H]PK11195 binding on blood cells seems to represent a useful addition to the few biochemical tools available for the study of anxiety disorders in humans.

REFERENCES

1. Olsen R, Venter C. *Benzodiazepine/GABA receptors and chloride channels: structural and functional properties*. New York: Alan R Liss, 1986.
2. Ninan PT, Insel TM, Cohen RM, Cook JM, Skolnick P, Paul SM. Benzodiazepine receptor-mediated experimental "anxiety" in primates. *Science* 1982;218:1332–4.
3. Corda MG, Biggio G. Stress and GABA-ergic transmission: biochemical and behavioral studies. In: Biggio G, Costa E, eds. *GABAergic transmission and anxiety*. New York: Raven Press, 1986:121–36. (Advances in Biochemical Psychopharmacology, Vol 41.)
4. Costa E, Guidotti A. Molecular mechanism in the receptor action of benzodiazepines. *Annu Rev Pharmacol Toxicol* 1979;19:531–45.
5. Tallmann JF, Paul SM, Skolnick P, Gallager DW. Receptor for age of anxiety. *Science* 1980;207:274–81.
6. Snyder SH, McEnery MW, Verma A. Molecular mechanism of peripheral benzodiazepine receptors. *Neurochem Res* 1990;15:119–23.
7. Drugan RC, Holmes PV. Central and peripheral benzodiazepine receptors: involvement in

an organism's response to physical and psychological stress. *Neurosci Biobehav Rev* 1991; 15:277–98.
8. Mukhin AG, Papadopoulos V, Costa E, Krueger KE. Mitochondrial benzodiazepine receptors regulate steroid biosynthesis. *Proc Natl Acad Sci USA* 1989;9813–6.
9. Papadopoulos V, Mukhin AG, Costa E, Krueger KE. The peripheral-type benzodiazepine receptor is functionally linked to Leydig cell steroidogenesis. *J Biol Chem* 1990;265:3772–9.
10. Schoemaker H, Boles RG, Horst WD, Yamamura HI. Specific high affinity binding sites for the (^{3}H)-Ro 5-4864 in rat brain and kidney. *J Pharmacol Exp Ther* 1983;225:61–9.
11. Rago L, Kiivet RA, Harro J, Pold M. Central- and peripheral-type benzodiazepine receptors. Similar regulation by stress and GABA receptor agonists. *Pharmacol Biochem Behav* 1989;32:879–83.
12. Weizman A, Fares F, Pick CG, Yanai J, Gavish M. Chronic phenobarbital administration affects GABA and benzodiazepine receptors in the brain and periphery. *Eur J Pharmacol* 1989;169:235–40.
13. Weissman BA, Cott J, Paul SM, Skolnick P. Ro 5-4864: a potent benzodiazepine convulsant. *Eur J Pharmacol* 1983;90:149–50.
14. Mizoule J, Gauthier A, Uzan A, et al. Opposite effects of two ligands for peripheral type benzodiazepine binding sites, PK11195 and RO5-4864 in a conflict situation in the rat. *Life Sci* 1985;36:1059–68.
15. Okun F, Weizman R, Kats Y, Bomzon A, Youdim MBH, Gavish M. Increase in central and peripheral benzodiazepine receptors following surgery. *Brain Res* 1988;458:31–6.
16. Karp L, Weizman A, Tyano S, Gavish M. Examination stress, platelet peripheral benzodiazepine binding sites, and plasma hormone levels. *Life Sci* 1989;44:1077–82.
17. Rago LK, Kiivet RA, Harro JE, Allikmets LH. Benzodiazepine binding sites in mice forebrain and kidneys: evidence for similar regulation by GABA receptor agonists. *Pharmacol Biochem Behav* 1986;24:1–3.
18. Benavides J, Fage D, Carter C, Scatton B. Peripheral type benzodiazepine binding sites are a sensitive indirect index of neuronal damage. *Brain Res* 1987;421:167–72.
19. Starosta–Rubistein S, Ciliax BJ, Penney JB, McKeever P, Young AB. Imaging of a glioma using peripheral benzodiazepine receptor binding. *Proc Natl Acad Sci USA* 1987;84:891–5.
20. Ferrarese C, Appollonio M, Gaini SM, Pialti R, Frattola L. Benzodiazepine receptors and diazepam binding inhibitor in human cerebral tumors. *Ann Neurol* 1989;26:564–9.
21. Surany–Cadotte B, Lafaille F, Dongier M, Dumas M, Quiron R. Decreased density of peripheral benzodiazepine binding sites on platelets of currently drinking but not abstinent alcoholics. *Neuropharmacology* 1988;27:443–5.
22. Gavish M, Weizman A, Karp L, Tyano S, Tanne Z. Decreased peripheral benzodiazepine binding sites in platelets of neuroleptic-treated schizophrenics. *Eur J Pharmacol* 1986;121: 275–9.
23. Weizman R, Tanne Z, Karp L, Tyano S, Gavish M. Peripheral-type benzodiazepine binding sites in platelets of schizophrenics with and without tardive dyskinesia. *Life Sci* 1986;39: 549–57.
24. Weizman R, Tanne Z, Granek M, et al. Peripheral benzodiazepine binding sites on platelet membranes are increased during diazepam treatment of anxious patients. *Eur J Pharmacol* 1987;138:289–92.
25. Ferrarese C, Appollonio I, Frigo M, et al. Decreased density of benzodiazepine receptors in lymphocytes of anxious patients: reversal after chronic diazepam treatment. *Acta Psychiatr Scand* 1990;82:169–73.
26. McKahnn G, Drachman D, Folstein M, Katzman R, Price D, Stadlan BM. Clinical diagnosis of Alzheimer's disease: report of the NIN-CDS-ADRDA work group under the auspices of Department of Health and Human Services Task Force on Alzheimer's disease. *Neurology* 1984;134:939–44.
27. Boyum A. Isolation of mononuclear cells and granulocytes from blood. *Scand J Lab Invest* 1968;21:77–85.
28. Moigeon PH, Bidart JM, Alberici GF, Bohuon C. Characterization of a peripheral type benzodiazepine binding site on human circulating lymphocytes. *Eur J Pharmacol* 1983;92: 147–9.
29. Ferrero P, Rocca P, Gualerzi A, et al. ^{3}H-PK11195 binding to lymphocyte peripheral type benzodiazepine receptors: evidence of decreased binding in hepatic encephalopathy. *J Neurol Sci* 1991;102:209–19.

30. Rocca P, Ferrero P, Gualerzi A, et al. Peripheral-type benzodiazepine receptors in anxiety disorders. *Acta Psychiatr Scand* 1991;84:537–44.

31. Dorow R, Horowski R, Paschelke G, Amin M, Braestrup C. Severe anxiety induced by FG 7142, a β-carboline ligand for benzodiazepine receptors. *Lancet* 1983;2:98–9.

32. Insel T, Ninan P, Aloi J, Jimerson D, Skolnick P, Paul S. A benzodiazepine receptor-mediated model of anxiety, studies in nonhuman primates and clinical applications. *Arch Gen Psychiatry* 1984;41:741–50.

33. Drugan RC, Basile AS, Crawley JN, Paul SM, Skolnick P. Inescapable shock reduces (^{3}H)-Ro 5-4864 binding to "peripheral-type" benzodiazepine receptors in the rat. *Pharmacol Biochem Behav* 1986;24:1673–7.

34. Novas ML, Medina JH, Calvo D, De Robertis E. Increase of peripheral type benzodiazepine binding sites in kidney and olfactory bulb in acutely stressed rats. *Eur J Pharmacol* 1987; 135:243–6.

35. Benavides J, Guilloux F, Allam DE, et al. Opposite effects of an agonist Ro5-4864 and an antagonist PK11195 of the peripheral type benzodiazepine binding sites on audiogenic seizure in DBA/2J mice. *Life Sci* 1984;34:2613–20.

36. Weissman BA, Cott J, Jackson JA, et al. "Peripheral-tipe" binding sites for benzodiazepines in brain: relationship to the convulsant actions of Ro5-4864. *J Neurochem* 1985;44: 1494–9.

37. Khansari DN, Murgo AJ, Faith RJ. Effects of stress on the immune system. *Immunol Today* 1990;11:170–5.

38. Klein DF. Anxiety reconceptualized. In: Klein DF, Rabkin J, eds. *Anxiety: new research and changing concepts*. New York: Raven Press, 1981:235–63.

39. Klein DF. Delineation of two drug-responsive anxiety syndromes. *Psychopharmacologia* 1984;5:397–408.

40. Breier A, Charney DS, Heninger GR. The diagnostic validity of anxiety disorders and their relationship to depressive illness. *Am J Psychiatr* 1985;142:787–97.

41. Roy–Byrne P, Uhde TW. Panic disorder and major depression: biological relationships. *Psychopharmacol Bull* 21:546:550.

42. Guidotti A, Berkovich A, Ferrarese C, Santi MR, Costa E. Neuronal-glial differential processing of DBI to yield ligands to central or peripheral benzodiazepine recognition sites. In: Sauvanet J, Langer SZ, Morselli PL, eds. *Imidazopyridine in sleep disorders*. New York: Raven Press, 1988:25–8.

43. Ravizza L, Rocca P, Ferrero P. Lymphocyte peripheral-type benzodiazepine receptors in neuropsychiatric diseases. In: Racagni G, Brunello N, Fukuda T, eds. *Biological Psychiatry*, Vol 1. Amsterdam: Elsevier Science Publisher BV, 1991:750–4.

Psychiatry and Advanced Technologies,
edited by L. Ravizza, F. Bogetto, and
E. Zanalda. Raven Press, Ltd.,
New York © 1993.

25

Excitatory Amino Acid Receptors as a Target for the Action of Nootropic Drugs

A.A. Genazzani, A. Copani, G. Casabona, E. Aronica,
*K.G. Reymann, *M. Krug, †P.L. Canonico, and F. Nicoletti

*Institute of Pharmacology, University of Catania, School of Medicine,
95125 Catania, Italy; *Institute of Neurobiology and Brain Research, University
of Magdeburg, Magdeburg, Germany; and †Department of Pharmacology,
University of Pavia, School of Dentistry, Pavia, Italy*

Activation of excitatory amino acid receptors is involved in the induction
and expression of long-term potentiation (LTP) of excitatory synaptic transmission, a putative substrate for learning and memory. In particular, although
activation of N-methyl-D-aspartate (NMDA) receptors is required for the
induction, an increased expression of α-amino-3-hydroxy-5-methyl-4-isoxa-
zolpropionic acid (AMPA) and perhaps metabotropic receptor may contribute to the late expression of LTP. Nootropic drugs (piracetam, aniracetam,
and oxiracetam) positively modulate AMPA receptors, as reflected by an
increase in AMPA-stimulated $^{45}Ca^{2+}$ influx in primary cultures of cerebellar
neurons. These results support the view that AMPA-sensitive glutamate receptors are putative targets for the action of nootropic drugs.

INTRODUCTION

Nootropic drugs, such as piracetam and its congeners oxiracetam and
aniracetam, are widely used in clinical practice for the treatment of dementia,
alcoholic mental disorders, dyslexia, and posttraumatic disturbance of consciousness, and exert positive effects on learning and memory in experimental animals (1–3). However, their mechanism of action is unknown at present.

A modern approach to the study of the mechanism of action of nootropic
drugs should be based on current knowledge of the molecular mechanisms
underlying the learning process in mammals. The LTP of excitatory synaptic
transmission is considered an experimental model for learning and memory
(4,5). Recent evidence implies a major role for excitatory amino acid (EAA)

receptors in the synaptic events that enable the induction, expression, and maintenance of LTP in the hippocampal formation (for review, see 6). Present results confirm the view (7) that nootropic drugs positively modulate a specific subtype of "ionotropic" EAA receptors activated by AMPA.

LTP AND EAA RECEPTORS

LTP of excitatory synaptic transmission refers to a long-lasting increase in synaptic response induced by high-frequency stimulation of excitatory afferent pathways (5). Because of its fundamental properties (associativity, cooperativity, and specificity), LTP is considered a putative substrate for associative learning. Although LTP is essentially an unitary phenomenon, it can be divided into three stages, i.e., induction, expression, and maintenance (reviewed in ref. 8). Induction of LTP in most (but not all) hippocampal pathways requires the activation of NMDA-sensitive glutamate receptors in the presence of an associative depolarizing stimulus (reviewed in ref. 6). Postsynaptic depolarization is needed to remove the Mg^{2+} blockade of the NMDA-gated ion channel (9,10). The influx of Ca^{2+} through the NMDA-receptor/ionophore complex triggers a cascade of intracellular reactions that leads to the "development" of LTP. A hyperactivity of AMPA-sensitive glutamate receptors underlies the potentiated response to the afferent input in postsynaptic neurons (reviewed in ref. 6). Two distinct mechanisms may account for the increased activity of AMPA receptors: (i) an enhanced release of glutamate (presynaptic component of LTP), which occurs during the early stages of LTP formation (reviewed in ref. 11); and (ii) an increased sensitivity of AMPA receptors, which develops 30 min–2 h after the induction of LTP (12,13). Although arachidonic acid has been implicated as a retrograde messenger responsible for the enhanced release of glutamate, the molecular mechanisms underlying the increased expression of AMPA receptors are unclear at present. The increased responsiveness to iontophoretically applied AMPA that occurs after LTP induction is prevented by the protein kinase C inhibitor K-252b (14). In addition, activation of phospholipase A_2 increases the affinity of [^{3}H]AMPA binding in hippocampal membranes (15). Hence, it has been suggested that activation of Ca^{2+}-dependent enzymes is required to maintain the increased sensitivity of AMPA receptors during the expression of LTP. Generation of diacylglycerol and inositol-1,4,5-triphosphate (Ins-1,4,5-P$_3$) from inositol phospholipids may contribute to sustaining the activity of Ca^{2+}-dependent enzymes during the expression of LTP. Accordingly, we have shown that the stimulation of inositol phospholipid hydrolysis by excitatory amino acids or norepinephrine (but not carbamylcholine) is enhanced after tetanic stimulation of the Schaffer collaterals projecting to the CA1 regions (in hippocampal slices) or the perforant

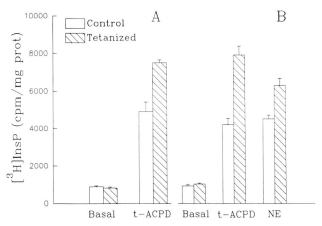

FIG. 1. Stimulation of inositol phospholipid hydrolysis by t-ACPD or norepinephrine in hippocampal slices after tetanic stimulation of excitatory afferent pathways. **(A)** Long-term potentiation (LTP) has been induced in CA1 pyramidal cells by stimulating the Schaffer collaterals in vitro, as described previously (27). Five hours after LTP induction, slices (450 μ*M*) were transferred (three per tube) in Krebs/Henseleit buffer containing 0.3 μ*M* 2-myo-[³H]inositol. Inositol phospholipid hydrolysis was estimated by measuring the accumulation of [³H]inositolmonophosphate (InsP) in the presence of Li⁺, as described previously (28). **(B)** LTP has been induced in the dentate gyrus by stimulating the perforant pathway in freely moving animals, essentially as described previously. Twelve hours after the induction of LTP, animals were sacrificed and transmitter-stimulated [³H]-InsP formation was measured in hippocampal slices, as described previously (18). Values are means ± SEM of 6–12 determinations.

pathway projecting to the dentate gyrus (in freely moving animals) (Fig. 1). This effect required a latency of more than 2 h and was abolished if slices were tetanized in the presence of NMDA-receptor antagonists, a condition in which LTP did not develop (16). These results suggest that an enhanced action of glutamate receptors coupled to inositol phospholipid hydrolysis ("metabotropic" receptors) contributes to the mechanisms that enable the late expression of LTP. Accordingly, both L-2-amino-3-phosphonopropionate (L-AP3) (Reymann et al., personal communication) and L-2-amino-4-phosphonobutanoate (L-AP4) (17) eliminate late phases of LTP induced by tetanic stimulation of the Schaffer collaterals in hippocampal slices. To confirm a role for metabotropic receptors in the expression of LTP, we have induced LTP in animals pretreated with Li⁺, a condition that reduced the extent of excitatory amino acid–stimulated inositol phospholipid hydrolysis in the hippocampus. In animals treated with Li⁺, tetanic stimulation of the perforant pathway induced a "decremental" form of LTP, which decayed back to normal within 5 h (16).

In summary, activation of different glutamate receptor subtypes is involved in the induction, expression, and maintenance of LTP. Hence, any drug that positively modulates NMDA, AMPA, or metabotropic receptors has potential value as a cognition and memory enhancer.

EAA RECEPTORS AS PUTATIVE TARGETS FOR THE ACTION OF NOOTROPIC DRUGS

We have used primary cultures of cerebellar neurons to study signal transduction at EAA receptors in the presence of various pyrrolidone derivatives (piracetam, oxiracetam, and aniracetam). These cultures consist of a homogeneous population of glutamatergic neurons (the granule cells) with few GABAergic neurons and a small number of glial and endothelial cells as contaminants (18). Cultured cerebellar neurons express both ionotropic and metabotropic glutamate receptor subtypes, the activation of which leads to an increased Ca^{2+} influx and inositol phospholipid hydrolysis, respectively (reviewed in 19). Addition of nootropic drugs enhanced the maximal stimulation of $^{45}Ca^{2+}$ influx induced by AMPA (Fig. 2). but not that induced by kainate or NMDA (Table 1). Nootropics did not influence quisqualate-induced phosphoinositide hydrolysis in cultured cerebellar granule cells, excluding an action at metabotropic receptors (Fig. 3). AMPA-stimulated Ca^{2+} influx is mostly mediated by a secondary activation of voltage-sensitive Ca^{2+} channels and or the Na^+/Ca^{2+} antiporter (20,21), although a small proportion of Ca^{2+} entry may follow the activation of high-conductance opening states of AMPA-gated ion channels (22,23). In cultured cerebellar neurons, stimulation of $^{45}Ca^{2+}$ influx by AMPA was substantially reduced in the presence of the voltage-sensitive Ca^{2+}-channel blocker nifedipine. Potentiation of AMPA-stimulated $^{45}Ca^{2+}$ influx by oxiracetam was not obliterated by nifedipine (data not shown), suggesting that the effect of nootropics was not secondary to an increased activity of voltage-sensitive Ca^{2+} channels. The selectivity of nootropic action for AMPA receptor-activated signal transduction confirms the original finding by Ito et al. (7). Accordingly, aniracetam has been found to increase current responses to AMPA and quisqualate, but not to NMDA or kainate, in *Xenopus* oocytes injected with rat brain mRNA (7).

Nootropics may act by unmasking a subset of AMPA receptors that are not normally available for synaptic transmission. [3H]AMPA binding measured in rat cortical membrane was resolvable into high- and low-affinity components with apparent K_D values of 16 and 114 nM, respectively. Piracetam, aniracetam, and oxiracetam increased the maximal density (B_{max}) of low-affinity binding sites for [3H]AMPA without affecting the high-affinity component of the binding (30).

The recruitment of a subpopulation of AMPA receptors may account for the electrophysiologic effects of nootropic drugs, including synaptic facilitation and LTP formation (7,24,25). In addition, recent evidence suggests

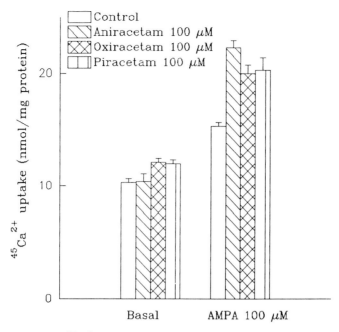

FIG. 2. Stimulation of $^{45}Ca^{2+}$ influx by α-amino-3-hydroxy-5-methyl-4-isoxazolpropionic acid (AMPA) in cultured cerebellar neurons incubated in the presence of aniracetam, oxiracetam, or piracetam. Primary cultures of cerebellar granule cells were prepared from 8-day-old rats, as described previously (28). In brief, cells were dissociated by trypsinization and then suspended in basal Eagle's medium (BME) containing 10% fetal calf serum, 25 mM KCl, 2 mM glutamine, and 0.05 mg/ml gentamicin, and plated (10^6/ml) onto 35-mm Nunc Petri dishes precoated with 10 μg/ml of poly-L-lysine. Cytosine arabinofuranoside (10 μM) was added 16–18 h later to avoid the replication of non-neuronal cells. After 7–9 days of maturation in vitro, these cultures contained over 90% granule cells, 4–6% GABAergic neurons, and a small amount (2–3%) of glial and endothelial cells as contaminants (28). Stimulation of $^{45}Ca^{2+}$ uptake was studied as described by Wroblewski et al. (29). Values are means ± SEM of 6–21 determinations.

TABLE 1. *Stimulation of $^{45}Ca^{2+}$ by AMPA and kainate in cultured cerebellar neurons incubated in the absence or presence of oxiracetam[a]*

	$^{45}Ca^{2+}$ influx (nmol/mg prot)	
	Control	Oxiracetam 100 μM
Basal	9.5 ± 0.9	11 ± 0.3
AMPA (100 μM)	13 ± 0.4	19 ± 1.6*
Kainate (100 μM)	21 ± 2.0	23 ± 1.1

AMPA, α-amino-3-hydroxy-5-methyl-4-isoxazolpropionic acid.
[a] Cultures were incubated in the presence of 1 μM MK-801 to exclude any indirect component mediated by the activation of N-methyl-D-asparate receptors. Values are means ± SEM of six determinations.
* $p < 0.01$ (Student's test) if compared with controls.

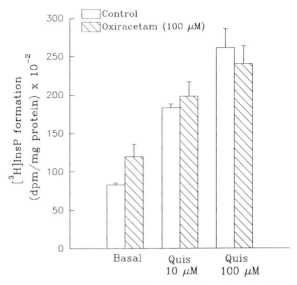

FIG. 3. Stimulation of inositol phospholipid hydrolysis by quisqualate in cultured cerebellar neurons incubated in the presence of oxiracetam. Transmitter-stimulated inositol phospholipid hydrolysis was estimated by measuring the accumulation of [³H]-InsP, as described previously (28). Values are means ± SEM of 6–9 determinations.

that oxiracetam increases glutamate release in depolarized hippocampal slices (26). Taken collectively, these data suggest that nootropic drugs may improve the learning process through a dual mechanism: by increasing the efficiency of postsynaptic AMPA receptors, and by enhancing glutamate release from presynaptic terminals. Further studies are needed to establish whether the effects of nootropic drugs are mediated by their interactions with specific high-affinity sites located on neuronal membranes.

REFERENCES

1. Giurgea CE. The nootropic concept and its prospectives implications. *Drug Rev Res* 1982; 2:441.
2. Branconnier RJE, Cole JO, Dessain EC, Spera KF, Ghazvinian S, DeVitt C. The therapeutic efficacy of pramiracetam in Alzheimer's disease: preliminary observations. *Psychopharm Bull* 1983;19:726.
3. Villardita C, Parini J, Grioli S, Quatropani N, Nicoletti F, Scapagnini U. Clinical and neuropsychological investigation on oxiracetam in patients with mild to moderate degree dementia. *Clin Neuropharmacol* 1986;9:301.
4. Bliss TVP, Gardner-Medwin AR. Long-lasting potentiation of synaptic transmission in the dentate area of anaesthetised rabbit following stimulation of the perforant path. *J Physiol* 1973;232:357.
5. Bliss TVP, Lomo T. Long-lasting potentiation of synaptic transmission in the dentate area of anaesthetised rabbit following stimulation of the perforant path. *J Physiol* 1973;232:331.
6. Collingridge GL, Lester RA. Excitatory aminoacids in the vertebrate central nervous system. *Pharmacol Rev* 1989;40:145.

7. Ito I, Tanabe S, Kohda A, Sugiyama H. Allosteric potentiation of quisqualate receptors by a nootropic drug aniracetam. *J Physiol* 1990;424:533.
8. Matthies H. Neurobiological aspects of learning and memory. *Annu Rev Psychol* 1989;40: 381.
9. Nowak L, Bregetowski J, Ascher P, Herbet A, Pronchiants A. Magnesium gates glutamate-activated channels in mouse central neurons. *Nature* 1983;307:492.
10. Mayer ML, Westbrook GL, Guthrie PD. Voltage-dependent block by Mg^{++} of NMDA responses in spinal cord neurons. *Nature* 1984;309:261.
11. Bliss TVP, Lynch MA. Long-term potentiation of synaptic transmission in the hippocampus: properties and mechanism. In: Landfield PW, Deadwyler SA, eds. *Long-term potentiation: from biophysics to behaviour.* New York: Alan R Liss, 1988:3.
12. Muller D, Lynch J. Long-term potentiation differentially affects two components of synaptic responses in hippocampus. *Proc Natl Acad Sci USA* 1988;85:9346.
13. Davies SN, Lester RAJ, Reymann KJ, Collingridge GL. Temporally distinct pre- and post-synaptic mechanisms maintain long-term potentiation. *Nature* 1989;338:500.
14. Reymann KG, Davies SN, Matthies H, Kase H, Collingridge GL. Activation of a k-252b-sensitive protein kinase is necessary for a post-synaptic phase of long-term potentiation in area CA1 of rat hippocampus. *Eur J Neurosci* 1990;2:481.
15. Massicotte G, Baudry M. Modulation of DL-α-amino-3-hydroxy-5-methylisoxazoleproprionate (AMPA)/quisqualatereceptors by phospholipase A2 treatment. *Neurosci Lett* 1990;118: 245.
16. Aronica E, Frey U, Wagner M, et al. Enhanced sensitivity of "metabotropic" glutamate receptors after induction of long-term potentiation in rat hippocampus. *J Neurochem* 1991; 57:376.
17. Reymann KG, Matthies H. 2-amino-4-phosphonobutyrate selectively eliminates late phase of long-term potentiation in rat hippocampus. *Neurosci Lett* 1989;98:166.
18. Nicoletti F, Wroblewski JT, Novelli A, Alho H, Guidotti A, Costa E. The activation of inositol phospholipid hydrolysis as a signal transducing system for excitatory aminoacids in primary cultures of cerebellar granule cells. *J Neurosci* 1986;6:1905.
19. Costa E, Fadda E, Kozikowski AP, Nicoletti F, Wroblewski JT. Classification and allosteric modulation of excitatory aminoacid signal transduction in brain slices and primary cultures of cerebellar neurons. In: Ferendelli J, Collins R, Johnson E, eds. *Neurobiology of aminoacids, peptides and trophic factors.* Boston: Martinus Nijhoff, 1988:35.
20. Murphy SN, Miller RJ. A glutamate receptor regulates Ca^{++} mobilization in hippocampal neurons. *Proc Natl Acad Sci USA* 1988;85:8737.
21. Weiss JH, Hartley DM, Koh J, Choi DW. The calcium channel blocker nifedipine attenuates slow excitatory aminoacid neurotoxicity. *Science* 1990;247:1474.
22. Cull-Candy SG, Usowicz MM. Multiple conductance channels activated by excitatory aminoacids in cerebellar neurons. *Nature* 1987;325:525.
23. Jahr CE, Stevens CF. Glutamate activates multiple single channel conductance in hippocampal neurons. *Nature* 1987;325:522.
24. Olpe HR, Linch G. The action of piracetam on the electrical activity of hippocampal slices preparation: a field potential analysis. *Eur J Pharmacol* 1982;80:415.
25. Satoh M, Ishihara K, Iwama T, Takagi H. Aniracetam augments and midazolam inhibits the long-term potentiation in guinea pig hippocampal slices. *Neurosci Lett* 1986;68:216.
26. Marchi M, Besana E, Raiteri M. Oxiracetam increases the release of endogenous glutamate from depolarized rat hippocampal slices. *Eur J Pharmacol* 1990;185:247.
27. Reymann KG, Malisch R, Schulzeck K, Brodemann R, Ott T, Matthies H. The duration of long-term potentiation in the CA1 region of the hippocampal slice preparation. *Brain Res Bull* 1985;15:249.
28. Nicoletti F, Iadarola MJ, Wroblewski JT, Costa E. Excitatory aminoacids recognition sites coupled with inositol phospholipid metabolism: developmental changes and interaction with α_1-adrenoreceptors. *Proc Natl Acad Sci USA* 1986;83:1931.
29. Wroblewski JT, Nicoletti F, Costa E. Different coupling of excitatory amino-acid receptors with Ca^{++} channels in primary cultures of granule cells. *Neuropharmacology* 1985;241: 919.
30. Copani A, Genazzani AA, Aleppo G, et al. Nootropic drugs positively modulate 4-amino-3-hydroxy-5-methyl-4-isoxazolepropionic acid-sensitive glutamate receptors in neuronal cultures. *J Neurochem* 1992;58:1199.

Psychiatry and Advanced Technologies,
edited by L. Ravizza, F. Bogetto, and
E. Zanalda. Raven Press, Ltd.,
New York © 1993.

26

A Linkage Study in Italian Schizophrenic Families: Testing the Chromosome 5 Hypothesis

F. Macciardi, *J.L. Kennedy, C. Cavallini, C. Marino,
†P. Carrera, †M. Ferrari, ‡V. Rinaldi, §A. Bussi,
‡D. Piacentini, and E. Smeraldi

*Department of Clinical Psychiatry III, Scientific Institute San Raffaele, University of Milan Medical School, 20127 Milan, Italy; *Clarke Institute of Psychiatry, University of Toronto, School of Medicine, Toronto, Canada; †Department of Molecular Biology, Scientific Institute San Raffaele, 20127 Milan, Italy; ‡USSL 27, Department of Psychiatry, Zogno (BG), Italy; and §USSL 32, Department of Psychiatry, Treviglio (BG), Italy*

The finding by some researchers (1) that schizophrenia co-segregated with a trisomy of a segment of the proximal long arm of chromosome 5 in an uncle–nephew pair prompted genetic linkage studies using the translocated region as a candidate area for susceptibility to schizophrenia. Sherrington et al. (2) found positive evidence for linkage, studying British and Icelandic families, whereas Kennedy et al. (3) found no evidence for linkage between a marker in the 5q11.2-13.3 region and schizophrenia in a geographically isolated Swedish kindred, nor did St. Clair et al. (4) in some Scottish families.

Similar studies from other laboratories have been carried out, but thus far the positive results of Sherrington et al. (2) have not been replicated (5,6). These results cannot be strictly comparable, primarily because of the different approach used in the collection of pedigrees: only the patients with narrowly-defined schizophrenia were selected as affected by Kennedy et al. (3) whereas all the other authors included a broader spectrum of diagnoses in addition to schizophrenia for the definition of the affected phenotype.

In our Institute we decided to further examine the "chromosome 5 hypothesis." We focused our attention on a South European population that had never been investigated before and have chosen pedigrees in which only schizophrenia segregates, tentatively to minimize the effect of a variable phenotypic expression.

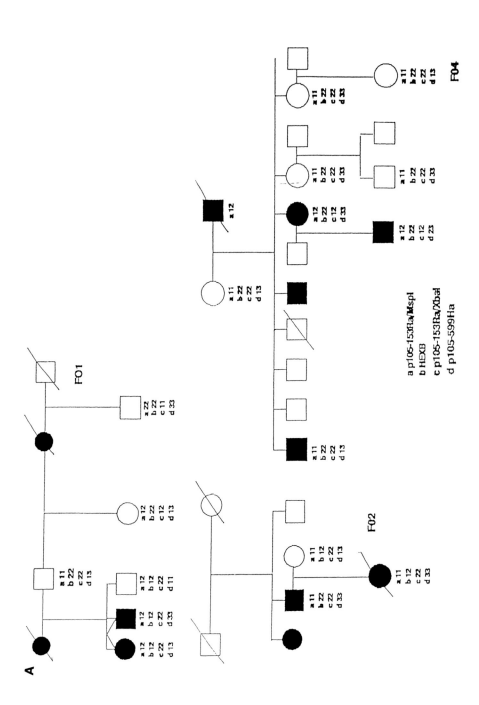

270

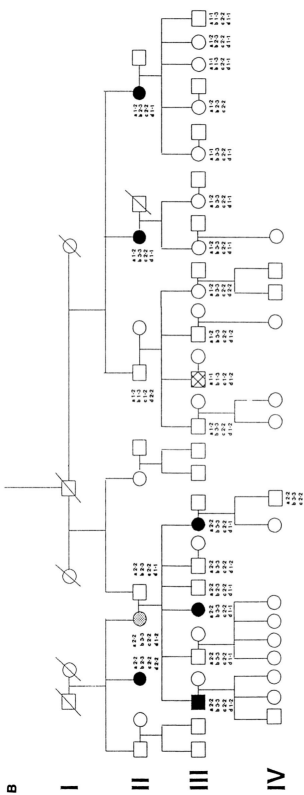

FIG. 1. (A) Pedigrees of families F01, F02, F03, F04 and marker data; ■, schizophrenia. **(B)** Pedigree of family F05 and marker data; ☒, recurrent depression; ●, schizophrenia; ◉, postpartum psychosis.

TABLE 1. Recombination fractions = θ: data of chromosome 5[a]

	0.0	0.1	0.2	0.3	0.4
D5S76	0.13431	0.09475	0.05798	0.02753	0.00717
D5S39 (Msp I)	−2.25314	−0.43178	−0.20454	−0.09810	−0.03762
D5S39 (Xba I)	−2.09271	−0.14219	0.00722	0.03939	0.02938
HEXB	−0.02773	−0.01738	0.00962	0.00423	0.00105

[a] Sum of lod score from F01, F02, F03 families.

MATERIALS AND METHODS

We studied four Italian families (F01, F02, F04, F05), and we personally interviewed most of the people represented in the pedigrees. Of the 73 subjects interviewed, we detected 20 schizophrenics, one subject with major depression recurrent, and one with episodes of atypic psychosis, according to DSM-III-R criteria (7). DNA extracted from blood samples of 44 subjects was digested with MspI, XbaI, BamHI, PstI, and TaqI restriction enzymes and traditional Southern blotting techniques were used to identify restriction fragment length polymorphisms (RFLPs). We have studied four marker loci mapped in the translocated 5q11.2-13.3 area: D5S39, D5S76, D5S6, and HEXB. Individuals were classified as "affected," for the linkage analyses, only when they presented a full clinical picture of schizophrenia. The pattern of the families and their marker distributions are shown in Fig. 1.

RESULTS

In our analyses, schizophrenia was treated as an autosomal dominant trait with equal penetrances of 72% for homozygotes and heterozygotes. The disease allele was given a frequency of 0.0085 to account for a morbid risk of about 1% in the Northern Italian population.

Tables 1 and 2 show the results for paired analyses, using the MLINK program (8), between three loci located on chromosome 5q and the putative locus controlling for schizophrenia. Data shown are the lod scores obtained from independent analyses of all families combined (Table 1) or for family F05 alone (Table 2). The 2-point lod scores obtained for loci D5S76, HEXB, and D5S39, reaching a minimum at θ = 0.0 for D5S39 (lod score −2.2), allowed us to exclude close linkage with these markers. Figure 2 shows the

TABLE 2. Recombination fractions: data of chromosome 5[a]

	0.0	0.1	0.2	0.3	0.4
D5S76	−0.36474	−0.18978	−0.08689	−0.03363	−0.01095
D5S6	−0.42267	−0.25364	−0.14859	−0.07806	−0.02342
D5S39 (Msp I)	−0.18279	−0.12086	−0.07115	−0.03417	−0.01056
HEXB	−0.39538	−0.28848	−0.18393	−0.09114	−0.02458

[a] Lod score of family F03.

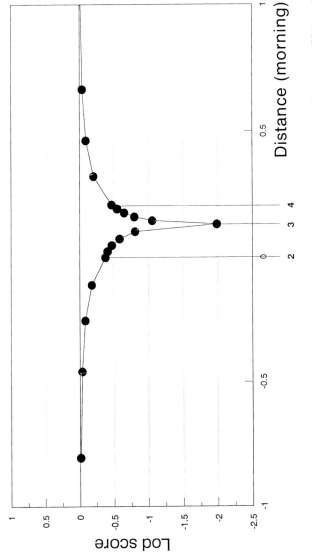

FIG. 2. Multipoint analysis: chromosome map D5S76–D5S39–HEXB. D5S76 = 2; D5S39 = 3; HEBX = 4; ——, F01 + F02 + F04 + F05.

result of a 4-point analysis for schizophrenia, using the LINKMAP program (8), which provides evidence against linkage of schizophrenia across the entire region examined, reaching a statistically significant minimum at D5S39. We then added the locus D5S6 and performed two different multipoint analyses using family F05 alone (Fig. 3). We obtained weak evidence against linkage throughout the region D5S76–D5S39 (lod score −0.17) and the same negative result throughout the map D5S6–D5S39–HEXB (lod score −1.1).

DISCUSSION

Our negative results are consistent with the majority of published reports in providing evidence against the presence of a susceptibility gene for schizophrenia in the 5q11.2-q13.3 region in our Northern Italian population. It has been proposed (9) that the positive linkage found by Sherrington could be related to the presence of a gene responsible for the general predisposition to the development of psychiatric disorders, since the best lod scores have been obtained with the inclusion of a broader range of affected phenotypes. The discrepancy between the results could also be explained by the heterogeneity of the disease, even though other explanations have been discussed elsewhere (10,11).

It is well known that the heterogeneity could be present either at a pure genetic level (i.e., a variability of the mode of transmission or of the parametric structure of the hypothetical gene controlling for the disease) or at a mixed genetic/phenotypic level (e.g., the true definition of the affected phenotype). When we controlled for the possible existence of a genetic form of the heterogeneity, comparing our findings with other published results, we did not find any statistical significance and we concluded, at least provisionally because only one paper produced positive lod scores, that apparently the differences among the various studies cannot be attributed to variability of the genetic parameters.

When we analyzed the effect of varying the definition of the affected phenotype as presented in the published reports, we found a statistically positive result. In this case, there is a large difference between the results for linkage presented by the different authors according to the various definitions of the affected phenotypes. It is of no matter that, in spite of the proposed assumption made by the majority of the authors that broadening the phenotype could not affect the linkage result except in a trivial way, the inclusion of different definitions of "affected status" introduces so many uncontrolled sources of variation that the different results obtained are no longer comparable (Figs. 4 and 5). One of the possible consequences, in addition to the confirmed heterogeneity, is that it is impossible to use the results derived by linkage studies to obtain a classification criterion for the clinical diagnosis of "affec-

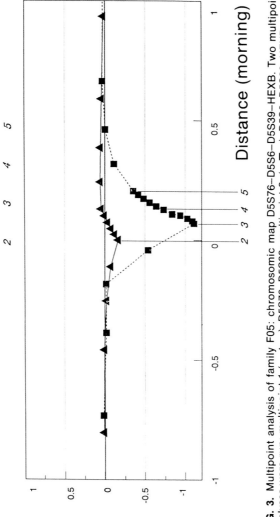

FIG. 3. Multipoint analysis of family F05: chromosomic map D5S76–D5S6–D5S39–HEXB. Two multipoint analyses were run: multipoint 1 (——▲——), D5S76–D5S39; multipoint 2, (---■---), D5S6–D5S39–HEXB.

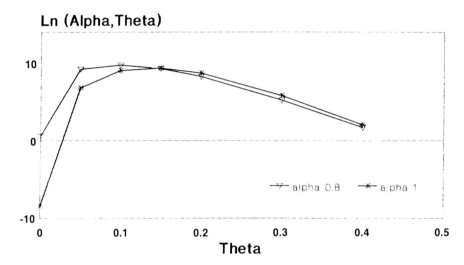

FIG. 4. Heterogeneity test for schizophrenia: no statistical differences for the genetic structure. (Combined data from refs. 2, 4, and present study.)

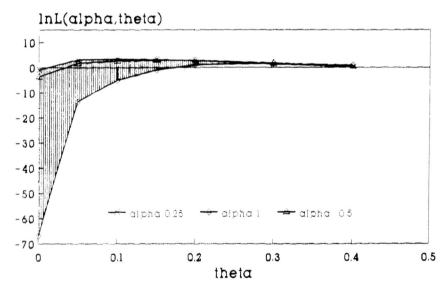

FIG. 5. Heterogeneity of schizophrenia: the effect of variable phenotype; diagnoses include bipolar patients. (Data from refs. 2, 4, 5, and present study.)

tion" because this implies a "circular" reasoning (we define a phenotype; then we test for a biological determinant of that phenotype; whether the result is satisfactory or not, we modify the definition of the phenotype and we do the test again; when we find the best result, we go back to the phenotype and state that "that" phenotype has been biologically demonstrated, hence it is true) that does not have any logical foundation.

Therefore, the diagnosis of schizophrenia still remains a central controversy in the field, and it is quite conceivable that reliable and comparable data will be found only when the schizophrenia phenotype has been unambiguously defined.

REFERENCES

1. Bassett A, Jones B, McGullivray B, Pantzar J. Partial trisomy chromosome 5 cosegregating with schizophrenia. *Lancet* 1988;1:799–801.
2. Sherrington R, Brynjolfsson J, Peturson H, et al. Localization of a susceptibility locus for schizophrenia on chromosome 5. *Nature* 1988;336:164–7.
3. Kennedy J, Giuffra L, Moises H, et al. Evidence against linkage of schizophrenia to markers on chromosome 5 in a northern Swedish pedigree. *Nature* 1988;336:167–70.
4. St. Clair D, Blackwood D, Muir W, et al. No linkage of chromosome 5q11-13 markers to schizophrenia in Scottish families. *Nature* 1989;339:305–7.
5. Detera–Wadleigh S, Goldin L, Sherrington R, et al. Exclusion of linkage to 5q11-13 in families with schizophrenia and other psychiatric disorders. *Nature* 1989;340:391–3.
6. Kaufmann C, De Lisi L, Lehner T, Gilliam C. Physical mapping, linkage analysis of a putative schizophrenia locus on chromosome 5q. *Schizophren Bull* 1989;15:3:441–52.
7. American Psychiatric Association. *Diagnostic and statistical manual of mental disorders*, 3rd ed., revised. Washington, DC: American Psychiatric Association, 1987.
8. Lathrop M, Lalouel JM, Julier C, Ott J. Multilocus linkage analysis in humans: detection of linkage and estimation of recombination. *Am J Hum Genet* 1985;37:482–98.
9. Byerley W. Genetic linkage revisited. *Nature* 1989;340:340–1.
10. Kennedy J, Giuffra L, Moises H, et al. Molecular genetic studies in schizophrenia. *Schizophren Bull* 1989;15:3:383–91.
11. Diehl S, Kendler K. Strategies for linkage studies of schizophrenia: pedigrees, DNA markers, and statistical analysis. *Schizophren Bull* 1989;15:403–19.

Psychiatry and Advanced Technologies,
edited by L. Ravizza, F. Bogetto, and
E. Zanalda. Raven Press, Ltd.,
New York © 1993.

27

Mapping Genes for Complex Diseases Such as Bipolar Illness: Issues and Problems

Maria Martinez

Department of Health and Human Services, National Institute of Mental Health, Bethesda, Maryland 20892

Linkage analysis can be a powerful method for detecting the effect of a major gene for complex diseases. However, identification of linkage of a disease susceptibility locus to marker loci for major psychiatric disorders (affective disorders and schizophrenia) is complicated by several factors such as reduced penetrance, variable age of onset, presence of phenocopies, and heterogeneity in etiology. Given these factors, it is important to know how the power of the linkage analysis is affected by complex inheritance and genetic heterogeneity. Given the current power to screen the entire genome for linkage, it is necessary to determine what sampling schemes are required to detect both linkage and heterogeneity. For simple mendelian diseases, the number of nuclear families needed to detect linkage and/or heterogeneity has been investigated by others (1–3). The joint segregation of the disease locus and a known map of two flanking markers has been investigated for the case of linkage-phase known and a fully penetrant disease gene (4).

In the context of psychiatric disorders (i.e., complex inheritance) we have examined the power to detect linkage in medium-sized pedigrees (11 individuals and three generations) under various modes of multiplex ascertainments and when heterogeneity exists both among and within families. We have considered a disorder caused by either one of two independent disease loci. A highly polymorphic marker locus is linked to the disease locus A and unlinked to the second disease locus B. A fraction α of the cases in the population are due to the disease locus A. We have shown that the power to detect linkage depends on the mode of ascertainment and therefore on the mode of transmission of both susceptibility loci (5). For example, when the rate of heterogeneity α is equal to 50% and when families are selected through vertical transmission (at least three affected), the power to detect linkage for a dominant disease locus with 50% penetrance in a sample of 50 families is equal to 45 and 79%, respectively, when the unlinked disease locus is dominant with either 90 or 50% penetrance. When families are selected with multiple affected members, the rate of heterogeneity within families increases. However, for the pedigree structure we have considered, the power of the linkage test is more affected by an increase of heterogeneity among families. Thus, optimal sampling strategies for common and complex traits are difficult to determine because the "correct" ascertainment does not always favor detection of the disease gene of interest when there is substantial heterogeneity.

Clearly, the linkage test can be improved by sampling large families and by increasing the linkage information (6), particularly when two flanking markers are used (7). We have compared the linkage information using a map of two linked markers vs. one single marker locus. Conservative approximations may be proposed: for linkage map intervals equal to or less than 20 cM, two flanking markers are roughly equivalent to a single marker that is twice as close to the disease locus. However, for tight linkage between the markers, single marker approaches tend to be as efficient as interval mapping analysis. Using the appropriate criterion for linkage (8), we have also compared efficiency of the lod score allowing for genetic heterogeneity (lod2) to the usual lod score (lod1) which assumes homogeneity, and by use of three-point linkage analysis in successive map intervals (9). We have shown that the lod1 test loses power relative to the lod2 test as the proportion of linked families decreases, as the flanking markers are more closely linked, and as more map intervals are tested. Moreover, the three-point linkage test is not robust to misspecification of genetic heterogeneity.

In conclusion, our results show that for low values of the rate of linked families, the sample sizes required for linkage detection remain large even when multipoint linkage analysis is used. Furthermore, when using dense linkage maps (i.e., chromosomes mapped with close markers), we have shown that the lod2 linkage test is more efficient for detecting a true linkage for a heterogeneous disorder and is less likely to falsely reject a true linkage from the entire linkage area.

REFERENCES

1. Cavalli–Sforza L, King MC. Detecting linkage for genetically heterogeneous diseases and detecting heterogeneity with linkage data. *Am J Hum Genet* 1986;38:599–616.
2. Ott J. The number of families required to detect or preclude linkage heterogeneity. *Am J Hum Genet* 1986;39:159–65.
3. Clerget–Darpoux F, Babron MC, Bonaiti–Pellie C. Power and robustness of the linkage homogeneity test in genetic analysis of common disorders. *J Psychiatr Res* 1987;21:625–30.
4. Lander ES, Botstein D. Strategies for studying heterogeneous genetic traits in humans by using a linkage map of restriction fragment length polymorphisms. *Proc Natl Acad Sci USA* 1986;83:7353–7.

5. Martinez M, Goldin LR. Power of the linkage test for a heterogeneous disorder due to two independent inherited causes: a simulation study. *Genet Epidemiol* 1990;7:219–30.
6. Gejman PB, Martinez M, Gershon ES. New strategies in linkage research in psychiatry. *Int Rev Psychiatry* 1989;1:307–14.
7. Martinez M Goldin LR. The detection of linkage and heterogeneity in nuclear families for complex disorders: one versus two linked marker loci. *Am J Hum Genet* 1989;44:552–9.
8. Risch N. Linkage detection tests under heterogeneity. *Genet Epidemiol* 1989;6:473–80.
9. Martinez M, Goldin LR. Systematic screening for heterogeneous disorders using map intervals. *Am J Hum Genet* 1990;47:A191.

Psychiatry and Advanced Technologies,
edited by L. Ravizza, F. Bogetto, and
E. Zanalda. Raven Press, Ltd.,
New York © 1993.

28

Genetic Linkage and Association Studies in Affective Disorders

A. Bocchetta, F. Bernardi, M. Pedditzi, C. Burrai,
*R. Corona, and M. Del Zompo

*Department of Neurosciences, University of Cagliari; and *Central Laboratory,
"S. Giovanni di Dio" Hospital, 09124 Cagliari, Italy*

The role of genetic factors in susceptibility to the major psychiatric disorders has been supported by family, twin, and adoption studies. However, the precise nature of the genetic defects remains unknown. The development of molecular genetic techniques has offered the opportunity for an accurate identification of linked marker loci. Nevertheless, linkage studies with restriction fragment length polymorphisms (RFLP) have thus far provided conflicting results. Well-known examples are the studies on linkage between bipolar affective disorder (BP) and markers on the tip of the short arm of chromosome 11 (11p15). In fact, the initially positive finding of linkage between BP and the Harvey-ras-1 oncogene and insulin loci in the Old Order Amish (1) was not confirmed in other ethnic groups (2,3) or even by a subsequent reevaluation of the original Amish pedigree (4). These and other inconsistencies in published linkage studies may in part depend on the many problems that can be anticipated in common and complex neuropsychiatric disorders, such as the probable presence of genetic heterogeneity, the presence of nongenetic forms (phenocopies), and the incomplete and age-related penetrance (the gene can be present also in some well individuals).

In addition to linkage, another approach to the genetics of psychiatric disorders is the study of associations between markers and illness in populations of patients and within families of patients. A recent promising example is the potential association found in a French population between BP and a locus on chromosome 11p15 (5). Such a locus is contiguous to the insulin gene and contains the gene for tyrosine hydroxylase, the rate-limiting enzyme for catecholamine synthesis.

In a previous preliminary study, we reported the potential association between BP, particularly of schizoaffective type, and heterozygous β-thalassemia (Th) in an outpatient psychiatric population in southern Sardinia (6). Because this hematologic disorder is due to mutations of the β-globin gene, which is closely linked to the insulin gene, and the Harvey-ras-1 oncogene loci, the establishment of an association can help to clarify the hypothesis of a gene on chromosome 11p15 involved in BP. The present study is an extension of our preliminary report and confirms the initial findings.

SUBJECTS AND METHODS

The subjects in this study were 348 psychiatric outpatients consecutively admitted to the Service of Clinical Pharmacology, Department of Neurosciences, University of Cagliari, given diagnoses according to modified Research Diagnostic Criteria. The sample included patients with schizoaffective disorder, bipolar subtype (SA-B); schizoaffective disorder, depressive subtype only (SA-D); bipolar I disorder (BP-I); bipolar II disorder (BP-II); and unipolar major depressive disorder (UP).

Individuals with a diagnosis of SA disorder, manic (or mixed) subtype, and individuals with diagnoses of both SA-D and BP-I were considered to have SA-B. Individuals with a diagnosis of mania (or hypomania) without an additional diagnosis of depression were classified as having BP-I (or BP-II). Patients with only drug-induced hypomania were included as having BP-II.

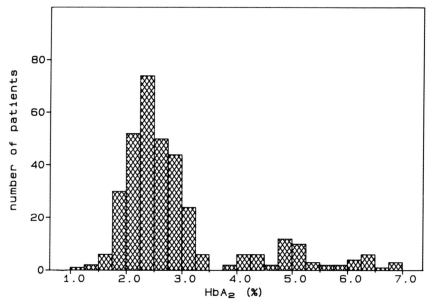

FIG. 1. Distribution of HbA_2 levels in 348 patients.

Hemoglobin (Hb) electrophoresis and chromatography were performed on red blood cell hemolysate from venous blood samples in EDTA. Test–retest reliability as well as correlation between electrophoresis and chromatography were high. The distribution of HbA$_2$ levels in the overall sample is shown in Fig. 1. Subjects with HbA$_2$ levels higher than 3.5% were considered to have Th. Hematologic and psychiatric diagnoses were always done blind to one another.

RESULTS AND DISCUSSION

Table 1 shows the prevalence of Th by diagnosis. The prevalence in the overall sample (17%) was similar to that reported in our preliminary survey in 180 patients (17.8%). The results are within the range found in the general population in different areas of southern Sardinia (7).

A disproportionately higher prevalence of the hematologic disorder ($p <$ 0.025) was found in subjects with SA-B (25/102 = 24.5%) compared with the remaining patients (34/246 = 13.8%). Moreover, the subgroup of patients with bipolar disorders (including SA-B) showed a significantly higher proportion of Th (44/220 = 20.0%) ($p < 0.05$) compared with those with non-bipolar disorders (15/128 = 11.7%). No sex differences were observed.

There are several explanations for the existence of an association between a genetic marker trait and a disease. First, such an association may be an artifact resulting from sampling bias. With regard to the psychiatric diagnosis, we paid particular attention to the material available for each patient. We applied longitudinal diagnostic criteria to medical records, direct interview, and information from relatives. It has been reported that syndrome shifts in the longterm course are frequently observed, but they usually occur within the first few episodes (8). Therefore, because the majority of our patients had a long history of recurrent episodes and records of their hospitalizations were often available, our assessment of bipolarity and/or schizoaffectivity should be accurate. Moreover, data on the rates of affective illness in relatives of a large sample of our patients confirm the bipolar–non-bipolar distinction as well as the specific familial risk for SA-B (9).

Another artifact may be due to population stratification. For example, SA-

TABLE 1. *Heterozygous β-thalassemia in 348 patients*

Diagnosis	No. heterozygotes/total	%
Bipolar I	12/71	16.9
Bipolar II	7/47	14.9
Bipolar schizoaffective	25/102	24.5
Depressive schizoaffective	6/51	11.8
Unipolar depression	9/67	13.4
Total	59/348	17.0

B or bipolar patients may come from an area that has a high incidence of Th and non-bipolar patients come from an area that has a low frequency. We controlled for areas of origin and no obvious stratifications were found. Moreover, we are studying whether Th and affective illness co-segregate within families to further control for population stratification, as all members of a family are part of the same population and co-segregation can exclude a spurious association.

In addition to possible artifacts, an explanation for the existence of an association is that Th itself may play a role in susceptibility to bipolar or schizoaffective illness. A direct effect may even act only in the presence of other genetic and environmental components. To our knowledge, the only reports in the literature of any relationship between Th and affective illness are those by Joffe et al. (10), who observed a possible association in members of a limited pedigree with BP or UP, and by Scherer and Eberle (11), who found that women with both depressive disorder and Th may show some peculiarities in symptoms (such as complaints of muscle weakness and bone pain).

A different explanation is that a gene closely linked to the β-globin locus on chromosome 11p15 may cause susceptibility and that there is a linkage disequilibrium. Disequilibrium refers to the case in which particular allele combinations of loci (haplotypes) occur in individuals more frequently than expected by chance. There are other examples of genetic disequilibrium in Sardinia that are most likely the result of an interaction between founder effect, selection, and close linkage (12). We can hypothesize that linkage disequilibrium with respect to the two chromosome 11p15 loci was present in the ancestor Sardinian populations and that selection (e.g., the higher adaptiveness of Th in a malarial environment) contributed to enhance the original condition of disequilibrium. Subsequent generations have not been sufficient to restore complete equilibrium because the recombination fractions were extremely small. If confirmed, such a possibility would be of great value in reducing the number of candidate genes for BP within this linkage region. Accordingly, we could exclude the involvement of either the gene for tyrosine hydroxylase, which is contiguous to the insulin locus (13), or the Harvey-ras-1 oncogene locus, because they show 12–13% recombination with the β-globin gene cluster (14). However, we cannot exclude that other mechanisms, such as epistatic interactions between the two genes or selection on the Th-BP haplotype, might have allowed the association to persist.

ACKNOWLEDGMENT

This study was supported by a grant from Regione Autonoma della Sardegna, Assessorato all'Igiene e Sanità. The authors thank Dr. Liliana Del

Zompo for the English version and Miss Maura Usai for typing the manuscript.

REFERENCES

1. Egeland JA, Gerhard DS, Pauls DL, et al. Bipolar affective disorders linked to DNA markers on chromosome 11. *Nature* 1987;325:783–7.
2. Hodgkinson S, Sherrington R, Gurling H, et al. Molecular genetic evidence for heterogeneity in manic depression. *Nature* 1987;325:805–6.
3. Detera–Wadleigh SD, Berrettini WH, Goldin LR, Boorman D, Anderson S, Gershon ES. Close linkage of C-Harvey-ras-1 and the insulin gene to affective disorder is ruled out in three North American pedigrees. *Nature* 1987;325:806–8.
4. Kelsoe JR, Ginns EI, Egeland JA, et al. Re-evaluation of the linkage relationship between chromosome 11p loci and the gene for bipolar affective disorder in the Old Order Amish. *Nature* 1989;342:238–43.
5. Leboyer M, Malafosse A, Boularand S, et al. Tyrosine hydroxylase polymorphisms associated with manic-depressive illness. *Lancet* 1990;1:335, 1219.
6. Bocchetta A, Del Zompo M. Bipolar-affective disorder and heterozygous β-thalassemia. *Am J Psychiatry* 1990;147:8, 1094.
7. Siniscalco M, Bernini L, Filippi G, et al. Population genetics of haemoglobin variants, thalassaemia and glucose-6-phosphate dehydrogenase deficiency, with particular reference to the malaria hypothesis. *Bull WHO* 1966;34:379–93.
8. Marneros A, Deister A, Rohde A. Syndrome shift in the long-term course of schizoaffective disorders. *Eur Arch Psychiatr Neurol Sci* 1988;238:97–104.
9. Bocchetta A, Bernardi F, Garau L, et al. Familial rates of affective illness in Sardinia with special reference to schizoaffective disorder. *Eur Arch Psychiatry Clin Neurosci* 1990;240: 1, 16–20.
10. Joffe RT, Horvath Z, Tarvydas I. Bipolar affective disorder and thalassemia minor. *Am J Psychiatry* 1986;143:933.
11. Scherer J, Eberle E. Major affective disorder and heterozygout beta-thalassaemia. *Psychopharmacology* 1988;96(suppl):145.
12. Filippi G, Rinaldi A, Palmarino R, Seravalli E, Siniscalco M. Linkage disequilibrium for two X-linked genes in Sardinia and its bearing on the statistical mapping of the human X-chromosome. *Genetics* 1977;86:199–212.
13. O'Malley K, Rotwein P. Human tyrosine hydroxylase and insulin genes are contiguous on chromosome 11. *Nucleic Acids Res* 1988;16:4437–45.
14. White R, Leppert M, Bishop DT, et al. Construction of linkage maps with DNA markers for human chromosomes. *Nature* 1985;313:101–5.

Psychiatry and Advanced Technologies,
edited by L. Ravizza, F. Bogetto, and
E. Zanalda. Raven Press, Ltd.,
New York © 1993.

29

Dopamine D_2 Receptor Heterogeneity and Neuroplasticity: Modulatory Effects of GM1

R. Dal Toso, M. Santi, S. Romanello, L. Cavicchioli,
A. Zanotti, *P.H. Seeburg, A. Leon, and G. Toffano

*Fidia Research Laboratories, 35031 Abano Terme (PD), Italy; and *Zentrum für Molekulare Biologie, 6900 Heidelberg, Germany*

Alterations of dopaminergic transmission have been associated with neurologic disorders such as Parkinson's disease and schizophrenia. The main therapeutic approach for these neuropathologies involves pharmacologic manipulation of dopamine receptors, either by administration of a dopamine precursor, such as L-dopa, in Parkinson's disease, or administration of neuroleptic drugs, such as haloperidol, in schizophrenia.

Dopamine receptors are classified into two pharmacologically distinct subtypes: D_1 receptors, which stimulate the production of cyclic AMP, and D_2 receptors, which inhibit the activity of adenylate cyclase (1). The two receptor subtypes also appear to be functionally associated with different populations of neurons in the striatum (2).

The antipsychotic activity of neuroleptic drugs has been suggested to be related to their antagonistic effects on D_2 receptors. However, one biochemical side effect induced by chronic neuroleptic drug administration, in humans as well as in animals, is a significant upregulation of D_2 receptor density in the caudate nucleus (3). This increased D_2 receptor density persists for long periods after drug withdrawal and is associated with typical behavioral supersensitivity to dopaminergic agonists. Nevertheless, young adult rats spontaneously recover normal D_2 receptor levels 3–4 months after drug withdrawal; administration of D_2 agonists can accelerate this process (4). These results suggest the existence of neuronal plastic mechanisms involved in recovery of normal D_2 receptor density, a process that can be pharmacologically modulated.

Several laboratories, including our own, have shown that monosialoganglioside (GM1) treatment reduces striatal D_2 receptor upregulation in rats, not

TABLE 1. *Effect of GM1 ganglioside treatment on specific [^{3}H]spiperone binding in rat striatal membranes after haloperidol withdrawal[a]*

| Treatment period | | B_{max} |
First (14 days)	Second (14 days)	(pmol/mg prot)
Vehicle	Vehicle	0.294 ± 0.044
Haloperidol	Vehicle	0.385 ± 0.003*
Haloperidol	GM1	0.305 ± 0.099**

[a] Specific [^{3}H]spiperone binding was assessed according to Creese et al. (10). The B_{max} reported is the mean ± SEM of four experiments, each consisting of triplicate values with or without (+)-butaclamol. Drug dosage: haloperidol (2 mg/kg/day, i.p.); GM1 (30 mg/kg/day, i.p.).
* $p < 0.01$ vs. vehicle-treated animals; ** $p < 0.01$ vs. haloperidol-treated animals.

only after dopaminergic depletion by mechanical hemitransection of the nigrostriatal pathway (3) or MPTP treatment but also after pharmacologic deafferentation with haloperidol (6–9). To further support the later studies and extend their physiologic relevance, we have investigated GM1 effects on striatal D_2 mRNA content and apomorphine-induced stereotyped behaviors.

MATERIALS AND METHODS

Male rats (Sprague–Dawley, 250 g) were treated daily with haloperidol (2 mg/kg) or vehicle for 2 weeks. After a 5-day washout period, they were further treated with either GM1 (30 mg/kg/day) or saline for another 2 weeks. The animals were then used for behavioral studies or killed, either for removal of caudate nuclei to prepare membranes for binding studies with [^{3}H]spiperone (10) or for extraction of total RNA and amplification by the polymerase chain reaction as previously described (11).

RESULTS AND DISCUSSION

D_2 Receptor Upregulation

Animals treated with haloperidol or saline after the washout period showed a significant 30–40% increase in the apparent B_{max} of [^{3}H]spiperone in striatal membranes. Likewise, D_2 receptor mRNA levels in the striatum (approximately 50% above control) were more elevated in the haloperidol- and saline-treated animals. The enhanced D_2 receptor protein and mRNA levels after haloperidol treatment are thus indicative of an increased rate of synthesis of D_2 receptor under our conditions.

On the other hand, animals that received GM1 after haloperidol had [^{3}H]spiperone binding levels significantly lower and comparable to those observed in control animals. GM1 administration alone did not modify D_2 receptor binding. No modifications in the apparent K_d value were seen among the different groups (Table 1). Rats treated with haloperidol and GM1 or with

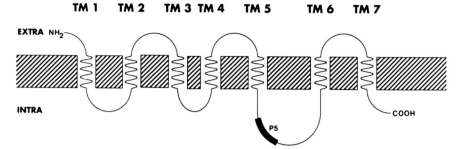

FIG. 1. Schematic diagram of the dopamine D_{2A} receptor showing the location of the additional exon (P5) in the third cytoplasmic loop. TM, transmembrane region; P5, 29-amino acid peptide coded by exon 5 of the D_2 receptor gene.

GM1 alone showed no significant difference in their content of D_2 receptor mRNA compared with control animals.

D_2 Receptor Heterogeneity

Recently, several laboratories have found that two isoforms of the D_2 receptor are generated by alternative splicing of the primary transcript of a single gene (12–14) and that both isoforms are present in the rat striatum. The two isoforms differ by a 29–amino acid insertion in the third intracellular loop of the receptor (Fig. 1), a region potentially important for G-protein coupling. The mRNA coding for the long receptor isoform is more abundant both in rat brain and pituitary (approximately fivefold). It has been speculated that variations in the isoform ratio might correlate with altered dopaminergic conditions.

To address the question of whether haloperidol treatment was able to modify the relative abundance of the two isoforms of the striatal D_2 receptor, the polymerase chain reaction (PCR) was used for amplification. The PCR primers were chosen to select for sequences spanning the third intracellular loop of the receptor (14), which contains the insertion site, so as to generate two fragments of different lengths separable by gel electrophoresis. The relative content of the two isoforms, however, did not appear to be modified by either haloperidol or GM1 administration, suggesting that the splicing mechanism of the D_2 receptor mRNA is not altered by these pharmacologic treatments.

Effect of Haloperidol and GM1 on the Enkephalinergic System in the Striatum

It is well documented that neuroleptic treatment also modifies peptidergic neurotransmitter systems in the striatum. Blockade of D_2 receptors is associated with a marked increase of both proenkephalin mRNA and protein content (15,16), and a decrease in the preprotachykinin mRNA content (2). The enkephalin and tachykinin peptidergic systems are known to be localized in GABAergic neurons projecting, respectively, to the external pallidum or the substantia nigra pars reticulata.

Consistent with the above observations, a significant increase in the levels of proenkephalin mRNA in the striatum was detected after chronic haloperidol treatment. GM1 administration also normalized levels of the mRNA coding for these neuropeptides. Therefore, several of the biochemical modifications induced by haloperidol can be restored to control levels by GM1 treatment, suggesting that the nigrostriatal neurotransmitter circuitry regains a normal balance.

Effect on Apomorphine-Induced Stereotyped Behavior

Upregulation of dopamine receptor density is correlated with characteristic apomorphine-induced motor behaviors which can be easily measured and quantified. When D_2 receptor upregulation is unilateral, apomorphine challenge produces a typical rotational behavior towards the contralateral side. After haloperidol treatment a bilateral up-regulation of D_2 receptor levels occurs. Apomorphine administration induces a stereotyped "sniffing" behavior in which the duration has been correlated with the level of D_2 receptor upregulation. Therefore, in our experiments haloperidol-treated animals were challenged with apomorphine and were examined 20 min later for the duration of the "sniffing" behavior. These animals showed a significant increase in the amount of time spent in the stereotyped activity even after 19 days of drug withdrawal, indicating the existence of persistent motor–behavioral alterations. Conversely, in animals treated with haloperidol and GM1 or with GM1 alone, the duration of sniffing behavior was comparable to that of control animals.

CONCLUSIONS

The present findings support the notion that several central nervous system neurotransmitter systems are affected by haloperidol treatment, although its primary pharmacologic sites of action are the D_2 receptors. Our working hypothesis is that GM1 administration can accelerate neuroplastic processes that, in D_2 receptor supersensitive rats, regulate the recovery of a normal physiologic neurotransmitter balance in the basal ganglia. These mechanisms might involve postsynaptic D_1–D_2 receptor interactions, D_2 receptor turnover rates, or effects on presynaptic dopaminergic terminals. Whether any or all of these possibilities plays a role in D_2 receptor upregulation (including associated behavioral supersensitivity) and in GM1 modulation remains to be established in future studies.

REFERENCES

1. Creese I, Sibley DR, Hamblin NW, Left SE. The classification of dopamine receptors: relationship to ligand binding. *Annu Rev Neurosci* 1983;6:43–71.
2. Gerfen CR, Engber TM, Mahan LC, et al. D₁ and D₂ dopamine-regulated gene expression in striatonigral and striatopallidal neurons. *Science* 1990;250:1429–32.
3. Burt DR, Creese I, Snyder SH. Antischizophrenic drugs: chronic treatment elevates dopamine receptor binding in brain. *Science* 1977;196:326–8.
4. List S, Seeman P. Neuroleptic dopamine receptors: elevation and reversal. In: F Cattabeni et al., eds. *Long term effects of neuroleptics.* New York: Raven Press, 1980;24:95–101. (Advances in Biochemical Psychopharmacology, Vol 24).
5. Toffano G, Savoini G, Moroni F, Lombardi G, Calzà L, Agnati LF. GM1 ganglioside stimulates the regeneration of dopaminergic neurons in the central nervous system. *Brain Res* 1983;261:163–6.
6. Agnati LF, Fuxe K, Benfenati F, Zini I, Toffano G. Chronic GM1 ganglioside treatment counteracts with biochemical signs of dopamine receptor supersensitivity induced by chronic haloperidol treatment. *Neurosci Lett* 1983;40:293–7.
7. Cavicchioli L, Zanotti A, Consolazione A, Leon A, Toffano G. Plasticity of dopaminergic nigro-striatal connection and post-synaptic receptor supersensitivity: effect of chronic GM₁ ganglioside treatment. *New Trends Clin Neuropharm* 1987;1:111–4.
8. Tilson HA, Harry GJ, Nanry K, Hudson PM, Hong GS. Ganglioside interactions with the dopaminergic system of rats. *J Neurosci Res* 1988;19:88–93.
9. Weihnmuller FB, Hadjiconstantinou M, Bruno JP, Neff NH. Continued administration of GM1 ganglioside is required to maintain recovery from neuroleptic-induced sensomotor deficits in MPTP-treated mice. *Life Sci* 1989;45:2495–502.
10. Creese J, Schneider R, Snyder SH. ³H-Spiperone labels dopamine receptors in pituitary and brain. *Eur J Pharmacol* 1977;46:377–81.
11. Cavicchioli L, Flanigan TP, Disckson JG, et al. Choline acetyltransferase messenger RNA expression in developing an adult rat brain: regulation by nerve growth factor. *Mol Brain Res* 1991;9:319–25.
12. Giros B, Sokoloff P, Martres MP, Riou JF, Emorine LJ, Schwartz JC. Alternative splicing directs the expression of two D₂ dopamine receptors isoforms. *Nature* 1989;342:923–6.
13. Monsma FJ, McVitties LD, Gerfen CR, Mahan C, Sibley DR. Multiple D₂ dopamine receptors produced by alternative RNA splicing. *Nature* 1989;342:926–9.
14. Dal Toso R, Ewert M, Sommer B, et al. The dopamine D₂ receptor: two molecular forms generated by alternative splicing. *Embo J* 1989;8:4025–34.
15. Sabol S, Yoshikawa K, Hong JS. Regulation of methionine-enkephalin precursor messenger RNA in rat striatum by haloperidol and lithium. *Bioch Biophys Res Comm* 1983;113:391–9.
16. Schwartz JP, Costa E. Hybridization approaches to the study of neuropeptides. *Annu Rev Neurosci* 1986;9:277–304.

Psychiatry and Advanced Technologies,
edited by L. Ravizza, F. Bogetto, and
E. Zanalda. Raven Press, Ltd.,
New York © 1993.

30

Application of Polymerase Chain Reaction Technology to Quantitate Specific RNA Transcripts in Cultured Neurons

Maurizio Memo

Institute of Pharmacology and Experimental Therapeutics, University of Brescia, 25124 Brescia, Italy

The polymerase chain reaction (PCR) is a recently developed technique for selectively amplifying polynucleotide sequences (1). Application of the basic PCR procedure has been valuable to molecular biologists, to medical researchers investigating both inherited and infectious diseases, and to forensic specialists.

POLYMERASE CHAIN REACTION TECHNOLOGY AND APPLICATIONS

The general application of PCR requires the availability of sequence-specific primers flanking the region to be amplified. Therefore, PCR is limited to targets whose sequence is known a priori. The first PCR report was published in 1985 (2). Since that time, PCR has become an increasingly powerful, versatile, and useful technique. The development of this technology in the late 1980s resulted from a combination of improvements and optimization of the methodology, introduction of new variations on the PCR theme, and use of the heat-stable "Thermus Aquaticus" (Taq) DNA polymerase (3). With PCR, tiny bits of embedded and often hidden genetic information can be amplified into large amounts of accessible, identifiable, and analyzable material. The starting material for PCR, the target sequence, is a gene or a segment of DNA. In a matter of hours, this target sequence can be amplified a millionfold according to the scheme shown in Fig. 1. A source of DNA including the desired sequence is denatured in the presence of a large molar excess of

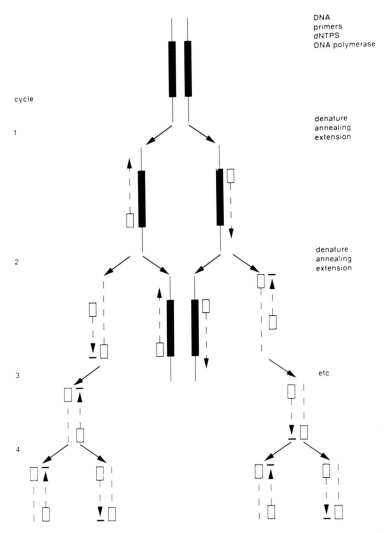

FIG. 1. DNA amplification by PCR. Target sequence (▬); PCR primer (☐); new DNA ----; dNTPS, deoxynucleotide triphosphates.

two oligonucleotides and the four deoxyribonucleoside triphosphates. The oligonucleotides are complementary to different strands of the desired sequence and at relative positions along the sequence, such that the DNA polymerase extension product of one, when denatured, can serve as a template for the other, and vice versa. DNA polymerase is added and reaction is allowed to occur. The reaction products are denatured and the process is repeated for many cycles until the desired amount of DNA fragment is obtained.

Many improvements to the original PCR method have been made. One of the most relevant is the substitution of a heat-stable enzyme for the original DNA polymerase, which was heat-labile and had to be replenished after each cycle. The stable Taq polymerase, which comes from bacteria that live in hot springs, continues working almost indefinitely despite the heating steps. Taq polymerase improved the yield, generated more specific and longer products, and facilitated automation (3–5).

The basic PCR procedure has been valuable in disease diagnosis because specific DNA sequences can be enormously amplified. One of the first uses led to improved diagnosis of a genetic disease (sickle-cell anemia), because the PCR technique required much less clinical material than standard procedures (6). PCR can also be used to amplify trace amounts of genetic materials of infectious agents in blood, cells, water, food, and other clinical and environmental samples (3). PCR-based tests are especially valuable for detecting pathogens that are difficult or impossible to culture, such as the agents for Lyme disease and AIDS (3,4). For cancer diagnosis and cancer research, PCR can indicate what genes are expressed or turned off and allow detection of gene deletions and point mutations, as well as chromosomal translocations, in inherited diseases (3,4,7,8). Finally, PCR technology has been used by molecular biologists for direct DNA targeting, sequencing, and cloning. PCR analysis has been also used for RNA blot analysis, mRNA phenotyping, and nuclease protection analysis for the study of short-lived, low–copy-number mRNA transcripts.

POLYMERASE CHAIN REACTION TO QUANTITATE mRNA TRANSCRIPTS

Many studies of gene expression are limited by the sensitivity of standard hybridization techniques, and for this reason several groups have recently made use of PCR for detection of specific mRNA after reverse transcription to DNA. We investigated the quantitative aspects of the assay. Quantitative PCR is based on the fact that, under defined experimental conditions, the amount of amplified product is exponentially proportional to the amount of original template. Critical to successful PCR quantitation of mRNA concentrations are the amount of original template used in the reaction and the number of cycles used in the amplification process. These conditions must be previously established to ensure that the amplification rate is in the exponential phase. This requires determination of the amount of amplified product generated as a function of original template concentration and number of amplification cycles used. In addition, it is necessary to use either an internal or an external standard to verify the RNA concentrations of samples to be compared.

We have adopted this technology for identification of the mRNAs that encode various subunits of the $GABA_A$ receptor in neurons in culture and for measurement of their relative abundance after treatment of the cells with various agents (9).

VALIDATION OF QUANTITATIVE POLYMERASE CHAIN REACTION

Validation of PCR for identification and quantitation of a given mRNA transcript was based on (i) the specificity of the primers, (ii) the size of the amplified band, and (iii) a correlation between amount of template and yield of amplified DNA product. The primers used to amplify the mRNAs encoding the various $GABA_A$ receptor subunits were 22 BP long, with a G + C content higher than 50%, and endowed with the lowest homology with comparable mRNA sequences. The sizes of the amplified bands were identical to those predicted from the corresponding published sequences and were 500 BP long.

To determine whether PCR could be used to quantitate the amount of a given transcript present in a RNA sample, a series of experiments to correlate the effect of different cDNA concentrations as function of the yield of PCR product were performed. In particular, PCR was performed with a pair of primers specific for each individual mRNA encoding the different $GABA_A$ receptor subunits, in the presence of ^{32}P-labeled dCTP. The amplified DNA fragment visualized in the 1.2% Agarose gel by ethidium bromide staining was removed and the radioactivity incorporated into the band was counted by scintillation spectrometry. We found that the amount of radioactivity incorporated into the amplified DNA product was proportional to the amount of original reverse-transcribed mRNA in a range between 0.1 and 2.0 ng. Increasing the amount of template over these values does not allow the detection of differences in the amplified product because of the plateau effect (10). For the most accurate quantification, 1.0 ng of cDNA were used to compare the amplified products from different sources.

Because the yield of amplification is very sensitive to small differences in the amount of template, two additional internal controls were adopted. First, the efficiency of the reverse transcription was evaluated by measuring the amount of reverse-transcribed cDNA. This enabled us to normalize the amount of DNA to be amplified by PCR. Second, PCR was performed with primers specific for the structural protein β-actin. Similar results in the yield of amplification reflected similar amounts of original template in the different experimental samples (data not shown). These two experimental controls gave an accurate evaluation of the amount of template to be amplified and enabled us to validate any possible changes detectable by priming PCR with pairs of primers specific for other mRNA transcripts.

DIFFERENTIAL EXPRESSION OF GABA$_A$ RECEPTOR SUBUNIT mRNAs IN NEURONS

The quantitative PCR was originally developed to both identify and determine the relative abundance of the different mRNAs encoding the different subunits of the GABA$_A$ receptor in primary culture of cerebellar granule cells (9,10). The aim of that project was to investigate the mechanism(s) by which the expression of the GABA$_A$ receptor genes is regulated. We found that exposure of granule cells to specific antagonists of the N-methyl-D-aspartate (NMDA)-selective glutamate receptor reduces the steady-state levels of mRNAs encoding various GABA$_A$ receptor subunits. The experimental protocol and the results are summarized in Fig. 2. These neurons are glutamatergic in nature and require a depolarizing concentration of potassium (25 mM) for optimal development and survival. When the neural differentiation rate is retarded by lowering the extracellular potassium concentrations (to 12.5 mM), persistent stimulation of the same glutamate receptors with NMDA increases the expression of these GABA$_A$ receptor subunits. These results indicate that the regulation of the GABA$_A$ receptor subunit genes may involve a complex interplay between continuously expressed neural genetic programs and signals generated through heterologous receptor stimulation. These data confirm earlier reports that, in addition to its role in neurotransmission and neurotoxicity, glutamate may regulate gene expression. Specifi-

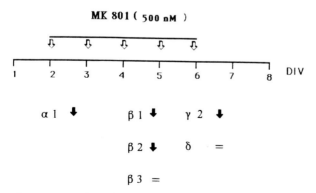

FIG. 2. Schematic representation of the experimental protocol and summary of the results. Cells were treated daily with MK 801 from the second day after plating for 5 consecutive days. mRNA was extracted at the seventh day of culture. Arrows indicate the qualitative change in the levels of the mRNAs encoding the various GABA$_A$ receptor subunits. Quantitatively, the reduction was in the magnitude of 60–70% in comparison with the corresponding GABA$_A$ receptor subunit mRNA levels in untreated cells.

cally, glutamate, via stimulation of the NMDA-selective glutamate receptor, has trophic influences on differentiating cerebellar granule cells in culture and regulates the expression of different subunits of the $GABA_A$ receptor.

REFERENCES

1. Herlich HA, Gibbs R, Kazazian HH Jr. *Polymerase chain reaction*. Current communication in molecular biology. Cold Spring Harbor, NY: CSHL Press, 1989.
2. Saiki RK, Sharf S, Faloona F, et al. Enzymatic amplification of B-globin genomic sequences and restriction site analysis for diagnosis of sickle cell anemia. *Science* 1985;230:1350–4.
3. Herlich HA. *PCR technology*. Stockton Press, 1989.
4. Innis MA, Gelfand DH, Sninski JJ, et al. *PCR protocols*. San Diego: Academic Press, 1990.
5. Gibbs RA, Chamberlain JS. Delation screening of the DMD locus via multiplex genomic DNA amplification. *Genes Dev* 1989;3:1095–8.
6. Saiki RK, Chang CA, Levenson TC, et al. Diagnosis of sickle cell anemia and B-thalassemia with enzymatically amplified DNA and nonradioactive allele-specific oligonucleotide probes. *N Engl J Med* 1988;319:537–41.
7. Gibbs RA, Nguyen PN, McBride LJ, et al. Identification of mutations leading to the Lesch-Nyhan syndrome by automated directed DNA sequencing of in vitro amplified cDNA. *Proc Natl Acad Sci USA* 1989;86:1919–23.
8. Chelly J, Kaplan JC, Maire P, et al. Transcription of the dystrophin gene in human muscle and non-muscle tissues. *Nature* 1988;33:858–60.
9. Memo M, Bovolin P, Costa E, et al. Regulation of aminobutyric acid-A receptor subunit expression by activation of N-methyl-D-aspartate-selective glutamate receptors. *Mol Pharmacol* 1991;39:599–603.
10. Memo M, Bovolin P, Costa E, et al. Expression of GABA-A receptor subunit mRNAs in neurons differentiating in culture. In: *Neurotransmitter regulation of gene expression*. New York: Raven Press, 1991;125–31. (Fidia Research Symposium Series, Vol 8).